DEVELOPMENTAL HEALTH
AND THE WEALTH OF NATIONS

MRC/CSO SPHSU
University of Glasgow
200 Renfield Street
Glasgow G2 3QB

Developmental Health and the Wealth of Nations

Social, Biological, and Educational Dynamics

DANIEL P. KEATING
CLYDE HERTZMAN

Editors

Foreword by J. Fraser Mustard and Lewis P. Lipsitt

THE GUILFORD PRESS
New York   London

© 1999 The Guilford Press
A Division of Guilford Publications, Inc.
72 Spring Street, New York, NY 10012
http://www.guilford.com

Printed in the United States of America

This book is printed on acid-free paper.

Last digit is print number: 9 8 7 6 5 4 3 2

Library of Congress Cataloging-in-Publication Data

Developmental health and the wealth of nations : social, biological,
   and educational dynamics / Daniel P. Keating, Clyde Hertzman,
   editors : foreword by J. Fraser Mustard and Lewis P. Lipsitt.
     p. cm.
   Includes bibliographical references and index.
   ISBN 1-57230-454-5 (hc.) ISBN 1-57230-455-3 (pbk.)
   1. Social medicine. 2. Public health. 3. Child development.
   4. Adjustment (Psychology) I. Keating, Daniel P., 1949–
   II. Hertzman, Clyde, 1953–
   RA418.D49 1999
   306.4'61—dc21   99-22408
                                          CIP

About the Editors

Daniel P. Keating, PhD, is a Royal Bank Fellow of the Canadian Institute for Advanced Research (CIAR) and Director of the CIAR Program in Human Development. He is also Professor and Chair of the Department of Human Development and Applied Psychology at the Ontario Institute for Studies in Education (OISE), University of Toronto. Prior to coming to OISE in 1987, he served on the faculties of the University of Minnesota (Institute for Child Development) and the University of Maryland, where he was the founding director of the doctoral program in applied developmental psychology. In 1985 he was a Visiting Scientist at the Max Planck Institute for Human Development and Education in Berlin. His research has focused on the cognitive, social, and emotional development of children and youth, and through CIAR, he has written on how social institutions need to change in order to promote human development in the face of emerging social and economic challenges.

Clyde Hertzman, MD, FRCPC, completed training in medicine, community medicine, and epidemiology at McMaster University in Hamilton, Ontario, between 1976 and 1985, and has been on faculty in the Department of Health Care and Epidemiology at the University of British Columbia since 1985. Currently, he is a full professor in the Department and Associate Director of the Centre for Health Services and Policy Research. Nationally, he is a Lawson Fellow of both the Population Health Program and the Human Development Program of the Canadian Institute for Advanced Research. He is also Director of the Program in Population Health. Through the Canadian Institute for Advanced Research, he has played a central role in developing the conceptual framework for the "determinants of health" and elucidating the special role of early childhood development as one of those key determinants.

Contributors

Carl Bereiter, PhD, Centre for Applied Cognitive Science, Ontario Institute for Studies in Education, University of Toronto, Toronto, Ontario, Canada

Camil Bouchard, PhD, Laboratoire de recherche en écologie humaine et sociale (LAREHS), Université du Québec à Montréal, Montréal, Québec, Canada

Pia Rebello Britto, PhD, Center for Young Children and Families, Teachers College, Columbia University, New York, New York

Jeanne Brooks-Gunn, PhD, Center for Young Children and Families, Teachers College, Columbia University, New York, New York

Robbie Case, PhD, Institute of Child Study, University of Toronto, Toronto, Ontario, Canada

Christopher L. Coe, PhD, Harlow Center for Biological Psychology, University of Wisconsin, Madison, Wisconsin

Max S. Cynader, PhD, FRSC, Department of Ophthalmology, University of British Columbia, Vancouver, British Columbia, Canada

Greg J. Duncan, PhD, Institute for Policy Research, Northwestern University, Evanston, Illinois

Barrie J. Frost, PhD, FRSC, Department of Psychology, Queen's University, Kingston, Ontario, Canada

J. Samuel Gardner, MA, Centre for Studies of Children at Risk, McMaster University/Hamilton Health Sciences Corporation, Hamilton, Ontario, Canada

Sharon Griffin, PhD, Department of Education, Clark University, Worcester, Massachusetts

Richard Harrington, MD, Child and Adolescent Psychiatry, Royal Manchester Children's Hospital, Manchester, United Kingdom

Clyde Hertzman, MD, FRCPC, Department of Health Care and Epidemiology, Faculty of Medicine, University of British Columbia, Vancouver, British Columbia, Canada

Peter S. Jensen, MD, Child and Adolescent Disorders Research Branch, National Institute of Mental Health, Rockville, Maryland

Alan E. Kazdin, PhD, Department of Psychology, Yale University, New Haven, Connecticut

Daniel P. Keating, PhD, Department of Human Development and Applied Psychology, Ontario Institute for Studies in Education, University of Toronto, Toronto, Ontario, Canada

Wendy M. Kelly, MA, Department of Psychology, Trent University, Peterborough, Ontario, Canada

Helena Chmura Kraemer, PhD, Department of Psychiatry, Stanford School of Medicine, Palo Alto, California

Fiona K. Miller, PhD (candidate), Department of Human Development and Applied Psychology, Ontario Institute for Studies in Education, University of Toronto, Toronto, Ontario, Canada

David R. Offord, MD, Department of Psychiatry, McMaster University, and Centre for Studies of Children at Risk, McMaster University/Hamilton Health Sciences Corporation, Hamilton, Ontario, Canada

Alan R. Pence, PhD, School of Child and Youth Care, Human and Social Development, University of Victoria, Victoria, British Columbia, Canada

Chris Power, PhD, Institute of Child Health, Department of Epidemiology and Public Health, University of London, London, United Kingdom

Thomas P. Rohlen, PhD, Institute for International Studies, Asia/Pacific Research Center, Stanford University, Stanford, California

Marlene Scardamalia, PhD, Centre for Applied Cognitive Science, Ontario Institute for Studies in Education, University of Toronto, Toronto, Ontario, Canada

Stephen J. Suomi, PhD, Laboratory of Comparative Ethology, National Institute of Child Health and Human Development, National Institutes of Health, Bethesda, Maryland

Richard E. Tremblay, PhD, Groupe de recherche sur l'inadaptation psychosociale chez l'enfant (GRIP), Université de Montréal, Montréal, Québec, Canada

J. Douglas Willms, PhD, Atlantic Centre for Policy Research, Faculty of Education, University of New Brunswick, Fredericton, New Brunswick, Canada

Foreword

The integration of knowledge about the determinants of health and human development is an important but difficult task. At a recent meeting in Stockholm, sponsored by the Wenner-Gren Foundation and the Natural Sciences and Engineering Council of Canada, the need for stronger interdisciplinary research endeavors was discussed, during which the director of the National Science Foundation in the United States, Rita Colwell, stated that "the departmental structure is a block. We need to tear down the walls that separate our funding agencies."

The Canadian Institute for Advanced Research has advanced programs in Population Health and Human Development that have broken down these disciplinary walls and have fostered collaborations between disciplines that do not customarily interact with each other. The structure of this Institute has made it possible for talented individuals of diverse academic origins to cross the boundaries of their disciplines and develop a common understanding of factors that have critical influences on learning, behavior, and health throughout the life cycle.

The Population Health Program recognized, early in its work, that a crucial factor for determining health is the environment in which people live and work throughout their life cycle, and how individuals cope with their varying environments. As the Program developed, it was increasingly apparent that the contributions of many specialties within the social sciences and epidemiology were not only relevant but were essential, and that health conditions present themselves as gradients when assessed against the social and economic circumstances of individuals.

The importance of these observations was twofold. First, because health status is a gradient, it follows that all sectors of society are affected by factors in the environments where people live and work. Although we know that people in poorer socioeconomic circumstances are not as healthy as those at the top, there is no cutoff point between those at the bottom and those at the next level in the social hierarchy. Furthermore, a large number at the bottom still develop into healthy and competent adults.

The second point is that these gradients in health are not disease specific. The causes of death range from accidents and suicides to cardiovascular diseases and cancer. One of the striking pieces of evidence comes from Michael Marmot's studies of individuals in Great Britain's Whitehall Civil Service, an educated middle-class population with a national health service. Clear health gradients appeared as measured by death and by absence from work due to sickness. Those at the bottom of the job hierarchy had the highest mortality rates and those at the top had the lowest, for all kinds of diseases and injuries. This work showed clearly that the circumstances in which people live, and with which they cope, are important in creating health gradients.

Clyde Hertzman and John Frank, early in the work of the Population Health Program, suggested to their colleagues that the health gradients might be related to the conditions of early childhood. Although there was a literature suggesting that early childhood conditions influence health in adult life, this was not yet a strongly held view in medicine, which was still driven by the disease-based assumption that each disease has a specific cause.

As the Population Health Program wrestled with how to explore this relationship in more detail, information about how the brain develops was becoming better understood through dramatic breakthroughs in the neurosciences. Fortunately, the Institute had in one of its other programs (the Artificial Intelligence and Robotics Program) two individuals, Max Cynader and Barrie Frost, who were actively conducting research in neuroscience. The hypothesis began to emerge that the conditions of early life influencing brain development could set coping skills for life and that the emerging fields of psychneuroendocrinology and psychoneuroimmunology might explain the biological pathways by which an individual's competence and coping skills set health risks throughout life.

The Institute, recognizing that the revolution in neuroscience also had huge implications for our understanding of learning and behavior, proceeded to bring together individuals from developmental psychology, education, anthropology, primatology, experimental biology, and the neurosciences to explore the establishment of a program in human development. As this Human Development Program emerged, under the leadership of Daniel Keating, cross-linkages were developed with the Program in Population Health. Chris Power, associated with the British Birth Cohort studies, was already a member of the Population Health group and had started to build, with Hertzman and Frank, an analysis of the relationship between early-life circumstances and health risks in later life. This emphasized the importance of being able to establish studies that allow for longitudinal analysis of human development and health over the life span.

The further implications of socioeconomic gradients for other critical domains of development besides health status and outcomes became clear through the work of David Offord, Richard Tremblay, Robbie Case, Jeanne Brooks-Gunn, and J. Douglas Willms. Moreover, explorations with comparative studies, organized and implemented by Stephen Suomi and Christopher Coe, have become showcase demonstrations of the importance of critical periods in neuroendocrine and neuroimmune development. These biobehavioral linkages have been extended further to sensitive periods in cognition and behavior, as in mathematics development (Case) and in the functioning of regulatory systems (Keating).

This volume presents an integrated synthesis of what has been learned through the cooperative work of these Institute individuals over the past decade. It establishes that the gradients in health, behavior, and cognitive functions such as mathematics and literacy are largely set in early life. Succeeding events over the life span also influence these characteristics and outcomes, but the weight of the evidence suggests that the quality of nourishment and nurturing in the early years is far reaching. An obvious further observation is that when societies undergo major socioeconomic change, one particularly vulnerable group is young children since they have the least political clout.

These societal implications deriving from the unfolding of the gradient theme became increasingly salient as the story on biological embedding and lifespan trajectories grew clearer. Exploring these connections led to a conception of "the learning society." Thomas Rohlen's work forged some central themes, which were further elaborated by Marlene Scardamalia, Camil Bouchard, Alan Pence, and others in the Human Development Program.

The material in this book raises pertinent questions for societies. Given what we now know about the factors influencing the development of the brain, the biological pathways that affect learned behavior and health, and the long-term effects of a poor early childhood, how do we minimize poor environments for early child development? Clearly, the quality of early childhood affects the quality of the future population and prosperity of the society in which these children are raised. The World Bank, in its endeavors to help the developing world, has adopted this verity as a crucial theme. Because it has been well established by now that the human newborn arrives with all sensory systems functioning, and is capable of learning at birth or even before, the starting point for involving families in child development programs must be very early. Lack of knowledge of infants' capabilities and of the environmental circumstances that best promote early growth and development is no longer a constraint to putting sound programs in place for enhancing children's development. Rather, in the words of the World Bank: "Transforming this knowledge into action is the major limiting factor in implementing early child development programs and requires the combined support of governments, non-government organizations, the private sector and the media" (Young, 1997, p. 330).

Despite the broad synthesis presented in this volume, it needed to be further expanded to include an understanding of the determinants of societies' economic growth. The quality of a population, including its psychological well-being and its capacity for production and intelligent consumerism, is an important factor in economic growth. Often, the narrowly based theories of economists do not embrace the reciprocating effects of economies on the social environment and, in turn, those socioenvironmental effects on human development over the life cycle.

In his Nobel Prize lecture, Robert Fogel, an economic historian, emphasized that the conditions of early childhood set health risks for adult life and have a major effect on economic growth. At the end of his lecture, Fogel pleaded with his economist colleagues to have a better understanding of the long-run dynamic processes and implications: "At the outset of the lecture I stressed the need for economists to take account of long-run dynamic processes through a study of history. Uncovering what actually happened in the past requires an enormous investment in time and effort. Fortunately for theorists, that burden is borne primarily by economic historians. Theorists only need to spend the time necessary to comprehend what the historians have discovered. A superficial knowledge of the work of economic historians is at least as dangerous as a superficial knowledge of theory."

Today, although much remains to be learned, we have enough information about the determinants of life destinies to suggest that it is important for economists and social theorists to acquire a deep knowledge about human development. Furthermore, the work of Robert Putnam has shown that the elements needed to support and sustain healthy societies also develop over the long term and are intimately associated with the economic dynamics of a community.

In this book, the challenge is set for Western societies. Given what we now know about the experiential and environmental determinants of health and human development, we must now meld this intelligence with knowledge about the determinants of economic growth. This effort should move us further toward equality of opportunity for children, in the absence of which we cannot foresee having a healthy, competent population at all socioeconomic levels. Without this, it will be difficult to sustain economic growth in the future, and to establish the basis for tolerant, democratic, sustainable civic societies. The challenge for society explored in this volume is timely and substantial, and it provides a valuable framework within which to address this challenge.

J. Fraser Mustard, MD, PhD
Founding President, Canadian Institute for
Advanced Research

Lewis P. Lipsitt, PhD
Professor Emeritus of Psychology, Medical Science,
and Human Development, Brown University

Preface

This book represents a collaborative effort of the Human Development Program of the Canadian Institute for Advanced Research (CIAR). The members of this program are research scientists and scholars based in Canada, the United States, and the United Kingdom. Under the auspices of CIAR, members have been meeting together since 1993 to discuss the ideas and the research presented in this volume. The conceptual framework reported here is the outcome of intense collaboration, and we have attempted to present the work as a coherent whole. Our goal is to communicate to many audiences, including researchers, policy specialists, students, community developers, and the general public, and to initiate a broad based discussion on the critical topic of human development in the modern world.

The overall argument for the book is summarized in Chapter 1, the Part introductions, and Chapter 18. We hope that readers will be sufficiently intrigued by this framework to explore the research from many disciplines that we use to support the general argument. We also invite readers to follow and to participate in the ongoing dialogue on these topics. Toward this end, we have established a website—the Learning Society Network (lsn.oise.utoronto.ca)—where we have begun to assemble additional background information and to organize web-based discussions for various groups. Future developments of the Learning Society Network will be announced at that site.

Organizing and supporting an international research network, and the members of the network, requires the efforts of many individuals and institutions. CIAR, and the Human Development Program, are indebted to these supporters, and we acknowledge that support with gratitude:

The Atkinson Charitable Foundation
The Lawson Foundation
Donner Canadian Foundation
Manulife Financial
Bank of Montreal
The Molson Foundation

Max Bell Foundation
Royal Bank of Canada Charitable Foundation
Bell Canada
Joseph E. Seagram & Sons Inc.
Canadian Imperial Bank of Commerce
Sun Life Assurance Company of Canada
General Motors of Canada
Tate & Lyle PLC
Great-West Life Assurance Company
The Toronto-Dominion Bank
Investors Group
The W. Garfield Weston Foundation

We are also grateful for the significant intellectual contributions of a number of advisors throughout the history of the program. Two individuals deserve special mention. J. Fraser Mustard, Founding President of CIAR, and Lewis P. Lipsitt, who has chaired the program's advisory committee, have provided invaluable support as senior scientists and scholars in health and human development. We thank them also for writing the Foreword for this volume. We have learned much from them and from other advisors to the program: Stephen Ceci, Doris Entwisle, David Grier, Peter Hicks, Michel Manciaux, Freda Martin, Senator Landon Pearson, Angele Petros-Barvazian, Robert Picard, Saul Schanberg, and Emmy Werner. The unfailing support from CIAR has of course been central to our work, and we particularly want to thank Stefan Dupré, President, and Kathryn Hough, Vice President for Programs.

We have discovered in the course of our conversations that any research network is in fact a network of networks. Too numerous to mention are the many colleagues at the host universities and research institutes where the program members carry out their work. Some of these individuals appear as coauthors of chapters in this volume, and acknowledgments of the contributions of other colleagues and of granting agencies appear after the relevant chapters.

Finally, we want to thank Denese Coulbeck, without whose administrative, editorial, and technical expertise the work of the program and the completion of this volume would have been impossible.

DANIEL P. KEATING
CLYDE HERTZMAN

Contents

1

Modernity's Paradox

Daniel P. Keating
Clyde Hertzman

A puzzling paradox confronts observers of modern society. We are witnesses to a dramatic expansion of market-based economies whose capacity for wealth generation is awesome in comparison to both the distant and the recent past. At the same time, there is a growing perception of substantial threats to the health and well-being of today's children and youth in the very societies that benefit most from this abundance. Urie Bronfenbrenner testified in 1969 to a U.S. congressional committee about the troubling scientific evidence that pointed to a societal breakdown in the process of "making human beings human": "The signs of this breakdown are seen in the growing rates of alienation, apathy, rebellion, delinquency and violence we have observed in youth in this nation in recent decades" (Bronfenbrenner, 1969, p. 1838). More than a quarter of a century later, Bronfenbrenner and several of his colleagues reviewed these trends since the time of his earlier testimony and arrived at a similarly stark conclusion: "Today they have reached a critical stage that is much more difficult to reverse. The main reason is that forces of disarray, increasingly being generated in the larger society, have been producing growing chaos in the lives of children and youth" (Bronfenbrenner, McClelland, Wethington, Moen, & Ceci, 1996, pp. viii–ix).

Nor are these exclusively American concerns. In a recent volume on the stresses facing Canadian families as they try to provide opportunities for the healthy development of their children, it was noted that

> during periods of profound social change, such as the present, some sectors of society are at high risk of encountering a decline of social support and hence an inadequate nurturing of developmental needs. Families with young children are often the most vulnerable, and this appears to be true in our contemporary society. Although economically poor families are at the

1

> highest risk for this form of family insecurity, the changes we are currently experiencing are so widespread that negative consequences are occurring even for the children of families that are moderately secure economically. In particular, labour market policies that do not recognize the extensive demands placed on families with young children, combined with the dearth of good, affordable child care, create a situation in which adequate nurturing of the next generation cannot be assured. (Keating & Mustard, 1993, p. 88)

These concerns, which have been expressed by numerous observers in and beyond North America, are sometimes met with dismissive responses. One of the most powerful is that, although observers have bemoaned the sorry state of youth since the dawn of history, things have always turned out all right in the end despite worried projections. There is another, more limited dismissal: Although the current trends may be real and worrisome, they are no more than phases we are going through as we adapt to new technologies and new social arrangements. Once this phase is past, so this argument goes, things will settle down and return to normal. From this view, the developmental risks are likely not severe but are in any case the cost of progress, common during the sometimes unruly growth of major economic transitions. Both of these dismissive arguments eliminate the paradox by denying that it exists: yes, modern economies are generating record wealth; no, there is nothing especially worrisome in the current trends in human development, because they are trivial, whether persistent or passing.

Yet there are reasons not to accept such dismissals, even if we were to accept their premises. The first arises from a wariness in equating change with progress. Past adaptability of human populations to dramatic social and economic change, even if it could be shown to be the usual case, is no assurance of continued adaptability. To be truly reassured by a claim of enduring adaptability, we would need to know what processes contributed to past success and whether those processes continue to operate effectively in the present. A second reason is that we don't have a ready metric by which to decide whether the current changes offer challenges to healthy human development similar to or different from those in the past. If we use an evolutionary yardstick, the sheer size of human populations, the increasing concentration of populations in urban centers, the sophistication required by new technologies, and the social disruptions experienced by families and communities are sudden, dramatic, and of unprecedented scope. Given this paradox of material abundance and apparent threats to healthy human development, is there any basis on which we might make a reasonable choice between blissful reassurance and grave social concern?

A few years ago, the group of researchers whose work appears in this book began a series of conversations about the state of human development in the modern world with these issues in mind. Like other research groups, public policy groups, and groups of concerned citizens, we talked about both worries and opportunities. Like many others, we saw that there was a good deal to be concerned about—whether today's children and youth are developing in a positive and healthy way, and how we might deal with the impact of rapid social and technological change on society's ability to support human development.

As a group of researchers from a range of scientific disciplines, we were also attuned to the opportunities arising from a growing base of knowledge about many aspects of human development. The explosion of knowledge about the impact of early developmental experiences on brain and behavioral development was one key focus, one which has entered popular discussion with considerable vigor in recent years. The captivating phrase that has been applied to this process is "neural sculpting," whereby the social and physical environments of the infant and young child organize the experiences that shape the networks and patterns of the brain (see Cynader & Frost, Chapter 8, this volume).

Less noted in popular discussions, but of great importance to our growing understanding, is the recognition that the development of health and well-being is a population phenomenon rather than a purely individual affair. Particularly striking is the discovery of a strong association between the health of a population and the size of the social distance between members of the population. We have come to describe this as "the gradient effect": In societies that have sharp social and economic differences among individuals in the population, the overall level of health and well-being is lower than in societies where these differences are less pronounced. We review some of the key data for this claim in Part I of this volume (particularly in Chapters 2 and 3).

As we looked more closely at this gradient effect, two other pieces of the puzzle came to light. The first is that we found this gradient effect not only for physical and mental health but also for a wide range of other developmental outcomes, from behavioral adjustment, to literacy, to mathematics achievement. We came to use the term "developmental health" to describe this full range of developmental outcomes, all of which seem to show the gradient effect on virtually all occasions. The second piece of the puzzle is that the gradient effect seems to hold equally well whether we look at differences in current social status or in the social status of the family of origin. These social status effects appear to be quite persistent, evident at birth and with effects that show up into old age.

Considering this pattern of findings, we were confronted with some critical questions. What can account for this gradient effect for developmental health? Why is it pervasive across so many different outcomes? Why does it show such durability, apparently covering the full lifespan of human development?

In both science and society, we have become more aware in recent years of the strength of diversity in many different arenas, from biodiversity to cultural diversity. Our experience has been that this applies equally well when we are seeking answers to complex questions. Engaging the methods and findings of diverse scientific fields may be an essential ingredient for success in identifying the core processes of systems as complex as human development. As we considered the powerful evidence for neural sculpting in early development and for the gradient effect in developmental health, a potentially important story began to emerge that linked these two sets of findings together, one on individual brain and behavioral development, and the other on lifespan gradient effects in the developmental health of populations.

Simply put, the developmental mechanisms that could generate such pervasive and enduring effects on developmental health may well be located in the fundamental processes of neural sculpting, broadly defined. We came to use the term "biological embedding" to capture this linkage. Variations in social status are associated with important differences in the quality of the social and physical environment that infants and young children encounter, and these differences in turn produce variability in the specific experiences that contribute to neural sculpting and thus potentially to enduring differences in health, coping, and competence. The developmental pathways through which these linkages occur are likely to engage many features of the brain–behavior system, from central processes in the sensorimotor cortex (Chapter 8) to key systems in the neuroendocrine system, which in turn impact hormonal and emotional functioning (Chapter 9), and so also the neuroimmune system, with considerable influence on disease resistance and ability to recover from injury and trauma (Chapter 10).

As with any new formulation, the story is only as good as the evidence to support it. In Parts I and II of this book, we take up these questions in some detail, and focus on the evidence for population gradients in developmental health, for neural sculpting, for biological embedding, and for the linkages among them. If this story is accurate in its broad form, the implications are substantial.

There is a growing recognition that the potential for future economic growth in the Information Age and for the sustenance of civil society is tightly linked to the quality of the human resources available. Exploring these linkages makes it clear that the ways in which societies organize themselves play a crucial role. In Parts III and IV of this book, we take up some of the implications for society arising from this framework on human development, exploring the broad issues of society and culture as well as the local issues of community supports for families and children.

Our interest is not merely academic. If future prosperity and well-being are at stake, then a coherent conceptual framework may be of central importance not only for understanding our circumstances but also for thoughtful and effective action to secure the outcomes we desire.

INVITATION TO A CONVERSATION

We have three related goals in this book. The first is to outline what we see as a coherent conceptual framework for understanding human development in the modern world. This framework has emerged from an ongoing conversation over several years and can be read as a record of that conversation to date. An overview of this conceptual framework can be obtained by reading this introductory chapter, the brief introductions to each of the four parts of this volume, and the concluding chapter.

But a framework without the details to support it is like a blueprint without building materials—intriguing, perhaps even imaginative, but insubstantial in the final analysis. The second goal is thus to present sufficiently detailed discussions of the key evidence that we found compelling in our conversation so that readers can evaluate it for themselves. The real story lies in the details, of course, so we invite readers to explore them.

The third goal emerges from the first two. If the framework on human development we present is persuasive and if we have gone some way toward establishing it, then the implications for our collective future are significant, perhaps even critical. Addressing them, however, is fundamentally a societal issue rather than a merely scientific one. Building a learning society—a society capable of adapting to technological and social change rapidly enough and well enough to maintain or re-create the supports for healthy human development—is a project that can be informed by our best scientific understanding of the underlying processes but cannot be achieved without the widespread engagement of all sectors of society. The final goal is thus by far the most important. Generating a social discussion in which the fundamental importance of human development is recognized and included in societal decisions may well be essential to societal adaptability, and our aim is to offer a framework for such a discussion. In short, this goal is perhaps best understood as an invitation to join the conversation and to act on the insights we gain through this extended discussion.

POPULATIONS AND GRADIENTS

The term "gradient" will be used in this volume to refer to the commonly observed pattern of a monotonic increase or decrease, among a defined population, in an "outcome" variable related to human well-being, in association with an increase or decrease in a measure of socioeconomic status, such as income, education, or occupation. The commonly observed gradients that will be discussed in detail here are, first, increasing health status and, second, increasing levels of cognitive and behavioral development, with socioeconomic status. The common shorthand for these are "the socioeconomic gradient in health status" and "the socioeconomic gradient in development," respectively. We use the comprehensive term "developmental health" to refer to the full set of these outcomes.

We start here because the evidence leads us to believe that the steepness of these gradients gives important clues as to whether a society is supporting or undermining the development of its population. Most significant is the finding that for all areas of developmental health, steep gradients are associated with overall poorer outcomes in comparisons among countries or regions. In particular, steep gradients together with lower levels of developmental health suggest that a society is failing as a collective entity, or that it is in a disruptive social transition due to technological, economic, or political change. In other words, the steepness of gradients may well be an important societal diagnostic to which we should pay attention in making important decisions. It is inconceivable that as a society we would make important decisions without an evaluation of their economic impact, and it is increasingly true that we do not make societal decisions without an understanding of their environmental impact. In contrast, the lack of any systematic way of evaluating the human development impact of the choices we make in the public sector, in the private sector, and in communities is an indication that we have not yet fully grasped the crucial point that these aspects of human development are central not only to our current well-being but also to our future prospects as a society.

FROM SOCIOECONOMIC GRADIENTS IN HEALTH TO HUMAN DEVELOPMENT

Our intellectual trajectory led us from the observation of socioeconomic gradients in health status to a concern with human development. In trying to understand the determinants of population health, three sets of "big facts" were identified which indicated that population health and overall human development were linked:

• Differences in equity of income distribution is one of the principal determinants of differing health status among wealthy societies. Countries with highly unequal income distributions have poorer health status than those with more equitable income distributions.

• From the available data, it seems as though the steepness of the socioeconomic gradient in health status correlates with the steepness of the income gradient, and drives health differences among wealthy societies. The shallower the socioeconomic gradient in health status, the higher the mean level of health. This pattern suggests that health status (as a measure of human well-being) may be embedded in collective factors in society, not just in individual factors.

• Socioeconomic gradients in health status have special characteristics that direct our attention to human development as a source of them: they have persisted across different historical eras in which different diseases have predominated in society; they cut across a wide range of disease processes, including some with an obvious behavioral component (e.g., lung cancer) and others without an obvious behavioral component (e.g., senile dementia); they are expressed in different ways in each stage of the life cycle; they include well-being as well as health narrowly defined; and they cannot be explained away by health selection.

SOCIAL CIRCUMSTANCES: DETERMINANTS OF POPULATION HEALTH

These findings led us to the conclusion that the underlying factors that determine health and well-being must be deeply embedded in social circumstances. There is a vast research literature on "social factors and health," regarding social support, psychosocial working conditions, and material factors that detail aspects of the social environment which are determinants of health and are also associated with socioeconomic status. But this research literature does not explain the full range of characteristics of the gradients in health described above. Thus, differing social circumstances at the time of disease expression are not a sufficient explanation for the robust population patterns connecting socioeconomic gradients to health outcomes.

These patterns of population gradients, especially their longitudinal nature, suggest a potentially important role for the organism's experience, particularly early experience, in shaping coping skills, resiliency, and thus neuroimmune and neuroendocrine response at the individual level, which can then show up later on as population effects. This naturally led us to search for underlying biological processes that have the capacity to affect a wide variety of different disease outcomes. The biology of human development, especially the neurobiology of early child development, has turned out to be a crucial link in this story, as will be discussed in Part II of this volume. Our particular interest is in how social circumstances systematically affect developmental trajectories; how these differences embed themselves in human biology; and how the process of biological embedding, in turn, affects well-being across the life cycle.

LATENT EFFECTS AND PATHWAY EFFECTS

Two different and sometimes conflicting explanatory models of this process have emerged. The first, called the "latency" model, emphasizes the prospect that psychosocial and socioeconomic conditions very early in life will have a strong impact later in life *independent of intervening experience.* It is closely tied to the twin notions of critical and sensitive periods in brain development, which are described in detail in Part II of this volume. Its corollary is that the specific competencies developed at discrete times early in life constitute a disproportionately important investment in lifelong well-being. The second, called the "pathways" model, emphasizes the *cumulative* effect of life events and the reinforcing effect of differing psychosocial and socioeconomic circumstances throughout the life cycle. The hypothesis underlying the pathways model is that, over time, the physiological aspects of less than optimal neurophysiological development, chronic stress and its physiological impacts, a sense of powerlessness and alienation, and a "social support" network made up of others who have been similarly marginalized will create a vicious cycle with short-term implications for education, criminality, drug use, and teen pregnancy, and with long-term implications for the quality of working life, social support, chronic disease in midlife, and degenerative conditions in late life.

In addition to the cumulative effects that pathway models illuminate, there is a second key feature of developmental pathways. Intervention and prevention strategies that are aimed at core developmental processes and that occur at important transition points in development have enhanced prospects for success. The research on early experience as the setting condition for neurophysiology supports the view that this is perhaps the most critical period in human development, but a pathways model affords the opportunity for investigating subsequent developmental transitions that may permit effective redirection of problematic pathways.

It is our intention to explore and understand the relative explanatory power of latency and pathway models, including evidence for cumulative effects and prevention or intervention effects. This, in turn, requires coordinated exploitation of insights from neurobiology and neurodevelopment; longitudinal epidemiology, especially birth cohort studies; primatology and comparative ethology; and international and subnational comparative studies of social functioning.

SOCIOECONOMIC GRADIENTS BEYOND HEALTH

Do we find gradient effects when we look at other kinds of developmental outcomes beyond health? We have found the "flatter equals better" phenomenon that we saw for population health, when we look at developmental outcomes like mathematics achievement, behavioral and school problems, general ability, mental health, and social adaptation. Generally speaking, these are of the same form as the health gradients, in that there do not appear to be major threshold effects. The effect, in other words, is not confined to the relatively poorer outcomes for members of the population at the lowest end. We have found similar patterns for health, competence, or coping—the totality of which we describe as developmental health. The strength of the gradient effect may vary somewhat by outcome, and we will have a clearer picture of the full pattern from the expanding research on this question. But if this pattern indeed holds true for such a wide range of developmental outcomes, as our current findings indicate, it would strongly suggest not only that there are common sources of the pattern but also that the steepness of socioeconomic gradients across different outcomes is an important indicator of population well-being and can thus be used as an important diagnostic of societal adaptation.

Thinking of these patterns as potential social diagnostics raises another important question: is the socioeconomic gradient for developmental health entirely dependent on the distribution of income and wealth in a society? Generally, we find that gradients are steeper in societies with greater wealth and income inequality. However, do such inequalities necessarily lead to steep socioeconomic gradients—that is, gradients in the outcomes of developmental health—or are there other "nurturing" processes which also affect socioeconomic gradients?

If socioeconomic gradients vary across national or regional groups that have comparable levels of wealth and income inequality, the possibility arises that they vary in their distributions of "developmental nurturance." Factors such as education, or stable communities, or stable families, or the opportunities for youth to participate in meaningful activities, may be driven by other social processes besides income. In other words, the social goods of nurturance might not be distributed in an identical way to the distribution of wealth in a given society. This is a very important question to consider, because it may suggest a range of developmentally effective social actions and policies beyond wealth distribution.

GRADIENTS IN SUPPORTS
FOR HUMAN DEVELOPMENT

If it is the case that the distribution of developmental resources rather than strictly the distribution of wealth is crucial, this may offer one possible route toward reducing the negative effects of steep gradients that we have been discovering. It seems unlikely on the evidence that the distribution of income and the distribution of developmental resources are independent. But societies that have discovered ways of disentangling them, to the advantage of higher levels of developmental health, may provide interesting opportunities for societal learning and adaptation.

Can we ask this question empirically so that there is solid evidence for alternative approaches? One method is to examine differences around the socioeconomic gradients to see if some groups or communities achieve better outcomes than would be expected by the gradient effect. It may well be the case that there are clusters of individuals or communities or schools that are outperforming what would be expected by the simple gradient that we have identified. If so, and in some cases it certainly does seem to occur, then it would be very important to understand what are the characteristics of those communities that are performing better than predicted. We often lose sight of this, because of course poorer communities in general fare worse than better-off communities. But in fact some poorer communities or families may be doing something that puts them above where we would expect them to be based on gradient information alone, and perhaps some of the better-off communities are doing worse than we would expect. If we can find these off-gradient clusters, we may be able to gain some important clues about the distribution of the social goods—the developmental resources—that are important to the task of improving outcomes.

This brings us back to a key question discussed above, namely, what are the underlying developmental processes that will help us to understand and unpack these pervasive socioeconomic gradients. Many of the identifiable developmental sources appear to be rooted in what we might call the quality of the social environment and how that operates, particularly during the early years of development. Identifying these sources as they affect children and youth, especially young children, is important due to the considerable staying power of these early influences at the population level across time. Recent work on the origins of antisocial and violent behavior in youth, for example, has clearly pointed to the preschool period as being one of the most crucial sources, suggesting that we may have more effective intervention or prevention activities at those earlier periods in development (discussed in more detail by Tremblay in Chapter 4, this volume).

UNPACKING THE GRADIENT EFFECT

To summarize, several core findings arise from our consideration of the gradients of health, coping, and competence as we move through various levels of socioeconomic status. One is that gradients are pervasive; they are virtually always found. A second feature is that when we compare across societies, the steepness of the gradient is in fact related to the overall functioning of that particular population. It is in the direction that we might expect: where we have steeper gradients, we have lower overall developmental health. Where there are relatively flatter gradients, there is better overall developmental health. This holds even after we remove some obvious factors that differ among societies, like GDP (gross domestic product) per capita. This is not then simply a main effect of differential wealth across societies. Note also that these factors appear to be substantially stronger in their explanatory power than, say, health care expenditures per capita (also adjusted for GDP per capita). The strong inference, therefore, is that the distribution of material or social goods has a substantial impact on developmental health.

We have noted some clues that point toward one promising hypothesis. One already mentioned is that these gradient effects are pervasive and are not disease specific. They occur across the board, including "health" outcomes we normally think of as behavioral, like homicide and suicide. Note also that these effects are not explained fully by lifestyle. Even after adjusting for factors like differential rates of alcohol consumption or smoking, the majority of the health effects still hold. Another clue is that there do not appear to be threshold effects; that is, these effects do not occur just because there is a poverty effect. Instead, these effects typically appear to be monotonic throughout different levels of the population—through the middle class and well into the professional classes. These and other clues led us to seek an answer to the question of how such gradients arise in the domain of early development, and particularly in which biologically based developments might establish patterns that would yield both latent and pathway effects on later developmental health.

BIOLOGICAL EMBEDDING OF GRADIENTS IN EARLY DEVELOPMENT

We saw the need for an approach we came to call "biological embedding" whereby systematic differences in psychosocial/material circumstances, from conception onward, embed themselves in human biology such that the characteristics of gradients in developmental health can be accounted for. In this sense, biological embedding is the key link between human development and health: gradients in health and well-being are therefore a function of human development and its interaction with social circumstances. In Parts I and II of this volume, we consider the evidence in favor of a notion of biological embedding as a useful account of both the gradient effects in developmental health and the longitudinal consequences of neural sculpting, broadly conceived, as a core developmental process that underlies these effects. There are a few key concepts that provide some clarifying context for this account, as discussed in the following subsections.

Biological Embedding Does Not Imply Developmental Determinism

It is crucial to note that biological embedding can be overinterpreted as meaning that there is no developmental flexibility after early development. This is clearly an overinterpretation because we know from current research that there is in fact considerable developmental flexibility and resiliency, even for children who grow up in adverse circumstances. Important developmental resources, such as other adults who can act as surrogate parents when there has been difficult parenting in the biological family, often have a significant positive impact. This suggests that we need to know more about the core processes underlying development, rather than only the identifiable social circumstances surrounding early development. Understanding more about the developmental trajectories of such resilient children can provide important insights for prevention and intervention programs that may be capable of redirecting otherwise problematic developmental pathways.

This observation, however, doesn't diminish the notion that the negative effects are harder to redirect later in development than they would be to prevent earlier in development. On a broad population scale, it has proved difficult to set up programs for redirecting problematic developmental pathways—from antisocial behavior to low educational achievement—that are highly reliable, effective with a substantial portion of the affected population, and affordable in the current economic climate (see Offord et al., Chapter 15, this volume, for a more detailed discussion).

Critical Periods in Early Development

The finding of critical periods in early development is central to the story of biological embedding. The long-term continuity of gradient effects means that we are observing more than simple behavioral continuity at the population level. Rather, the generalizability of the effects, and their longitudinal patterns, point toward a set of developmental mechanisms that incorporate these patterns biologically. Critical periods are defined as periods during which the experiences of the organism will be encoded, especially in the neural system. Before and after critical periods, the same experiences will have little or no effect on the developing organism. The existence of such critical periods increases the likelihood that biological embedding may be a key feature of the observed population patterns in developmental health.

In the sensory cortex, the evidence for critical periods yields a well-established story (see Cynader & Frost, Chapter 8, this volume). For some biological systems, there are very narrow and well-identified critical periods. If the right kind of stimulation is not available at the right time, that system will simply not get hooked up. If the visual system, for example, is deprived of visual input during the critical period, the eye continues to function, the optic nerve continues to function, there is no damage to the visual cortex—but the outcome is that the visual system does not work. If the right kind of stimulation is not available at that critical period in time, then functional vision does not occur, even though the pieces of the system are intact and can function. Evidence for similar critical periods continues to accumulate for neural systems beyond the visual cortex, including other aspects of the sensory cortex, as well as other systems of the brain. Indeed, some fundamental features of social interaction may be related to systems in the brain that are subject to critical periods.

Biology and Experience Interact

Consider one example that emphasizes the importance of experience in shaping the biological systems (which is taken up in more detail by Suomi in Chapter 9). A proportion of rhesus monkeys are genetically hyperreactive; that is, they overreact to stress and novelty. These hyperreactive monkeys actually occur naturally in the population at about the same proportion that hyperreactive individuals apparently occur in human populations—roughly 10% of the population in both primate groups.

The outcome for hyperreactive rhesus monkeys in the wild is not good. They are much less likely to survive to adulthood. If they do survive, they are much less likely to be reproductively fit and they are much less likely to have high status within the troop hierarchy. In general, they have a very rough time of it in normal circumstances. Given all this, one might wonder why hyperreactivity continues to be part of the gene pool. Apparently, in some circumstances, being overreactive is a good thing. If your territory is suddenly flooded with predators, it may be a good idea to run first and think later. On the other hand, in normal circumstances, being hyperreactive in interactions with others in the troop has some very negative consequences.

Physiologically, these individuals are quite different from others, in that the physiological markers of response to stress show very different patterns: hyperreactive monkeys compared to normal monkeys are quicker to respond; they respond more frequently, and to less threatening stimuli; they respond with greater intensity; and they take much longer to return to baseline. When those stress-released chemicals that help animals (including primates) to flee or to fight remain in the system, they have substantial negative impacts on immune system functioning and consequently on the organism's health.

In experimental studies, a hyperreactive monkey (who is known to be so by genetic breeding) can be cross-fostered to be raised by a highly experienced and highly nurturant mother. In those cases, hyperreactive monkeys become physiologically much less distinguishable from normal monkeys; that is, their stress response is generally in the normal range. In terms of behavioral outcomes, they appear to overcome many of the known risk factors and indeed are no less likely to survive, or to reproduce, or to have high status in the troop.

In fact, the one behavioral outcome that does show a significant difference is that hyperreactive monkeys who have been cross-fostered are more likely to become troop leaders. This interesting anomaly may suggest that hyperreactivity, in conjunction with a highly supportive early upbringing, may be recruited in the service of heightened sensitivity to contextual social cues but be able to operate from a sufficiently secure base so as to function well in the very complex social situation of troop life.

We should note that critical periods for social development and for emotional responsivity occur not only in primates but also in other nonprimate organisms. Thus, biological embedding appears to be a fairly widespread developmental phenomenon. The evidence arising from recent work in neural development (Chapter 8), neuroendocrine development (Chapter 9), and neuroimmune development (Chapter 10) suggests that there is a close interplay between biology and experience, especially in early development.

The patterns that get established have important consequences across the board for the organism. Individual experience sculpts the neural pathways that play a key role in shaping later development. They help to establish key pathways between the neural system, the endocrine system, and the immune system. What emerges, then, is not only a strong suspicion based on our longitudinal studies of populations and individuals but a sound biological story that helps us to understand why these effects might be obtained. It increases the likelihood that early experience plays a very major role in individual and population health, coping, and competence.

Sensitive Periods in Early Development

In addition to these biologically critical periods, it is likely that there are developmentally sensitive periods in the construction of human cognitive, social, and emotional systems. Although these are likely to have less of the "all-or-nothing" characteristics of some critical periods, they may operate in a similar fashion in setting important dispositional aspects and bases for future development. A good example is the work on early conceptual structures for mathematics, without which it becomes very difficult for individuals to benefit from typical educational activities in mathematics (see Case, Griffin, & Kelly, Chapter 7, this volume). Lags in achieving these core conceptual structures may not be completely irreversible, but they do make it difficult for the child to catch up or to restructure at a later point in time. In contrast, a solid grasp of these structures early on affords a sound basis for moving toward more complex mathematical concepts.

In a wide range of social and behavioral systems, other sensitive periods have been noted. The early origins of patterns of behavior that lead to subsequent antisocial and aggressive behavior have been well documented (see Tremblay, Chapter 4, this volume). We also have some evidence for sensitive periods in regulatory systems, that is, in emotion regulation, attention regulation, and social regulation, which show longitudinal continuity from the first year of life, to how well the individual will be able to function in school-related cognitive and behavioral skills as he/she enters first grade (see Keating & Miller, Chapter 11, this volume). These findings support the notion that we can understand population gradient effects in terms of underlying developmental processes at the individual level. The biological embedding of early experience in neural and behavioral development may offer the crucial link that explains the complex patterns of population effects.

RESOLVING MODERNITY'S PARADOX

We can return to the central paradox of economically prosperous modern societies: on the one hand, material abundance and the ability to generate wealth unimaginable even by our recent ancestors; on the other hand, grave concern about the deterioration of the quality of the human environment required for high levels of developmental health and about the consequences of this deterioration as seen in increasing developmental problems among children and youth.

The conceptual framework outlined above and explored throughout this volume identifies some elements that help us to see this paradox more clearly. Among prosperous modern societies, the steepness of the social and economic gradients is a key indicator of the overall developmental health of the population. Moreover, these gradients in developmental health likely arise from differential experiences during early development, which become pervasive and enduring due to processes we have identified as biological embedding. The twin notions of neural sculpting and critical or sensitive periods provide key support for such an interpretation. The long-term population consequences of these processes are of potentially great magnitude, due to their considerable reach into the future.

If the health and adaptability of a population do arise in this fashion, then the consequences for the society as a whole may also be considerable. Two centuries ago, at the dawn of the first industrial revolution, Adam Smith (1776/1952) noted two central factors that regulate the wealth of nations. The first is the "skill, dexterity, and judgment with which its labour is generally applied" (p. 1), and the second, the "proportion between the number of those who are employed in useful labour, and that of those who are not so employed" (p. 1). These explanatory factors have endured remarkably well, although we might employ modern economic idioms such as the "social organization of human capital" and "labor productivity."

These factors are worthy of reconsideration at the dawn of the information revolution and in light of the new economies being shaped by this revolution. An often-noted characteristic of the emerging economic order is that wealth generation will be increasingly knowledge driven and less dependent on the massive exploitation of natural and physical resources. An understanding of this innovation dynamic, which arises from the feedback between technological and social innovation (considered in more detail by Keating in Chapter 12, this volume), highlights the central role of human resources, such as human ingenuity, in future economic prosperity.

From this perspective, society's investments in developmental health are also its most significant economic investments. The ability to "apply labor" with skill and judgment presumes that high levels of health, competence, and coping exist in the population, so that human resources are available for use in knowledge-based economies that rely upon an innovation dynamic. The larger the proportion of the population able to participate productively in such innovation-oriented economies—that is, engaged in "useful labor"—the greater the likelihood of increased economic prosperity.

In short, the wealth of nations in the Information Age may depend heavily, perhaps primarily, upon their ability to promote the developmental health of their populations. This, in turn, requires them to create the capacity for providing the necessary developmental resources, which is a significant challenge during the period of rapid social and technological change we are now experiencing. To achieve this level of persistent societal adaptability, it may become advantageous to construct "learning societies" capable of organizing and acting on behalf of human development.

In Parts III and IV of this volume, we take up these questions in two related ways. We first examine the broad historical, cultural, and social terrain upon which a contemporary learning society would need to function (see Chapters 12–14). Within these constraints, we then look at particular issues and local contexts that present opportunities and obstacles for building a learning society (see Chapters 15–18). We found that the conceptual framework on human development with which we have been working provides a useful base for this consideration of society and community issues, and indeed the framework is readily extended to include aspects of human social organization.

We emphasize that this is an evolving framework on human development. At its best, a conceptual framework of any complex system is a way of describing the system's core dynamics and the links between them. Understanding how a system as complex as human development—from biology to society—functions dynamically requires that we observe it in motion.

Influencing its direction requires more than observation, however. It requires discussion among many individuals and groups, and consciously coordinated action among them. We are all, of necessity, both observers and participants in this system, and it is perhaps only through such an extended conversation, open to all observers, that we will be able to grasp the core dynamics of the system and move it toward greater prosperity and developmental health—which, we suspect, may become fundamentally the same in the not too distant future.

Societies that discover this identity at the heart of modernity's paradox—that future prosperity is a direct function of current investment in the developmental health of their populations—and that are capable of acting on this discovery by becoming learning societies seem far more likely to enjoy the benefits of both abundance and social well-being. Nor should the currently prosperous societies feel safe in presuming that they are better able to make the transition to a learning society. The cultural and social resources such a transformation may require are hard to specify in advance. But currently less economically advanced societies may suffer less from complacency about their current status, and so may see themselves as having less to lose and more to gain through substantial transformations.

In contrast to previous experiments in civilization, however, the information revolution may afford more widespread, even global, prosperity, because its knowledge-driven innovation dynamic places fewer demands on control of physical territory and natural resources for economic growth (see Keating, Chapter 12, this volume, for a more detailed discussion). Affordances are not, however, assurances. It is possible to conceive a future in which information technologies further centralize economic and political decisions in the hands of ever smaller and more sophisticated elites, as envisioned in some current science fiction dystopias.

One's estimate of the relative likelihood of these alternate pathways for societal adaptability probably arise from many sources, including evaluations of economic or demographic trends, perspectives on basic qualities in human nature, or personal dispositions. More to the point, however, would be an assessment of the prospects and the means for moving society toward one pathway or the other. For this task, a coherent conceptual framework on human development seems more useful than prognostications, if it can identify the core dynamics of human development and thus the points of leverage for change. These considerations give rise to our three goals: conveying a framework on human development that we have found useful; establishing it insofar as possible with current scientific evidence; and launching a conversation whose aim is to enhance our ability to choose developmental health.

Part I

The Gradient Effect in Developmental Health

I n Part I, we explore the gradient effect in developmental health from several related perspectives. Through an examination of the gradient effect in health, behavior, and achievement, it is clear that developmental health at the population level is at least in large part a function of differences in the steepness of those gradients across nations and regions. In addition, a number of factors that may help to unpack these gradients are identified through these analyses.

In Chapter 2, Clyde Hertzman notes that in wealthy societies the psychosocial and socioeconomic conditions of early childhood are a powerful determinant of health and well-being across the life cycle. Systematic differences in health status and well-being by socioeconomic status (the "gradient effect") in adulthood have their origins in early childhood. Less healthy societies have steep socioeconomic gradients in health status. More healthy societies have shallow gradients. He proposes a process, biological embedding, whereby conditions of early childhood contribute to the gradients. Understanding how these processes work is central to our development as a society.

In Chapter 3, Chris Power and Clyde Hertzman take this story several steps further. The connections between early child development and the socioeconomic gradient in health status operate through latent and pathway effects. Evidence from longitudinal studies shows that both apply. That is, circumstances in early childhood can affect health status later in life independent of intervening experience (i.e., latent effects), and also through the life pathways that individuals get set on. Pathway effects are closely related to cumulative risk, wherein the duration of "exposure" to at-risk living conditions has a dose–response effect on subsequent health and well-being. The effectiveness of early intervention programs is evidence of pathway effects up to the age of intervention and of latent effects thereafter.

Focusing on a behavioral domain of developmental health in Chapter 4, Richard E. Tremblay notes that longitudinal research also shows that the roots of juvenile delinquency and adult criminality are in early childhood. Somewhat counterintuitively, young children are quite physically aggressive but this declines in time for most. Among boys, direct physical aggression is most important. It is a powerful predictor of school success or failure. Among girls, indirect aggression predominates. Both phenomena show social class gradients. However, Canadian data show that, among low socioeconomic groups, the family can serve as a powerful buffer. Early interventions have been shown to successfully alter trajectories that begin with aggression and lead to grade failure and criminality.

In Chapter 5, J. Douglas Willms shows that on an international basis, literacy patterns parallel health status in a very important way: each country shows a socioeconomic gradient in literacy such that the countries with the highest level of literacy have the shallowest gradient. In other words, relative equality is good for both vulnerable and privileged elements in society. Between-province comparisons of literacy in Canada show the same pattern, and a socioeconomic gradient is found for the Peabody Picture Vocabulary Test (PPVT) at the age of entry to school. Studies of school performance in Scotland show that a socioeconomic mixture of students at a school is a powerful predictor of its collective academic standing. Attempts to improve school performance through parental choice are shown to be futile since they exacerbate, rather than mitigate, this effect.

In Chapter 6, Jeanne Brooks-Gunn, Greg J. Duncan, and Pia Rebello Britto take a closer look at early cognitive development and find that there are effects from a variety of sources: income, maternal education, single parenthood home environment, and neighborhood. Income is a significant independent predictor of cognitive development that functions in a gradient fashion. Most significant, it shows a "duration of exposure" effect as well as an "intensity" effect, based upon the depth of poverty. This analysis helps to identify the relative strengths of some of the most potent effects on developmental health and offers important insights on how they will need to be addressed.

In Chapter 7, Robbie Case, Sharon Griffin, and Wendy Kelly extend this gradient analysis to the domain of mathematics. Mathematics achievement, like literacy and health status, show socioeconomic gradients internationally that, like the others, are steeper in countries with lower average achievement and shallower in countries with higher achievement. Cognitive psychology studies demonstrate that competence in math is a function of the development of "central conceptual structures" whose neural substrate is currently under investigation. In the absence of intervention they show a socioeconomic gradient, likely based on the degree of exposure to quantitative concepts early in life. However, these conceptual structures can be put in place by appropriate interventions before school age such that the relative disadvantage on this dimension can be removed.

2

Population Health and Human Development

Clyde Hertzman

Health status differs markedly among individuals within a given population. Yet, it does not necessarily follow that the factors determining the health status of large populations are the same as the factors operating at the individual level. In recent years an impressive body of evidence has emerged that shows how population health is influenced by social/economic relations within society, by the psychosocial impact of these relations, and by experiences during sensitive periods in human development (the social/economic/psychosocial conjunction is herein referred to as SEP conditions). It is the purpose of this chapter to explore the determinants of health of populations, highlighting the complex relationship between human development and the SEP conditions that produce or undermine health from the beginning to the end of the human life cycle.

The notion that SEP conditions are the principal determinant of population health in wealthy societies is supported by country-by-country comparisons of health status. For these purposes health status is represented by longevity, as measured by life expectancy. At the level of international comparisons, longevity is the most useful health status indicator because it is well measured and recorded over time, and because it is not biased by cultural differences that affect other indexes based upon self-reported perceptions of well-being.

EMERGENCE OF THE "FLAT OF THE HEALTH–WEALTH CURVE"

The role of the SEP conditions is highlighted by the relationship between health and wealth in different countries over time. Superficially, international differences in per capita income appear to correlate positively with differences in longevity. Early in this century the relationship was simple: life expectancy was greater in countries with higher per capita incomes. Figure 2.1 shows that the longest-lived and richest country had a life expectancy of approximately 54 years (World Bank, 1993). However, in recent decades the relationship between health and wealth has become more complex as rich nations have grown increasingly rich.

The health–wealth curves for 1930 and 1960 are similar to those for 1900, but, as average life expectancies and national incomes increased over the century, the simple monotonic relationship between health and wealth broke down among the high-income countries. By 1990, the world's richest nations had achieved levels of national wealth unprecedented in history. At the same time, a distinct "flat of the health–wealth curve" had emerged, such that increasing income among those countries with per capita incomes greater than U.S. $10,000 was no longer associated with further increases in life expectancy (World Bank, 1993). Yet, the traditional monotonic relationship between health and wealth persisted among the world's poorer countries.

Why does the health–wealth curve flatten at the wealthy end? A closer look at the trends helps us to answer this question. Among the Organization for Economic Cooperation and Development (OECD) countries, which make up virtually all of the countries on the flat of the curve, increases in per capita income from 1970 to 1990 did not correlate with increases in life expectancy. In other words, not only has the "one point in time" relationship between health and wealth broken down among wealthy countries, but the temporal dynamic between health and wealth has broken

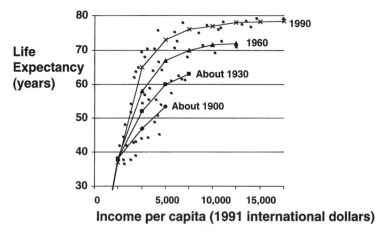

FIGURE 2.1. Life expectancy and income per capita for selected countries and periods. Adapted from *World Development Report 1993* by World Bank. Copyright 1993 by The International Bank for Reconstruction and Development/The World Bank. Used by permission of Oxford University Press, Inc.

down, too. This does not mean, however, that all the world's wealthy countries have health statuses that are similar to one another. In fact, there are large variations in health status among them and, also, there are large differences in the rate of increase in health status over time. An understanding of the basis of these variations should help to uncover the principal determinants of health in wealthy societies.

Useful insights come from studies of the relationship between income equality and life expectancy in wealthy societies (Wilkinson, 1992a, 1992b). These studies show that the proportion of national income being received by the least well-off families (after taxes and transfers) in each country is a strong positive correlate of life expectancy differences between them. Those countries with relatively equal income distributions are healthier than those with relatively unequal distributions. Furthermore, those countries that were able to preserve or increase their level of income equality during the 1970s and 1980s enjoyed greater gains in life expectancy than did those countries with increasingly unequal income distributions. Wealthy countries with the largest income gap from richest to poorest do show improvements in health status over time, but their gains are smaller than among wealthy countries with narrower income gradients.[1]

The validity of this relationship has been challenged (Judge, 1995) based upon concerns about the comparability of data on income distribution between countries, the arbitrariness of the income cutoffs used, and problems in reproducing the results. But these concerns have largely been answered by the work of Kaplan, Pamuk, Lynch, Cohen, and Balfour (1996), who compared income distribution and life expectancy among the 50 U.S. states and found that those with higher levels of income equality had populations with longer life expectancies. Because this study was done within one country, income data for each state came from a common data source. Also, the design passively controlled for national level effects. The observation that relative income equality predicts improved population health status serves as a valid starting point for understanding the determinants of health in wealthy societies.

SOCIOECONOMIC GRADIENTS IN HEALTH STATUS

Why does health status vary with income distribution in wealthy countries? No one has a precise answer to this question, but it is clear that it has something to do with the way in which different societies handle the tendency for market forces to produce social inequalities and reinforce social hierarchies. There is a large fact that supports this observation: health status increases with increasing socioeconomic status (Kunst, Guerts, & Berg, 1992; Kunst & Mackenbach, 1992) in every wealthy society on earth. The pattern is typically not a simple difference between the healthy rich and the unhealthy poor. Rather, the health status of each class within the population seems to be better than that of the classes below and worse than that of the classes above. In other words, middle class people may live longer and healthier lives than do the poor, as we would expect, but they also live shorter, less healthy lives than do the rich. The pattern just described is remarkably consistent across OECD countries, regardless of whether the classes are defined by levels of income, education, or occupation—so much so that this pattern has been canonized as the "socioeconomic gradient" in health status.

The socioeconomic gradient in health status is not new. It has remained largely unchanged since the beginning of the 20th century *despite the fact that the principal causes of death have changed completely since 1900.* In fact the socioeconomic gradient in health status seems to be able to replicate itself on the principal diseases of each era, despite the fact that their pathological basis varies greatly. For instance, at the turn of the century the gradient was found among the infectious diseases that were the principal causes of death at the time. By late in the century, the socioeconomic gradient had replicated itself in heart disease, injuries, and almost all prevalent cancers, which are the current major causes of death.

With respect to international differences in health status, the leading hypothesis is that differences in the magnitude of the socioeconomic gradient in health status within each country drive the difference in average health status between them. International comparisons to validate or refute this hypothesis are hard to make for largely technical reasons. However, the work of Vagero and Lundberg (1989), comparing socioeconomic gradients in health status between Sweden (a country with a relatively equal income distribution) and the United Kingdom (a country with a relatively unequal income distribution) is useful in this regard. They applied the British occupational classification system to the working populations of both countries in order to compare early mortality among adult males. Three important observations emerged. First, the socioeconomic gradient in mortality was steeper in the United Kingdom than in Sweden. Second, mortality was lower in Sweden for both the high and low occupational classes compared to their British counterparts. Third, mortality among the lowest occupational group in Sweden was, in fact, lower than that of the highest occupational group in the United Kingdom.

Since the United Kingdom is a comparatively low life expectancy country on the flat of the curve and Sweden is a high life expectancy country, Vagero and Lundberg's (1989) work suggests that societies which minimize the socioeconomic gradient in life expectancy maintain better health status for all social classes than societies which do not. The same pattern is seen in relation to socioeconomic gradients in mathematics achievement. Case, Griffin, and Kelly (Chapter 7, this volume) show that scores of grade school pupils from five countries participating in the Second International Mathematics Study display a gradient by father's occupation. A country-by-country comparison of these gradients shows the same three characteristics as those of the mortality analysis of Sweden and the United Kingdom.

The country with the highest average score (Japan) had the flattest gradient, and the superiority of Japanese scores over other countries was found across all occupational classes. Japan is also the country with the greatest longevity in the world. A general impression is created that equality is good, not only for the vulnerable but for the privileged, too.

With respect to health it has long been accepted that national economic factors mattered, and the question has always been, how much? But the belief was that economic factors operated through the consumption of items affecting health, such as food, housing, and medical care. The debate seemed to end with the notion that, beyond a certain level of individual income necessary to buy healthful goods and services, no more health gains could be expected from increasing prosperity. It is now clear that there is much more at stake and that the socioeconomic effect is not confined to those too poor to buy health-enhancing goods. The prospect that socioeconomic gradients in both mortality and mathematics achievement underlie between-country differences, and do so in similar ways, suggests that socioeconomic gradient functions tap attributes that are deeply embedded in the psychosocial character of human societies.

EXPLAINING SOCIOECONOMIC GRADIENT IN HEALTH STATUS

From a health status perspective, populations can be partitioned according to any number of different characteristics, but the interesting partitions are those that demonstrate important differences in health status across population subgroups in many diverse settings. The concern here is not the rather obvious fact that groups of people differ in their health status but in the fact that there are systematic partitions of the population that consistently define subgroups differing from one another with respect to health. For instance, when socioeconomic status is divided into quartiles based on income, occupation, or education (or combinations thereof) a gradient in health status is found at all ages but is embedded in different health outcomes at different stages of the life cycle.

The life cycle is fundamental to the study of health status because it is the basis of biological change in all individual organisms. It can be divided into age segments during which different types of diseases or conditions are predominant. The perinatal period is a subdivision of the life cycle so important that its statistics have often been used as major health indicators for populations (e.g., perinatal mortality rate and birth weight distribution). The period of "misadventure" extends from less than 1 year of age to the age at which chronic diseases of midlife begin to have significant impact. During this time, the principal threats to health are not disease based but rather accidents, violence, and suicide. The period from 45 to 74 years may be called the period of "premature" chronic degenerative disease. During this period, heart disease, stroke, arthritis, and cancer are the principal diseases that threaten health, function, and life. These chronic conditions are so prevalent in the later years of this age range that one may rightly term their occurrence by midlife as premature—reflecting an accelerated natural history in such individuals. The age of 75 is arbitrarily identified as the onset of the period of more generalized senescence, during which time health status is often determined by the late and usually less specific effects of chronic degenerative disease throughout the body, leading to multiple organ system dysfunction.

Early in life there is a gradient in infant mortality and low birth weight; during childhood and adolescence there is a gradient in injurious deaths, as well as in cognitive and socioemotional development; in early adulthood the gradient is found among deaths from injuries and mental health problems; in late middle age early chronic disease mortality and morbidity show a gradient; and in late life a similar pattern is seen for dementia and other degenerative conditions.

The largest component of the socioeconomic gradient in health status is differential mortality and morbidity at one specific stage of the life cycle: the period of premature chronic degenerative disease. But this is not the time at which the principal determinants of differential mortality and morbidity begin to have their biological effect. It is necessary to work backwards in time to find their origin. This issue has been addressed by population health researchers through a conceptual framework that accounts for "sources of heterogeneity" across the life cycle. In this context, heterogeneity is meant to be a value-free term for variations/inequalities in health status. Sources of heterogeneity are the basic types of causal pathways or mechanisms that might lead to the differences in health status observed across population partitions and stages of the life cycle. Each type of causal pathway has radically different implications for how we think about the origins of health and disease, and about policies to address them. Six mechanisms encompass all the relevant pathways. The first two of these explain away the gradient as an artifact; and the latter four are causal explanations. The artifactual explanations are as follows:

• *Health selection.* This is best explained with reference to a hypothetical example. If it were found that the prevalence of persons with mental health problems was higher in the city than in the suburbs, an investigator using the health selection approach would ask, "To what extent do persons with mental health problems migrate to cities?" rather than "Are cities a source of threat to a person's mental health?" In other words, the actual causal pathway is posed in reverse of what is initially supposed.

• *Differential susceptibility.* This is the propensity of different individuals to upward or downward social mobility determined by heritable (not acquired) characteristics that also determine better or worse health. For instance, the argument may be made that upward social mobility is itself based on inherently favorable genetic characteristics that also determine better prospects for health status.

The causal explanations are as follows:

- *Individual lifestyle.* In this account, the health habits and behaviors of those in different subgroups lead them to have different risks of particular life-threatening and/or disabling conditions. In particular, health-promoting behaviors may tend to be practiced more frequently among those in higher socioeconomic groups, and health-damaging behaviors, the reverse.
- *Physical environment.* Differential exposures to physical, chemical, and biological agents at home, at work, and in the community lead to differences in health status in this explanation. This category would include all the diverse influences of the built environment on health.
- *SEP conditions.* This includes the effects of access to material resources, social isolation, civil society functions, income distribution, and the panoply of psychosocial stresses of daily living.
- *Differential access to and/or response to health care services.* This encompasses differences in health status that are related to differences in care-seeking behavior, differences in the quality of health services and access to them, and differential outcomes for a given treatment.

The evidence regarding the socioeconomic gradient in health status has been evaluated according to this framework and can be summarized as follows. The reverse causality hypothesis is refuted by the fact that the socioeconomic gradient is as strong when social class is based upon education as it is when based upon income or occupation. After all, educational status does not decline with health status, as is possible with income or occupational category. Differential susceptibility can only be evaluated through evidence from longitudinal studies. When this has been done, as it was in a series of longitudinal studies in the United Kingdom, it turns out that factors such as height, which are developmental markers of future health, are also markers for upward social mobility. However, these factors' contribution to the gradient is not large and partially reflect the quality of the SEP environment (Power, Manor, & Fox, 1991).

Similarly, those in lower socioeconomic groups are exposed, on average, to more toxic chemicals and more unsafe physical environments than are those in higher socioeconomic groups. However, the proportion of deaths in OECD countries that can be attributed to the physical and chemical environment is small and does not explain a large percentage of the gradient (Hertzman, 1995). The same thing can be said for access to and/or response to health care services. Even in countries like Canada and the United Kingdom, where universal access to "medically necessary" services is the rule, there are social/economic differences in how individuals use the system. There are also differences in survival following treatment. But "medically avoidable death," that is, life-threatening disease for which there is effective *life-saving* treatment, represents a small proportion of all deaths and also a small proportion of the overall gradient in health status.

By exclusion, this leaves lifestyle and SEP conditions per se. There is no question that lifestyle factors play a significant role in the socioeconomic gradient in health status. Mortality from diseases with a large lifestyle/behavioral component, such as lung cancer, do have a steep socioeconomic gradient. But the socioeconomic gradient is not confined to diseases with a lifestyle or behavioral component. Among those with such a component most of the gradient in mortality survives after the contribution of social class differences in the behavior of interest has been taken into account.

The first Whitehall Study, which was a longitudinal follow-up of mortality by rank in the British civil service, illustrates this point best (Marmot, 1986; Marmot, Rose, Shipley, & Hamilton, 1987). In this study mortality from heart disease and all other causes was analyzed according to occupational rank within the civil service, as well as by each of the traditional cardiac risk factors, including smoking, blood pressure, and cholesterol level. The outcome was a large gradient in cardiac mortality by grade in the civil service. Mortality was lowest for the administrative grades of the civil service, higher for the professional and executive group, higher still for the clerical grades, and highest for those in the unskilled grades. The traditional risk factors explained only a small fraction of the gradient. Instead, most of the gradient was a function of the attributes of occupational grade per se (Marmot, Rose, et al., 1987).

In the end, a robust assessment emerges. Income gradients are a principal correlate of differences in health status among wealthy societies. Income gradients are, in turn, associated with socioeconomic gradients in health status within countries. Countries with relatively unequal income distributions tend to have relatively steep socioeconomic gradients in health status. Steep gradients in health status involve large effects at the low end of the socioeconomic spectrum but measurable negative effects at the high end, too. The primary component of the socioeconomic gradient in health status is SEP conditions per se. There is a secondary component, based upon the socioeconomic gradient in health-related behavior and lifestyle, that begins early in life and augments the underlying gradient.

A detailed understanding of how the socioeconomic gradient comes about depends upon an understanding of the complex mixture of psychosocial and material influences operating at various levels of social aggregation, and the series of biological responses whose character and significance varies from stage to stage across the life cycle. In humans, such a study of the determinants of health would be limited by money, time, and the supply of useful natural experiments. But these limitations do not apply as much to studies of certain other primate populations, which nevertheless show remarkable similarities to human populations. Their usefulness derives from the fact that the investigators are able to juxtapose measurements of well-being against a detailed understanding of the identities of individual primates, as well as the social dynamics and living conditions of the primate population "in the wild." One of the most useful of these has been the study of free-ranging baboon populations of the Serengeti Plains of Northern Tanzania (Sapolsky, 1992), from which a preliminary model of the determinants of health has been abstracted. This model, in turn, has become the basis of a framework for understanding the necessarily fragmentary information from human studies.

AN ANIMAL MODEL OF THE DETERMINANTS OF HEALTH IN WHOLE SOCIETIES

The model, which has four elements, is presented below:

1. *Rank.* When all other factors are held constant, higher rank in the baboon community means higher levels of well-being.

2. *Social stability and its enforcement.* When baboon societies are stable, those in dominant positions have higher levels of well-being than they do during periods of instability. When stability is imposed by high levels of violence and coercion, the nondominant baboons have lower levels of well-being than when it is maintained with low levels of violence and coercion.

3. *The experience of rank, stability, and enforcement.* When social instability occurs, some nondominant baboons will actually experience increases in well-being. This is because their relationships with those higher in the hierarchy are traditionally stressful. These relationships may be interrupted by the preoccupations the more dominant baboons have with each other during fights for supremacy. Other low-ranked baboons, however, will do worse if they become the victims of displaced aggression from the losers in the fight for social dominance.

4. *Personality and coping styles.* Individual characteristics matter, too. The ability to distinguish seriously threatening situations from ruses; to distinguish winning from losing a fight; to relieve stress by displacing aggression; and to be able to develop friendships and strategic alliances—all lead to increased well-being. Each of these characteristics has a component that is related to circumstances of upbringing and mentorship.

With one eye on nonhuman primates and the other on people, it is possible to identify the analogous elements of human society that may determine health and well-being. It also becomes easier than it was, in the absence of the primate model, to create a preliminary model of the relationships between these elements. This is described below.

The primate studies suggest that all levels of societal aggregation need to be considered simultaneously in order to adequately explain heterogeneities in health and well-being. Fundamentally, hierarchy and social stability are characteristics of whole societies, although they may be encoded either within society as a whole (social stability) or in the individual (place in hierarchy). There is a parallel between, on the one hand, the pattern of increased well-being in baboon communities with low levels of violence and coercion and, on the other, the findings (described earlier) showing that relative income equality (Wilkinson, 1992a, 1992b) and shallow social class gradients in health (Vagero & Lundberg, 1989) are determinants of longevity in human societies. The experience of hierarchy, stability, and enforcement (e.g., the day-to-day stresses of good times, such as a positive workplace and home life, and bad times, such as loss of control at work, layoffs, or long-term unemployment) are, by current terminology, "civil society" functions that reside in an intermediate zone between the individual and the state. Personality and coping styles are embedded in the individual but have both a social network aspect and a longitudinal, developmental aspect.

These relationships are summarized by the model in Figure 2.2, which represents the individual life cycle as an arrow, piercing a bull's-eye, which represents society. Society is shown to have three classes of factors, represented by three concentric circles, which represent determinants of health and well-being at three levels of social aggregation. At the most intimate level are the factors associated with social support. At the next level out are the factors at the level of the civil society that can buffer or exacerbate the stresses of daily living. Finally, at the broadest level of aggregation are state factors—in particular, national wealth, income distribution, and the structure of opportunity created by history, geography, and fortune—that support or undermine health and well-being.

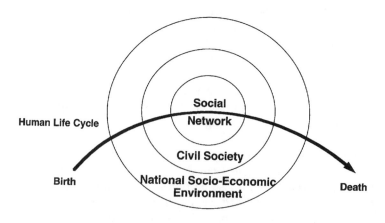

FIGURE 2.2. Framework for human development and the social determinants of health.

The picture that emerges is of a lifelong interaction between the cognitive and socioemotional capabilities of the *developing* individual and SEP conditions as they present themselves at the intimate, civic, and state level. The dimension of human development emerges as one of the principal components of the SEP conditions that determine health throughout the life cycle.

BIOLOGICAL EMBEDDING, LATENCY, AND PATHWAYS

By invoking insights into nonhuman primate and human biology, it is possible to tender a hypothesis that spending one's early years in an unstimulating, emotionally and physically unsupportive environment will affect the sculpting and neurochemistry of the central nervous system in adverse ways, leading to cognitive and socioemotional delays. The problems that children so affected will display early in school will lead them to experience much more acute and chronic stress than others, which will have both physiological and life path consequences. Because the central nervous system, which is the center of human consciousness, "talks to" the immune, hormone, and clotting systems, systematic differences in the experience of life will increase or decrease levels of resistance to disease. This will change the long-term function of vital organs of the body and lead to socioeconomic differentials in morbidity and mortality. This process, whereby human experience affects the healthfulness of life across the life cycle, is herein called "biological embedding" (Hertzman & Wiens, 1996).

Insights into biological embedding come from a variety of sources, including nonhuman primate studies, studies of critical periods in brain development, and the emergent fields of psychoneuroimmunology and psychoneuroendocrinology. For instance, the observation that the neurological system can talk to the immune and endocrine systems provides biological plausibility to the notion that the conditions of life, filtered through a perceptual screen, could affect vitality through a wide variety of pathological mechanisms. From the perspective of modern biomedicine and public health this is more than just a little bit counterintuitive, because it challenges the importance of specific disease labels and of the utility of pathophysiological characterization as the foundation of health care.

Consider dementia of the Alzheimer's type (DAT) as an example of how the population health perspective can transform our view of an "organic" condition. This example relates to the role of education in early life and the development of DAT in late life. When it first emerged that better-educated people scored better on the screening mental status exam for DAT than those who are less educated, the response of biomedical traditionalists was to presume that people who are better educated are generally better test takers and can "fool" screening tests (Kittner et al., 1986). If one did a complete Alzheimer's workup, they argued, this pattern of lower risk among the better educated would disappear. Since then several studies of the risk of fully diagnosed DAT in relation to education have been done. For example, the Canadian Study of Health and Aging involved a full Alzheimer's work up of a population-based sample of community living seniors. After adjustment for various confounds, there was a fourfold gradient of risk for DAT across the range of education received by those who came of age in the 1930s (D'Arcy, 1994). This study is not unique. There are other studies that have produced consistent results (Fratiglioni et al., 1993; Mortimer & Graves, 1993; Stern et al., 1994), and several longitudinal studies showing that the rate of decline of mental status with increasing age is greater among those with lower levels of education than it is among those with higher levels of education (Evans et al., 1993).

Learning and memory depend upon connections between nerve cells in various parts of the brain. Dementia involves the loss and disorganization of these connections. Education likely enriches the network of interconnections—creating reserve capacity that can compensate for the inevitable losses that occur with aging—and postpone the onset of dementia. Although a "use it or lose it" principle may apply to learning and memory capacity, there is evidence that, once capacity has been created, it may confer lifelong benefit. In one study, the written autobiographies of 93 young women entering convent life were analyzed for idea density and grammatical complexity 58 years later, when the women were 75–95 years old. Among the 14 who died with pathologically confirmed Alzheimer's disease, all had shown low idea density as young women. Low linguistic ability in early life was also a strong predictor of poor cognitive function in late life (Snowdon et al., 1996).

What is begged by observations like this is an understanding of how differing SEP conditions, unfolding over time, initiate and sustain processes that lead to differing levels of health, well-being, and competence across the life cycle. A developmental perspective that begins at the very beginning of life would seem indispensable here. In practice, this means paying particularly close attention to insights gleaned from longitudinal studies, especially those that begin at birth and follow large population samples for decades thereafter.

Two different and sometimes conflicting explanatory models emerge of the impact of childhood experiences in later life. The first, called the "latency" model, emphasizes the prospect that SEP conditions very early in life will have a strong effect later in life *independent of intervening experience*. The second, called the "pathways" model, emphasizes the *cumulative* effect of life events and the ongoing importance of SEP conditions throughout the life cycle. The empirical relationship between latent effects, pathway effects, cumulating risk, and a putative "outcome" (arbitrarily occurring at age 35) are presented graphically in Figure 2.3.

The Latency Model

The essence of the latency model can be illustrated with an example from animal research. A series of studies has been carried out that examined the lifelong impact of "handling" newborn rats (Meaney, Aitken, Bhatnager, van Berkel, & Sapolsky, 1988). Handling involves removing the mother from the litter, placing individual pups into a new cage for 15 minutes, then returning both mother and pups to their cage. This is done once per day for the first 3 weeks of life. When compared to nonhandled pups, this simple intervention was associated with improved function of the "stress system" throughout the life cycle (i.e., lower basal corticosterone concentrations and faster physiological recovery in stressful situations). These changes reduced the total lifetime exposure of the brain to corticosterone, which is toxic to nerve cells in a brain structure known as the hippocampus, and thus the rate of loss of nerve cells in the hippocampus was reduced in the handled rats over their lifespan.

Cognitive functions are sensitive to relatively small degrees of hippocampal damage, and so by 24 months of age, elderly by rat standards, the handled rats had been spared some of the cognitive deterioration typical of aging. The significance of this was demonstrated by performance on a learning task wherein rats had to find a submerged platform in a pool of opaque water, relying entirely upon visuospatial cues from the surrounding room. Nonhandled rats had a progressive deterioration in their performance with age; in contrast, no deterioration occurred in aged handled rats. *Most relevant in this context is the final observation: the handling phenomenon could not be induced by carrying out the handling paradigm at a later age* (Meaney et al., 1988).

This example clearly illustrates the notion of a critical period in development. For the purposes of understanding the latency model its essence is

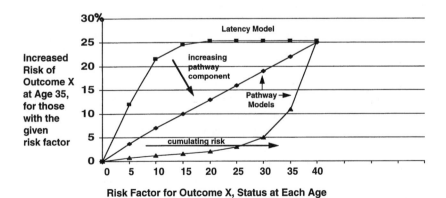

FIGURE 2.3. Latent effects, pathway effects, and cumulative risk.

an opportunity to develop a competence which occurs at a discrete and unique time in (early) life, and has a lifelong impact on well-being, independent of intervening experience. Figure 2.3 illustrates this in negative terms, with a risk factor rather than a protective one. It shows that the risk is associated with the status of the factor at an early age and does not increase thereafter. For instance, the risk of death from heart disease in the fifth decade of life is strongly associated with the size of an individual's placenta at birth and weight gain during the first year of life (Barker, 1991; Barker, Meade, et al., 1992; Barker, Bull, Osmond, & Simmonds, 1990; Barker, Godfrey, Osmond, & Bull, 1992; Barker & Martyn, 1992; Barker & Osmond, 1986; Barker, Osmond, Golding, Kuh, & Wadsworth, 1989; Barker, Osmond, Winter, Margetts, & Simmonds, 1989; Barker, Osmond, Simmonds, & Wield, 1993). Certain early childhood stimulation programs have been effective in improving the life trajectories of disadvantaged children (Palmer, 1979; Schweinhart, Barnes, & Weikart, 1993) even without any attempt to provide them with ongoing support. The common theme here is the notion of a discrete time, early in life, when the right things must happen, or else it is "all over."

The Pathways Model

The hypothesis underlying the pathways model is that, over time, the physiological aspects of less than optimal neurophysiological development, chronic stress and its physiological impacts, a sense of powerlessness and alienation, and a "social support" network made up of others who have been marginalized will create a vicious cycle with short-term implications for education, criminality, drug use, and teen pregnancy, as well as long-term implications for the quality of working life, social support, chronic disease in midlife, and degenerative conditions in late life. It is most closely associated with the findings from long-term follow-up studies of newborns, adolescents, working populations, and the elderly. These studies can be put together in a time sequence to reconstruct the life cycle. A pattern then emerges that highlights the enduring impact of status on health, well-being, and competence from cradle to grave. In highly abbreviated form, it goes something like this:

Status differences at birth are associated with different levels of stability and security in early childhood, which are, in turn, associated with different levels of readiness for schooling (Case & Griffin, 1991). Lack of school readiness leads to an increased risk of behavioral problems in school and ultimate school failure (Pulkkinen & Tremblay, 1992). Behavioral problems and failure in school lead to low levels of mental well-being in early adulthood (Power et al., 1991). Meanwhile, the status of one's parents helps to determine the community where one grows up, which, by the early school years, starts to influence the child's life chances through the social networks, community values, and opportunities that present them-selves (Haan, Kaplan, & Camacho, 1987).

By early adulthood individuals start to define their own status. Already, differences begin to emerge wherein those who are doing better report higher levels of well-being. As adulthood unfolds, lower-status individuals tend to end up in jobs that make relatively high demands on them but which offer low levels of control of the pace and character of the work (Karasek & Theorell, 1990). A good example of this is bus driving, which could be contrasted with conducting an orchestra. By the fifth decade of life, those who are stuck in such jobs first develop high rates of disability and absenteeism (Marmot, 1993; Marmot et al., 1991), and then they begin to die prematurely and from the full range of major causes of death (Marmot, Kogevinas, & Elston, 1987). This general pattern, which is more pronounced among those who are also socially isolated, persists into the eighth decade of life (Wolfson, Rowe, Gentleman, & Tomiak, 1991). Figure 2.3 shows a range of ways in which life pathways could link risk factors to cumulating risk to negative outcomes over the life course.

At first glance, it would appear commonsensical to view the latency and pathway models as complementary to one another. After all, there is no reason to suppose that latent factors only act independently, because any early life event that could exert a latent effect could also be the first step along a lifelong pathway that might have implications for health, well-being, or competence in the future. Conversely, any early childhood intervention designed to improve health and well-being in the long run will occur within a specific context that will provide a mixture of opportunities or barriers. Indeed, the closer the correlation between early life events and subsequent lifelong pathways, the more difficult the statistical problem of estimating the partial contribution of each.

Consider, for example, the findings of the longitudinal follow-up of subjects from the High/Scope Perry Preschool Project study (Schweinhart, Barnes, & Weikart, 1993), to age 27 (Figure 2.4). This study is significant because it was based upon one of the most comprehensive of the early intervention programs for children in American inner cities and because it was evaluated by comparing outcomes among children who were randomly assigned to "preschool" and "no preschool" (control) groups. The data can be interpreted in two ways. One interpretation would emphasize the remarkable improvements experienced by the preschool group in relation to the controls: higher rates of high school graduation, higher earnings, a higher proportion of home ownership, fewer receiving social services, and fewer with frequent arrests. The alternate viewpoint would emphasize the fact that most of the achievements of the preschool group, although impressive when compared with the controls, do not nearly match those of middle class children who have been presented with better opportunities but no special preschool intervention programs. After all, 7% of the inter-

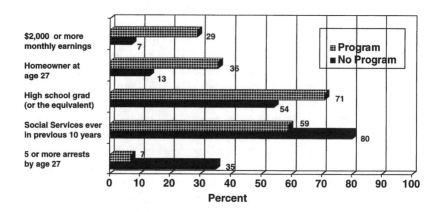

FIGURE 2.4. High/Scope Perry Preschool Project: Major findings at age 27. All findings are significant at $p < .05$, two-tailed. Adapted from Schweinhart, Barnes, and Weikart (1993). Copyright 1993 by High/Scope Educational Research Foundation. Adapted by permission.

vention group had still been arrested or detained at least five times and 59% had received social services in the 10 years prior to follow-up.

At first, this example seems to illustrate the complementary nature of the power of latency, as demonstrated by the elements of effectiveness of the targeted "early life" intervention, and the power of the pathway, as demonstrated by the strict limitations to success that existed in the specific context of the study community. Yet, despite the conceptual complementarity, the two approaches end up in ideological conflict. The latency model, on the one hand, leads easily to a "vaccination" approach to policy, through the following reasoning: the more important that critical periods are, the more important latent effects are. The more important latent effects are, the more important targeted strategies for child stimulation and social support are, at critical periods in the development of the human brain.

According to this approach, socioeconomic influences on health, well-being, and competence throughout the life cycle ought to be addressed through a series of "magic bullet" social, emotional, and/or educational strategies—highly focused in time and very specific in content. Deeper challenges to the nature of society can be blissfully ignored. The pathways model, on the other hand, leads directly to the prying open of social policy questions from cradle to grave and the pursuit of a broad agenda of social reform.

Can sophisticated measurements, in particular from longitudinal studies, overcome this nascent ideological debate? Insights from analyses of birth cohort studies are useful in refining our understanding of the relative contributions of latent and pathway effects. (Chapter 3 by Power & Herzman, this volume, on the 1958 British birth cohort study is useful in this regard.)

FROM INDIVIDUAL TO SOCIETY

The model of biological embedding would predict that, if childhood prevention or intervention efforts were to improve health and well-being throughout the life cycle and fundamentally address the socioeconomic gradient in health status, they would be more likely to be social or educational interventions than health interventions per se. The body of evidence that can be derived from intervention studies in the postneonatal and preschool period suggests that performance in two basic domains of child development, the cognitive and the social–emotional, can be modified in ways which should improve long-term outcomes. Moreover, evidence from such long-term follow-up studies as we have (see Chapter 3, this volume) strongly support the view that they *do* improve long-term outcomes.

But can the effects of individual intervention studies be scaled up to improve society as a whole? This question is motivated by comparison between Sweden, Canada, and the United States, which defined a very large "potential space" for improvement in competence in Canada and the United States (Organization for Economic Cooperation and Development [OECD] & Statistics Canada, 1995). Table 2.1 compares the level of literacy and numeracy among the *least well-educated* segments of the Swedish, Canadian, and American populations. Sweden is a high life expectancy OECD country with a shallow socioeconomic gradient in health status and a high level of income equality. Canada is a moderately high life expectancy country with a steeper socioeconomic gradient in health status and an intermediate level of income equality. The United States is a low life expectancy country with a steep socioeconomic gradient in health status and a low level of income equity. In addition, both Canada and the United States tolerate much higher levels of child poverty than do any countries in Western Europe. Table 2.1 shows that literacy and numeracy skills, even among the least-educated parts of Swedish society, are vastly better than in Canada or the United States.

This conjunction of levels of competence, health, and income equality is central to the relationship between population health and human development in wealthy societies. As an exercise in international comparison, the differences found could not necessarily be construed as being due to differences in child stimulation regimes, or any other specific factor for that matter. Factors at all levels of society may have played a role. The problem

TABLE 2.1. Percentage of Those with Primary Education Only Who Are at Each Literacy Level

		Document scale		
	Lowest	2	3	Highest
Canada	73.6	15.4	9.7	1.3
United States	74.0	18.8	6.3	1.0
Sweden	22.5	38.1	33.2	6.2
		Quantitative scale		
Canada	69.4	18.5	11.3	0.8
United States	66.8	23.2	9.1	0.8
Sweden	21.7	32.0	35.3	11.1

Note. Data from Organization for Economic Cooperation and Development (OECD) and Statistics Canada (1995).

of scale begs a deeper understanding of the dynamics of health, well-being, and competence in society.

HUMAN DEVELOPMENT AND POPULATION HEALTH IN CONTEXT: THE CASE OF CENTRAL AND EASTERN EUROPE

After 1989, changes occurred in Central and Eastern European society that amounted to the most massive experiment in social stress imaginable, short of war and mass starvation. Within 4 years of the sudden political changes of 1989, real wages in countries of the former Warsaw Pact had fallen significantly; between 18 and 54% (UNICEF, 1994). There was also marked disruption of the social environment, as demonstrated by 19–35% declines in crude marriage rates and reductions in pre-primary school enrollment (UNICEF, 1993). According to sample surveys of 10 countries in the region conducted in the winter of 1993/1994, between 20 and 53% of households reported that they could not cope economically; even when resources gleaned from the informal economy were considered (Rose, 1995; Rose & Haerpfer, 1994).

At the same time, there were dramatic increases in mortality among males and females of working age. Among young males aged 30–49, mortality rose as much as 70–80% in Russia; 30-50% in Ukraine; and 10–20% in Hungary, Bulgaria, and Romania. Among females, mortality in the same age range rose 30–60% in Russia; 20–30% in Ukraine; and more modestly in Hungary, Bulgaria, and Romania (UNICEF, 1994). Stresses in the socioeconomic/psychosocial environment would seem to be the principal determinant of the dramatic rise in mortality. This conclusion has been reached by thorough investigation and exclusion of the competing hypotheses and has been well documented elsewhere (Hertzman, Kelly, & Bobak, 1996).

How much of the life expectancy gap can be explained by the long-term effects of early life experiences, and how much has to do with current circumstances? Since mortality increased rapidly concurrently with rapidly deteriorating socioeconomic circumstances, it would seem at first glance that current circumstances must be more important than the long-term effects of early life experiences. However, as P. Watson has pointed out (see Hertzman et al., 1996), the mortality effect is not evenly distributed. In particular, single and divorced people are more affected than married people. Although this may be a current-time social support effect, the ability to create and maintain a marriage under recent Central and Eastern European conditions may also reflect a high level of capacity and coping skills brought forward from earlier in life.

One could think of the post-1989 period in terms of a giant interaction effect between increasing levels of unavoidable stress across society and individuals with markedly heterogeneous coping skills and stress responses. The expected result would be an unequal distribution of increased mortality, according to known vulnerability factors, such as marriage, education, social support, and income. The fact that the largest increase in mortality took place during the young-to-middle adult period would suggest that the greatest stresses were being exerted on those in the early stages of labor force participation and family formation. In this interactive model, the individual's coping skills represent the contribution of latent factors and the changing environment of stress represents the pathway contribution.

An existing model of this interaction between individual capacity and changing social stress comes from the work of Glen H. Elder (1979), who compared the life trajectories of cohorts born in the early and late 1920s in the United States. Up until the mass mobilization of World War II, those born in the early 1920s seemed to show developmental advantages of growing up during the economic prosperity of that decade, compared to those who spent their first decade of life living through the Great Depression. However, the effect of World War II, which brought new opportunities and renewed prosperity to the United States, was to ameliorate these differences. In other words, a societywide reduction in negative stress, due to mobilization, created an opportunity for individuals to overcome their vulnerabilities.

Is there an analogy, such that the stresses of the post-1989 period in Central and Eastern Europe had the opposite effect from the benefits to Americans of mobilization during the "good war"? In other words, does increasing social stress create the conditions under which differences in vulnerability among individuals are expressed? This is among the most compelling questions generated by the experience of Central and Eastern Europe; it is central to the relationship between population health and human development in wealthy societies.

NOTE

1. The term "gradient" will be used in this chapter to refer to a monotonic increase or decrease between an outcome variable, such as health status or level of cognitive development, and a measure of socioeconomic status, such as income, education, or occupation. In the case considered above, income gradients are based upon estimating the proportion of national income received by the poorest $X\%$ of the population, the next poorest $X\%$, and so forth.

3

Health, Well-Being, and Coping Skills

Chris Power
Clyde Hertzman

In Chapter 2 it was argued that the social environment has a profound effect on human development in general and health in particular. Evidence on the universality of socioeconomic gradients in health is especially important in this regard. But the extent of socioeconomic health differences is variable across societies, suggesting that reductions in these gradients might be achieved and that these reductions would be accompanied by health gains within a given population. Understanding the causes of health differences is therefore of relevance to health and social policy. For this reason it is fortunate that research to understand socioeconomic differences in health has developed in parallel with that focusing on explaining health differences among individuals.

It has also been appreciated, increasingly over the last decade or so, that circumstances in childhood can have long-term health effects. As described in the previous chapter, there are alternative ways in which such long-term health effects can occur. One is the latency model, illustrated with the early life rat "handling" experiment (see Chapter 2), in which discrete events early in life have a strong independent effect later in life. Evidence supporting the existence of critical or sensitive periods in brain development is taken to support this model (Cynader, 1994), as are the associations between birthweight, placenta size, and weight gain in the first year of life with cardiovascular disease in the fifth decade (Barker, 1992, 1994).

A second is the pathways model, emphasizing the role of early environment on subsequent life trajectories, which in turn influence adult health. In other words the pathways model focuses on the cumulative effect of life events along developmental trajectories, and it thereby implicates conditions of life throughout the life cycle in adult disease causation (Hertzman, 1994). Evidence for differential pathways and related health effects is most widely seen in relation to socioeconomic status, as supported by the findings of studies of working populations and the elderly, that highlight the enduring impact of social position on health.

The relative contribution of latent versus pathway effects in explaining long-term socioeconomic gradients in health and well-being can only be elucidated with detailed information on individuals followed over time. Longitudinal studies (both observational and interventional) are indispensable in this endeavor. Given that it is particularly in relation to development *in utero* and in infancy that latency models have been proposed, it is also of importance that follow up studies commence at birth, if not before. Thus longitudinal studies starting at birth, namely, birth cohorts, are of particular importance, especially when follow-ups extend far enough into adult life to include the chronic and degenerative conditions of middle and late life. Typically intervention studies have had shorter periods of follow-up, but their importance lies in their ability to demonstrate long-term impacts through altered life trajectories.

This chapter presents data from a birth cohort study that commenced in Great Britain in 1958 (hereafter the 1958 birth cohort) to provide insight into the relationship between latent and pathway effects. These insights will be supplemented with information from intervention studies that illustrate the significance of the timing and character of modifiable events during the first decade of life.

THE 1958 BRITISH BIRTH COHORT STUDY

The 1958 study is one of three British birth cohort studies (the other two being studies of births in 1946 and 1970). The 1958 cohort is especially useful for the purpose of investigating latency and pathway effects because of its large sample size: more than 17,000 subjects were included in the original study population of all births in 1 week in 1958 (March 3–9) in England, Scotland, and Wales (Butler & Bonham, 1963). Subsequent follow-up of survivors has been undertaken at ages 7, 11, 16, 23, and most recently in 1991, at 33 years (Ferri, 1993). At ages 7, 11, and 16 immigrants to Great Britain born during the same week were included in the study; 11,407 subjects (69% of the target) remained in the study at the most recent follow-up at age 33. During the adult years (ages 23 and 33) information was obtained through a personal interview with the study subject, whereas previously several sources were used, including parents and schools (teachers and doctors) and cohort members. Table 3.1 summarizes the basic study details.

With regard to birth and childhood, the study has recorded family and socioeconomic circumstances (such as family composition, housing ameni-

TABLE 3.1. Summary of the 1958 British Birth Cohort Study

	1958 Birth	1965 Age 7	1969 Age 11	1974 Age 16	1981 Age 23	1991 Age 33
Target sample[a]	17,773	16,883	16,835	16,915	16,457	16,455
Data sources	Parents	Parents School Tests Medical	Parents School Tests Medical Subject	Parents School Tests Medical Subject	Subject Census	Subject Census Spouse/ partner Children
Achieved sample	17,414	15,458	15,503	14,761	12,537	11,407

Note. From Power and Hertzman (1997). Copyright 1997 by The Royal Society of Medicine Press. Reprinted by permission.
[a]All living in Great Britain born March 3–9, 1958 (including immigrants 1958–1974).

ties, and level of crowding), health and social development and educational attainment. For example, details of occupation have been recorded for the parents during the child and adolescent sweeps and then of the subjects themselves at ages 23 and 33. In this chapter we refer to occupational class as grouped into four categories: (1) classes I and II (professional and managerial); (2) class IIInm (skilled nonmanual); (3) class IIIm (skilled manual); and (4) classes IV and V (unskilled manual). Information on educational qualifications achieved by early adulthood (age 23) is also used. There are five categories of qualifications: above A level, A level or equivalent, O level or equivalent, less than O level, and no qualifications. These are broadly comparable with U.S. groups: above high school diploma, high school diploma/grade 12, grade 10, less than grade 10, and no qualifications.

Health status in early adulthood is represented by a range of measures (mainly self-reported) that fulfill at least one of two criteria. They are particularly prevalent among young adults, and also they predict future disease risk. Measures include the following: self-assessed health rating; longstanding conditions that limit activities of daily life; psychological distress (as indicated by the Malaise Inventory symptom checklist); back pain; respiratory symptoms (cough and phlegm); and obesity, as derived from the body mass index (>30 for men and >28.6 for women).

LATENCY AND PATHWAY EFFECTS IN THE 1958 BRITISH COHORT

Table 3.2 shows the relationship between social class at birth (as defined by father's occupation in 1958) and selected health measures at age 33. The relationships are summarized as odds ratios of classes IV and V versus classes I and II. Odds ratios describe the increased probability of a particular outcome that can be attributed to a specific factor. An odds ratio of 2.0, for example, means that the risk is doubled.

It is evident that the lowest social classes at birth have elevated risks for almost all health measures, especially for psychiatric distress and poor self-health rating for both sexes. While each of these measures might be regarded as "soft" (despite their predictive value for subsequent mortality), the same general pattern emerges for "harder" health measures such as obesity and reports of respiratory symptoms. Table 3.2 therefore suggests a latent effect of social circumstances at birth and health in early adulthood.

However, a latency effect of early life social circumstances is difficult to establish from this information alone, and a latency model may be an incomplete explanation because there is no representation of intervening experience in Table 3.2. It is possible that social class at birth predisposes the individual to a series of social and biological events that evolve over time and are similarly related to social position. If so, social class at birth would be a marker for subsequent experience and the data in Table 3.2 could instead be explained by a pathway model.

The prospect at issue is that early life social origins and the experiences which go with them serve to differentiate subsequent life trajectories in a way that influences adult health. To study this proposition, we have examined how risks accumulate over time in relation to social class of origin.

TABLE 3.2. Relationship between Health at Age 33 and Social Class at Birth, Expressed as Odds Ratios (Classes IV and V vs. I and II)

Health measure	Men		Women	
	OR	CI	OR	CI
Poor self-rated health	2.30	1.69, 3.15	2.74	2.00, 3.75
Limiting long-standing illness	1.45	0.97, 2.16	1.94	1.30, 2.90
Psychological distress[b]	1.86	1.18, 2.91	3.03	2.15, 4.29
Respiratory symptoms	1.61	1.26, 2.06	1.97	1.51, 2.56
Obese[c]	1.85	1.33, 2.60	1.81	1.36, 2.40
Back pain[d]	1.12	0.92, 1.36	1.59	1.31, 1.94

Note. OR, odds ratio; CI, 95% confidence intervals.

[a]For a fuller definition of health measures see Power and Bartley (1993).

[b]Scoring 7 or more on the malaise inventory.

[c]Body mass index >30 (men); >28.6 (women).

[d]Back pain in the last 12 months.

TABLE 3.3. Social and Biological Risk Factors for Adult Disease, According to Social Class at Birth

| Risk factors | Sex | Social class at birth | | | | | Total sample | χ^2 trend |
		I & II	IIIn	IIIm	IV & V	All		
Birthweight	M	3,433	3,415	3,357	3,354	3,371	7,635	$p < .05$
(mean g)	F	3,295	3,277	3,237	3,207	3,239	7,154	$p < .05$
Childhood conditions[a]								
Crowding (%)	M	10.6	21.5	34.1	47.6	31.7	6,573	444.4*
	F	9.5	23.3	35.0	46.1	31.8	6,242	417.4*
Amenities (%)	M	2.7	5.3	8.8	12.8	8.3	6,641	95.5*
	F	3.0	4.8	9.1	13.1	8.5	6,305	92.5*
Parental	M	12.8	22.6	18.7	23.0	18.9	5,001	24.92*
divorce (%)	F	14.4	16.4	18.2	24.0	18.6	5,097	28.62*
Height age	M	1.78	1.77	1.77	1.76	1.77	6,388	$p < .05$
33 (mean m)	F	1.64	1.63	1.62	1.62	1.63	6,700	$p < .05$
Educational	M	5.2	10.0	14.7	27.9	15.3	5,645	212.3*
qualifications[b]	F	3.7	7.6	15.6	25.6	14.8	5,670	225.6*
Regular	M	20.3	23.2	27.2	30.4	26.1	4,239	25.48*
smoking ages 23–33 (%)	F	17.5	20.4	26.4	35.2	26.0	4,542	75.00*
Job demand/	M	14.5	17.6	21.8	27.1	21.0	4,655	46.88*
control[c] (%)	F	25.1	33.9	34.8	37.8	33.5	4,942	34.89*

Note. From Power and Hertzman (1997). Copyright 1997 by The Royal Society of Medicine Press. Reprinted by permission.
[a]Childhood material conditions, indicated by overcrowding (>1 person/room) at any two ages at 7, 11, or 16; and sharing or lacking household amenities (either hot water, bathroom, indoor toilet) at any two ages at 7, 11, or 16.
[b]Qualifications obtained by age 23, none versus 1 or more.
[c]High negative work attributes, such as no ability to vary the pace of work or timing of breaks; monotonous tasks; no requirement for learning new skills.
*$p < .001$.

This is illustrated in Table 3.3, which gives the distribution of seven social and biological risk factors according to social class at birth. Risk factors are presented in order of the age at which they occur. Each factor was selected because it had been suggested as having an independent predictive effect on adult disease: birthweight (Barker, 1992, 1994); childhood material circumstances (Forsdahl, 1977; Gliksman et al., 1995; Lundberg, 1993; Nystrom Peck, 1994); parental divorce (Amato & Keith, 1991; Parker, 1992; Schwartz et al., 1995; Tennant, 1988); height (Leon, Davey-Smith, Shipley, & Strachan, 1995; Marmot, Shipley, & Rose, 1984; Nystrom Peck & Vagero, 1989; Waaler, 1984); educational attainment (Doornbos & Kromhout, 1990; Elo & Preston, 1996; Feldman, Makuc, Kleinman, & Cornoni-Huntley, 1989; Pappas, Queen, Hadden, & Fisher, 1993; Valkonen, 1989); smoking behavior (Wald & Hackshaw, 1996); and demand and control relationships at work (notably work stressors and the range of decision making freedom) (Karasek & Theorell, 1990; Lerner, Levine, Malpeis, & Dagostino, 1994; North, Syme, Feeney, Shipley, & Marmot, 1996).

Strong gradients are observed according to social class at birth for each of these factors (Table 3.3). This confirms that class at birth, whatever else it represents, is systematically associated with several principal determinants of adult disease. Furthermore, Table 3.3 also provides evidence that the selected factors accumulate differentially by social group, such that by adulthood those born into successively lower social classes have experienced more bio- logical and psychosocial risk, have received fewer educational investments, and have poorer working environments and worse health behaviors than those with higher social origins (Power & Matthews, 1997).

The most parsimonious explanation of these findings is that pathway ef- fects are the dominant source of variation in health status in adulthood. This is because the opportunities, obstacles, and experiences that differ systemati- cally across social classes are the pathways through which systematic differ- ences in risk accumulate. Even so, the relationships in Table 3.3 may be misleading, in that what appear to be accumulating risks may merely be time- dependent markers that have been largely predetermined by early social ori- gins. Further evidence is needed to disentangle early and later life factors.

For example, if the pathway model were important, then adult health risk would be more strongly related to factors that accumulate over time than to social class at birth. One test of this is provided by a comparison of the relationships for educational attainment and adult health (Table 3.4)

TABLE 3.4. Relationship between Health at Age 33 and Educational Qualifications, Expressed as Odds Ratios (No Qualifications vs. above A Level)

Health measure[a]	Men		Women	
	OR	CI	OR	CI
Poor self-rated health	4.35	3.15, 6.00	4.76	3.48, 6.50
Limiting long- standing illness	3.33	2.22, 5.00	2.42	1.65, 3.56
Psychological dis- tress[b]	4.34	2.74, 6.88	6.96	4.88, 9.92
Respiratory symp- toms	3.82	2.95, 4.94	3.75	2.86, 4.91
Obese[c]	2.72	1.92, 3.84	2.11	1.61, 2.78
Back pain[d]	1.75	1.39, 2.19	1.66	1.33, 2.07

Note. OR, odds ratio; CI, 95% confidence intervals.
[a]For a fuller definition of health measures see Power and Bartley (1993).
[b]Scoring 7 or more on the malaise inventory.
[c]Body mass index >30 (men); >28.6 (women).
[d]Back pain in the last 12 months.

with those for social class at birth and adult health (Table 3.2). It appears that gradients of health outcome, at this stage in the life course, are stronger in general in relation to educational attainment than to social class at birth (Manor, Matthews, & Power, 1997).

Educational attainment is strongly influenced by social background, but it is not equivalent to it. Indeed, social measures such as occupational class and education may be related but they are theoretically distinct, with occupation representing working and living conditions, and education representing cultural, or human, capital (Dahl, 1994). This distinction is validated by the observation that health behaviors such as smoking and diet are more closely associated with education than they are with income and occupation (Winkleby, 1992). In the present context, educational attainment is likely to be representing aspects of readiness for school, social and behavioral adjustment, social investment opportunities made available, social stability, and health-related behaviors. Thus, it is an excellent marker of the "healthfulness" of accumulated childhood experience. That educational attainment is more strongly associated with adult health status than class at birth suggests that pathway effects may be operating, but it does not rule out latent effects because educational attainment may merely be an indicator of the quality of early life circumstances.

DISENTANGLING LATENCY AND PATHWAY EFFECTS

Is the implication of the above discussion that latency and pathway effects cannot be disentangled in the context of longitudinal studies? In Chapter 2 it was suggested that, whereas latency and pathway models are easy to differentiate in the abstract, the available evidence is difficult to attribute unequivocally to one or the other. Nonetheless, in relative terms, some pieces of evidence support one model more than the other.

For example, recent studies of the 1958 birth cohort, on the long-term effects of parental divorce, show contrasting patterns for symptoms of psychological distress (indicated by the Malaise Inventory score) and for heavy drinking (Hope, Power, & Rodgers, 1998; Rodgers, Power, & Hope, 1997). Table 3.5 presents odds ratios for study subjects whose parents divorced during their childhoods (i.e., before age 16). These data show that the sequellae of parental divorce in terms of psychological distress are already apparent by age 23 and that these persist to age 33. For heavy drinking, associations with parental divorce are weak at age 23, but adverse relationships have emerged 10 years later. There was no variation in these effects by the age at which parental separation occurred for either psychological distress or alcohol consumption.

This suggests that the latency model fits the relationships between parental divorce and heavy drinking better than that for psychological distress. In this case parental divorce is taken to represent childhood adversity

TABLE 3.5. Odds Ratios (95% Confidence Intervals) of Psychological Distress and Heavy Drinking and at Ages 23 and 33 by Parental Separation

	Men			Women		
	N	Age 23	Age 33	N	Age 23	Age 33
		Psychological distress				
No separation	3,818	1.00	1.00	3,947	1.00	1.00
Separation	390	2.54	2.03	480	1.69	1.82
		(1.80, 3.60)	(1.43, 2.89)		(1.34, 2.14)	(1.41, 2.35)
		Heavy drinking				
No separation	3,813	1.00	1.00	3,945	1.00	1.00
Separation	387	1.28	1.59	483	1.18	1.85
		(1.00, 1.63)	(1.21, 2.10)		(0.82, 1.70)	(1.21, 2.82)

Note. Psychological distress is indicated by a Malaise Inentory score of more than 7. Heavy drinking is defined as over 35 units of alcohol for men and over 20 units for women. Data from Rodgers et al. (1997) and Hope et al. (1998).

more generally, and psychological distress and heavy drinking in adulthood are long-term health outcomes. Thus, there is clear evidence of a latent period between the time of divorce and the onset of risk for heavy drinking, but there is less support for a latency effect for psychological distress. This observation, however, is not unequivocal. A skeptic could argue that heavy drinking at age 23 and age 33 are not the same phenomenon. At age 23, heavy drinking is generally accepted by society, albeit reluctantly, as a normal social activity of young adulthood, whereas heavy drinking by age 33 stands out as an inappropriate response to underlying psychosocial strain, which strain likely had its origins earlier in life.

Another example, in this case predominantly fitting a pathways model, comes from an analysis of cumulative risk in relation to a poor self-rating of health among cohort members at age 33 (Table 3.6). A cumulative score of socioeconomic circumstances, ranging from 4 (most favorable) to 16 (least favorable), was derived from parental occupational class at birth and age 16, and from own occupational class at ages 23 and 33. Thus, the cumulative score represents duration and intensity of material/psychosocial privilege or deprivation. The range in the percentages rating their health as poor is between four- and fivefold from the lowest to the highest cumulative risk category. This difference is greater than that which is apparent for any occupational class measure at a single point in time, indicating that cumulative exposure matters a great deal. Moreover, for both men and women the risk increases monotonically with increasing cumulative score, suggesting the absence of a timing effect in relation to socioeconomic circumstances. In other words, circumstances at each life stage add to one another; early exposures do not seem to preempt the effect of later exposures.

Studies with more limited information on lifetime socioeconomic cir-

TABLE 3.6. Percentage with Poor Health Rating at Age 33 According to
Cumulative Socioeconomic Circumstances (Birth to Age 33)

Cumulative socioeconomic score[a]		Men (3,461)	Women (3,602)
Best	4	4.1	3.9
	5	6.5	9.5
	6	5.8	3.9
	7	7.1	7.5
	8	11.4	9.8
	9	8.3	9.0
	10	10.4	13.9
	11	13.0	14.1
	12	16.0	14.5
	13	13.4	20.1
	14	18.3	23.2
	15	22.4	20.4
Worst	16	17.6	19.4

[a]Based on social class at birth, ages 16, 23, and 33.

cumstances, but whose follow-ups include later life disease risk and mortality are in support of cumulative socioeconomic effects. Within the British regional heart study, for example, the relative odds (adjusted for age) of myocardial infarction increased from 1.0 in men in a nonmanual occupational class both at birth and in their adult life, to 1.6 in men who had a manual class either at birth or in adulthood, to 1.7 in men who had a manual class on both occasions (Wannamethee, Whincup, Shaper, & Walker, 1996). Similarly, within the Paisley–Renfrew study based in Scotland, socioeconomic circumstances were examined at three life stages (birth, labor market entry, and later in adulthood) in relation to subsequent mortality risk, with men in the highest social class on every occasion having the lowest risk and those in the lowest social class on each occasion having the highest risk (C. Hart et al., 1995).

MODIFICATION OF EARLY LIFE INSULTS

None of the above discounts the prospect that early-life exposures will predispose individuals and groups to systematically differing subsequent life trajectories. In the Kauai birth cohort study, for example, it was found that severe perinatal stresses (i.e., complications of pregnancy, labor, and delivery) compromised the physical and psychological development of children from low socioeconomic status families but were successfully buffered in higher status families (Werner, 1989). By 20 months of age, the average "developmental quotient" for low socioeconomic status children who had experienced severe perinatal stress was much below that for similarly stressed children from higher socioeconomic status families. In contrast, low socioeconomic status children who had experienced mild or moderate perinatal trauma were developmentally much closer to their more affluent counterparts. High socioeconomic status, in this case, represents a series of ongoing investments that not only protect healthy children from future risks but can reverse the impact of existing risks.

Intervention studies are important because they evaluate investment strategies in early childhood that are designed specifically to modify life trajectories. After all, the "high socioeconomic status" investment described above pays off when children reach school age. Those who are less ready, intellectually and emotionally, to cope with the school environment quickly enter a spiral of behavioral acting out and academic failure that may lead to early dropout and delinquent behavior in both boys and girls (Tremblay, Mâsse, Perron, & LeBlanc, 1992).

Evidence showing that early life experiences can be altered, and in ways which affect subsequent health and well-being, is in effect support for a complex interaction between latent and pathway effects. If an intervention at a given age modifies subsequent trajectories and thereby alters a long-term outcome, then the pathway model clearly applies up to the age of the intervention and the latency model applies thereafter. This is because evidence of an effective intervention at a given age is also evidence that the long-term outcome had not yet been predetermined by that age. From the standpoint of social policy, evidence that earlier interventions are more effective than later ones supports the relative importance of the latency model. If late interventions are effective this provides support for pathway effects.

The model of biological embedding (Chapter 2, this volume) would predict that, if childhood interventions were to improve health and well-being throughout the life cycle and fundamentally address the socioeconomic gradient in health status, they would be more likely to be social or educational interventions than health interventions per se. There is now an extensive body of research showing that well-designed stimulation programs can improve the cognitive and social–emotional development of children. The focus on cognitive and social–emotional functioning is relevant because of its connection to school readiness. School readiness, in turn, is important because the complex web of early academic failure and early school misbehavior is associated with lack of school readiness and, in turn, strongly predictive of school failure, employability, criminality (Tremblay et al., 1992), and psychological morbidity in young adulthood (Power, Manor, & Fox, 1991).

Programs Beginning in Infancy

The search for ways to improve health, well-being, and competence throughout the life cycle begins with "parent–infant stimulation" programs. These programs usually start in the first few months or years of life.

The specific details of the programs vary, but they share certain common characteristics: the activities take place at home, with or without a separate learning center focus; there is voluntary involvement of at least one parent; the role of the parent in the process of child development is actively reinforced (Bromwick & Parmelee, 1979; Levenstein, O'Hara, & Madden, 1983), and positive role models from the local community are promoted (Jester & Guinagh, 1983); contact with program staff is frequent (i.e., at least twice monthly); and the programs consciously focus on both cognitive and social–emotional factors.

Most but not all of the parent–infant stimulation programs deal with "high-risk" children. Those considered high risk fall into two categories. In the first, aspects of the economic, educational, and/or psychosocial environment at home are considered disadvantageous for normal child development. In the second, high-risk status is due to low birth weight, prematurity, or malnutrition in the infant. Of this latter group, those deemed high risk by virtue of low birth weight or prematurity are often not socioeconomically disadvantaged.

The essence of the parent–infant stimulation family of programs is found in the Parent–Child Development Center model (Andrews et al., 1982), which was applied in three U.S. cities in the 1970s. The programs were designed to observe five major guidelines: service to low-income populations; primary participants to be mothers or other primary caregivers; the target age for children to be from birth to 3 years; programs to be of sufficient duration and intensity to maximize their potential effectiveness; and programs to be directed at the complex of problems of poor families by including a broad range of support services. By graduation at age 3, significant gains in cognitive and social–emotional development were found among children in all three cities compared with their respective controls.

Parent–infant stimulation programs are not the only ones that effectively improve cognitive and social–emotional functioning in the preschool period. There is evidence, starting at age 6 months, that programs based exclusively in education centers may be helpful for children in the socioeconomic/psychosocial category of high risk. Some of the effective programs have been particularly "high powered," involving very low child-to-instructor ratios (C. T. Ramey & Haskins, 1981), but others simply fall into the category of good community day care. One cannot conclude from this, however, that program content does not matter. When alternate programs are studied using a common evaluation protocol, differences in outcome are found between programs (Wasik, Ramey, Bryant, & Sparling, 1990) and by sex between programs (L. B. Miller & Bizzell, 1983). Project CARE, in particular, showed that intensive center-based educational day care combined with family support groups starting at age 6 months was superior to family support only in improving a variety of cognitive outcomes by age 54 months in socioeconomically disadvantaged children (Wasik et al., 1990).

An approach that was implicitly designed to prevent the effects of cumulative risk was the Family Rehabilitation Program (H. L. Garber & Heber, 1981). Compared to their peers, children of mothers having low-socioeconomic status and low IQ tend to lose ground in cognitive development over time and are at risk of developing into mentally challenged adults. The interaction of a mentally challenged mother and a slum environment was seen as the source of a home environment that was socially and psychologically different from home environments in slum communities with mothers of normal intelligence. The basis of intervention was an 8-year program for the mother in addition to an educational intervention for the children. The mothers' program involved vocational training and evening educational programs, followed by counseling as needed at work and in the home. The child educational program began at age 3–6 months and lasted until age 6 years. By 10 years of age, virtually none of the children in the experimental group were more than 1 standard deviation below the norm on a full-scale IQ test, compared to nearly 60% of control children. Thus, in terms of preventing mental retardation, the program appeared to be exceedingly effective. There was evidence that the experimental mothers' parenting style also improved over time, but the relative contribution of this aspect to the overall result was unmeasureable in this study.

Programs Beginning in the Preschool Period

The literature on school success following preschool and school-age intervention is divided between those studies that seem to show improvements primarily due to gains in cognitive development (Horacek, Ramey, Campbell, Hoffman, & Fletcher, 1987) and those which seem to suggest that the social–emotional effects may be more durable and may have a longer lasting impact (e.g., Syracuse) (Lally, 1988; Lally, Mangione, & Honig, 1988). Notwithstanding this dichotomy, most of the effective programs attempt to intervene in both cognitive and social–emotional domains. In fact, gains may occur in the opposite domains from which they were intended. One program (D. L. Johnson, 1988; D. L. Johnson & Breckenridge, 1982; D. L. Johnson & Walker, 1987) designed specifically to prevent behavior problems in low-income Mexican-American children showed cognitive benefits in addition to the expected declines in antisocial behavior.

In at least five cases, there is evidence that gains in cognitive development increased with increasing longevity of the program. In one preschool intervention program for socioeconomically disadvantaged children aged 4 years (Irvine, 1982), gains in cognitive development increased with increased parental time commitment to the program and other measures of school readiness, such as task orientation, extroversion, and verbal facility, increased with student participation time. In the Verbal Interaction Project (Levenstein et al., 1983) reading and arithmetic scores were higher by grade

3 in the 2-year intervention group (at ages 2–4) than in the 1-year intervention group, and both were higher than the controls.

In the Carolina Abecedarian Project (Horacek et al., 1987), socioeconomically disadvantaged subjects were randomly assigned to the control or experimental group in two time periods: the day care program and the school-age program. The first part of the project was entirely based in day care, and did not have a home intervention component. In fact, there was no evidence that the home environments of the intervention group improved over time compared to the control home environments (Martin, Ramey, & Ramey, 1990). Nonetheless, the intervention group made significant gains in cognitive development by 54 months of age. By grade 3, the pass rate was highest for those children who were part of both the day care and the school-aged educational interventions. Their success rate (84%) was virtually the same as that of the local school system as a whole (87%). The next most successful group comprised those who were given the preschool but not the school-age program (71%), followed by those given the school-age program only (62%), and then those given neither program (50%). By age 12, there was still a preschool but not a school-age treatment effect on IQ of approximately 5 points (Campbell & Ramey, 1994). The effects upon the distribution of IQ were more impressive: 87.2% of the preschool group had IQs above 85, compared with 55.8% of those in the school-age and control groups. It is striking that the intervention offered in the preschool period alone seemed to have more effect on the pass rate than did the intervention in the years immediately preceding the outcome evaluation (Horacek et al., 1987). Yet it is not possible to infer from one study that the difference in success between the "preschool only" and the "school-age only" groups is a reliable indication that earlier interventions are more effective than later ones.

It turns out that subsequent research is inconclusive on this point. There is evidence that special nutritional, health, and educational interventions for chronically undernourished children are more effective in improving cognitive development when they begin before age 4 years than at school age (Irvine, 1982). On the other hand, the Harlem study (Palmer, 1979, 1983) did not find any significant differences in school performance and cognitive development between intervention groups who received training at age 2 years and at age 3 years, but both groups showed improvements over the controls that lasted until age 13. Also, there is evidence that Head Start programs in the preschool period are more effective in creating long-term gains in cognitive and social–emotional outcomes when they were supplemented with primary school follow-throughs (Abelson, Zigler, & DeBlasi, 1974). Also, an 8-week kindergarten-based intervention to improve behavior was more effective when it was repeated over 2 years for a total of 12 weeks intervention (Shure & Spivack, 1982, 1988).

As children get older, the array of influences on their lives becomes more complex. Early cognitive gains may have a continuing effect not through sustained improvements in cognitive function but through the long-term effects of successful adjustment to school: academic success, placement in nonremedial classrooms, and avoidance of frustration and acting out behaviors. The 10-year follow-up of the Syracuse University family development research program (Lally, 1988; Lally et al., 1988) showed that girls in the experimental group were achieving more academically at school than girls in the control group but also had fewer absences and a higher level of social–emotional function. Both boys and girls in the experimental group enjoyed higher levels of family functioning, more positive self-perception, and more positive perceptions of school than the controls. The males also had fewer juvenile offenses. These results are consistent with the Ypsilanti study (Schweinhart et al., 1993), wherein it has been suggested that the impressive long-term benefits were largely due to positive attitudes to school which were engendered by the initial successes that the intervention group children had at school.

CONCLUSION

This chapter has shown that latent effects, pathway effects, and cumulative exposures are all fundamental to successful development. In turn, we have argued that child development is a powerful determinant of health in adult life, as indicated by the strong relationship between measures of educational attainment and adult disease. Because of the role of latency, early life experiences are important and effective early life interventions can make a contribution to subsequent health and well-being. Because of the importance of pathways, ongoing investments in development need to extend throughout childhood and adolescence.

However, as children age, the range of influences on them broadens such that classroom and home take up an ever-shrinking fraction of their time and their consciousness. Community characteristics, labor market forces, and peer relationships begin to predominate. This is where the evidence presented on cumulative effects becomes significant, because ameliorating social class gradients in health and well-being requires broad social and economic change and not just targeted interventions designed to improve the individual life course.

ACKNOWLEDGMENTS

Chris Power (Weston Fellow) and Clyde Hertzman (Lawson Fellow) are with the Canadian Institute for Advanced Research. Chris Power is grateful to the Department of Health (England and Wales) for financial support, and to Sharon Matthews, supported by the UK Economic and Social Research Council (ESRC) (Award No. L128251024).

4

When Children's Social Development Fails

Richard E. Tremblay

There is a budget which is paid with frightening regularity, it is that of prisons, hulks, and gallows; it is that one especially which it would be necessary to strive to reduce.
—QUETELET (1833)

In our "civilized" nations antisocial and violent behavior is still an important problem. Over the past 40 years the crime rate has increased by 91% in the United Kingdom, by 71.1% in Germany, and by 61.7% in France (French-American Foundation, 1996). This increase in crime is not only due to an increase in theft, drug use, or fraud. Rather, violent crimes appear to be increasing in most European and North American countries. For example, in France the rate of violent offenses went from 1.4 per 1,000 in 1952 to 1.6 in 1972, and 2.6 in 1992, an increase of 57% (French-American Foundation, 1996). The increase in violent crimes is especially true among youth.

Violent crimes get a large share of the attention from the media, especially when they are committed by youth. To a certain extent this media attention distorts reality. For example, of the 487 homicides committed in 1994 in Canada, only 51 were committed by youth. However, the reason youth account for only a fraction of crimes is that they represent only a fraction of the total population. Most cross-sectional and longitudinal studies of the prevalence of violent offenses from early adolescence to adulthood have shown that the risk of committing a violent offense is highest during middle adolescence. Data from the National Youth Survey (NYS) in the United States show that up to 25% of white males and 36% of black males report having committed a violent offense over a 12-month period at 17 years of age. The incidence curve is similar for females, but with much lower levels. At 17 years of age 10% of white females and 18% of black females report having committed a violent offense in the past year (Elliott, 1994).

Finding the causes for this increase in violence during the teenage years should help identify the means of preventing its appearance, or at least reducing its intensity. Because adult violence is generally linked to a history of youth violence (Farrington, 1994; Huesmann, Eron, Lefkowitz, & Walder, 1984; Serbin, Peters, McAffer, & Schwartzman, 1991; Serbin, Schwartzman, Moskowitz, & Ledingham, 1991) and because all adults are former youth, one would expect that reducing youth violence would also reduce adult violence. Thus, the reduction of youth violence should in the long run have a very large impact on total violence in a given society.

Most criminological studies of youth violence have focused on 12- to 18-year-old youth. This corresponds to the period of life when children have their last physical growth spurt to reach adult size. During that period they become stronger physically, their cognitive competence increases (e.g., they are better at hiding their intentions), they become sexually mature, they ask and obtain a greater freedom to use their time without adult supervision, and they have access to more resources such as money and transportation, which increases their capacity to satisfy their needs.

This rapid biopsychosocial development might be sufficient to explain why adolescence is a period of life when there are more opportunities and motives for antisocial behavior. The pressures to perform in school, to perform within the peer group, to perform with possible sexual partners, and to use their newly acquired freedoms could explain why proportionally more adolescents than adults resort to violent behavior. However, although a majority of adolescents will commit some delinquent acts, most of these are minor legal infractions (Farrington, 1987). Population-based surveys have systematically shown that a small proportion of adolescents (approximately 6%) account for the majority of violent acts and arrests (Baron, 1995; Farrington, 1987). In a recent study of the 7,101 males born in Stockholm in 1953, Hodgins and Kratzer (1996) have shown that 6.2% of the males (N = 441) had committed 70% of all the offenses, and 71% of all the violent offenses committed by this cohort up to age 30 years.

Of the total number of cases that proceed annually to youth courts across Canada, only 21% involve violence, and in nearly half of these cases the principal charge is minor assault (Youth Court Statistics, 1996). The major problem is to explain why some adolescents and some adults frequently resort to physically aggressive behavior while others do not. Although they are only a small proportion of the population, they represent a heavy burden of suffering for their victims, their families, and themselves. As shown by Power et al. (1991), adolescents with behavior problems are not only at high risk of criminal behavior, they are also at highest risk of unemployment, poor physical health, and mental health problems.

PHYSICAL AGGRESSION DURING CHILDHOOD

Longitudinal studies of children from early childhood to adolescence and adulthood have started to trace the developmental course of these deviant behaviors. There have been sufficient cases of extremely violent behavior by young children to understand that physically aggressive behavior does not suddenly appear with adolescence. For example, in February 1993 two 10-year-old boys bludgeoned to death a 2-year-old boy they had lured from his mother in a Liverpool shopping center ("Killing of Child Shocks Britain: Brutal Slaying Sparks Anger and Soul-Searching," 1993). In 1994 the world was again shocked to hear that in peaceful Norway a 5-year-old and two 6-year-old boys had kicked and stoned to death a 5-year-old girl (Associated Press, 1994). These and a few other more recent cases serve as a reminder that young children can be extremely violent. However, longitudinal studies of large samples of boys and girls followed from school entry to the end of adolescence show clearly that as children grow older they generally resort to less and less physically aggressive behavior (Cairns & Cairns, 1994; Choquet, 1996). Recent cross-sectional data from a random sample of 16,038 Canadian children aged 4–11 years old (National Longitudinal Survey of Children and Youth, NLSCY) confirms this developmental pattern. As seen from Figure 4.1, 4-year-old boys and girls have the highest

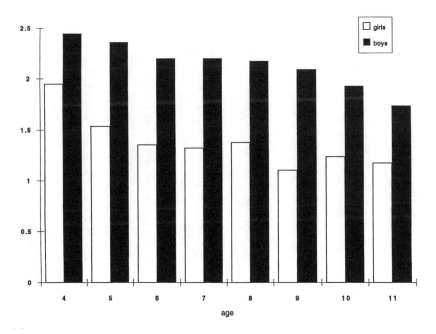

FIGURE 4.1. Physical aggression of boys and girls from 4 to 11 years of age.

levels of physical aggression whereas 11-year-old boys and girls have the lowest levels of physical aggression. As expected, at each age girls have lower levels of physical aggression compared to boys. These data are based on mothers' reports of their children's behavior. However, studies using teachers, peers, and self-reports have all found the same developmental trends (Cairns, Cairns, Neckerman, Ferguson, & Gariépy, 1989).

Interestingly, these patterns are completely reversed when indirect aggression is considered. Indirect aggression is defined as a behavior that aims to hurt someone without the use of physical aggression. For example, when a child is mad at someone he/she will say bad things behind the other's back or will try to get others to dislike that person. As shown in Figure 4.2, girls have higher levels of indirect aggression at each age from 4 to 11, and the level of indirect aggression increases with age for girls and boys (Björkqvist, Österman, & Kaukiainen, 1992). Thus, it appears that part of the effects of the socialization process is to bring some children to use indirect means of aggression in their interpersonal relationships rather than physical aggression.

Although this appears to be the representative developmental pattern

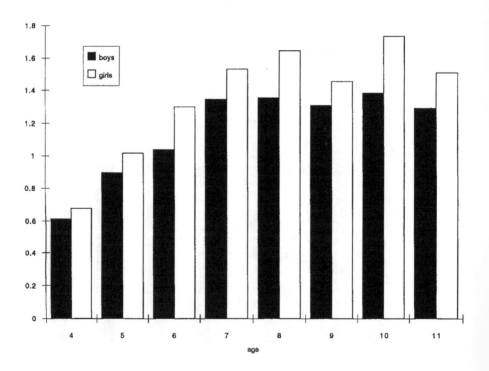

FIGURE 4.2. Indirect aggression of boys and girls from 4 to 11 years of age.

for the majority of children, there are children who maintain a high level of physical aggression as they grow older. Haapasalo and Tremblay (1994) found that 8.3% of kindergarten boys from lower socioeconomic areas of Montréal were constantly rated among the most physically aggressive by their teachers from 6 to 12 years of age. They also found that 9.3% of these boys from low socioeconomic areas went from low physical aggression in kindergarten to high stable physical aggression at the end of elementary school. These two groups of boys were the most at risk for being placed out of an age-appropriate regular classroom during elementary and secondary school.

Figure 4.3 shows the survival curves (i.e., survival in an age-appropriate regular classroom) from age 7 years, when the children should be in grade 1 of elementary school, to age 16 years, when they should be in grade 4 of high school. Five curves are shown for five groups of boys; these curves are created from the boys' pattern of physical aggression between 6 and 12 years of age. We can see that by age 10 years, 50% of the boys who were rated high fighters by their teachers from 6 to 12 years of age (stable high fighters, SHF) had been placed out of an age-appropriate regular class-

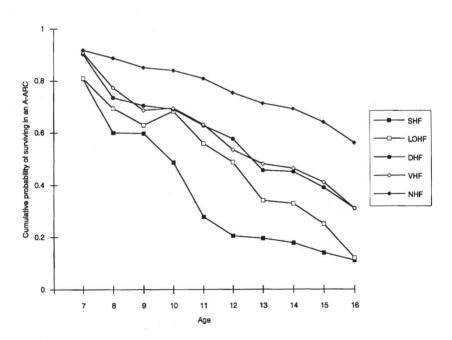

FIGURE 4.3. Survival rate of boys in an age-appropriate regular classroom (A-ARC) according to their history of physical aggression between 6 and 12 years of age.

room. By age 16 years only 18% had survived in an age-appropriate regular classroom. The boys who were not rated physically aggressive in kindergarten but were rated as such every year from age 10 to 12 years (late-onset high fighters, LOHF) had a similar fate. Although the survival rate was somewhat higher between age 10 and 12 years, by age 16 their survival rate was the same as the SHF group.

The boys who were rated highly physically aggressive only in kindergarten (desisting high fighters, DHF) and those who were rated highly physically aggressive off and on (variable high fighters, VHF) had a higher survival rate compared to the SHF and the LOHF groups, but by age 16 years less than 40% had survived. The difference between the SHF and the DHF survival curves may be an indication of the effect we can expect from an intervention that would help highly aggressive kindergarten boys reduce their aggressive behavior. We would double the survival rate. The survival curve for the boys who were never rated high fighters (NHF) may be an indication of the effect one would expect if preschool interventions helped boys from low socioeconomic environments to control their aggressive behavior. The relatively large rate of NHF boys who do not follow the school curriculum as planned (more than 40% by age 16) is a clear indication that the school curriculum needs to be adjusted for boys from low socioeconomic environments.

The boys who fail to learn alternatives to physical aggression are at very high risk of many other problems: they tend to be hyperactive, inattentive, anxious, and not prosocial (Tremblay, Mâsse, Pagani, & Vitaro, 1996); they are rejected by the majority of their classmates (Vitaro, Tremblay, & Gagnon, 1992); and their behavior disrupts the classroom activities as well as recess and transitions. They are thus swiftly taken out of their "natural" peer group and placed in special classes, special schools, and institutions with other "deviants," ironically the ideal situation to reinforce marginal behavior. They are among the most delinquent from age 10 years onward (Haapasalo & Tremblay, 1994). They are the first to initiate substance use (Dobkin, Tremblay, Mâsse, & Vitaro, 1995), the first to initiate sexual intercourse, the most at risk of dropping out of school, the most at risk of being placed under supervision or in custody under the Young Offenders Act, and the most at risk of being diagnosed as having a psychiatric disorder during adolescence (see Table 4.1).

From this perspective, failure to learn alternatives to physical aggression appears to have long-term negative consequences on the social adjustment of an individual. The studies that have followed aggressive children into their adult years have indeed shown that there are extremely negative consequences not only for the aggressive individuals but also for their mates, their children, and the communities in which they live (Farrington, 1994; Huesmann et al., 1984; Serbin, Schwartzman, et al., 1991). The stage is set for early parenthood, unemployment, family violence, and a second generation of poor children brought up in a disorganized environment.

TABLE 4.1. Percentage of Stable, Unstable, and Nonaggressive Boys in Each Outcome Category at Age 16

	Stable aggressive (SHF–LOHF) (N = 165)	Unstable aggressive (DHF–UHF) (N = 282)	Nonaggressive (N = 504)
Delinquent (above 90% on total delinquency scale)	18.5	13.5	7.8
Initiated sexual relations	54.5	46.5	30.2
Dropped out of school	19.4	11.3	3.0
Placed under supervision or in custody under the Young Offenders Act	7.3	3.5	0.6
Has a psychiatric diagnosis	49.2	32.7	20.4

SOCIOECONOMIC GRADIENTS FOR PHYSICALLY AGGRESSIVE BEHAVIOR

The 19th century pioneering epidemiological studies of crimes in France and Belgium by Quetelet (1833) and of poverty in London by Booth (1889) showed that criminality and social class were associated. Most 20th century sociological theories of criminality have attempted to explain this association (Gottfredson & Hirschi, 1990). Theories such as cultural deviance (Sutherland, 1939), strain (Merton, 1938), and social disorganization (C. R. Shaw & McKay, 1942) tried to explain why crime and criminals are more prevalent in poor communities.

If chronic childhood physical aggression leads to juvenile delinquency and adult criminality, one would expect that children's physical aggression would also be associated with social class. From teacher ratings of physical aggression in a random sample of boys and girls in kindergarten classes in the province of Québec, Tremblay, Mâsse, et al. (1996) showed large differences in the percentage of highly physically aggressive children when comparing children in schools of low socioeconomic areas and higher socioeconomic areas. A strong social class gradient was also observed when parents' socioeconomic status was used to classify the children. Data from the first wave of the Canadian NLSCY confirms the social class gradients for physical and indirect aggression. As can be seen from Figures 4.4 and 4.5, the levels of mother-reported physical and indirect aggression are highest for boys and girls from lower socieconomic status families and lowest for boys and girls from higher socioeconomic status families. These results are independent of age of the children.

In Chapter 6 of this volume, Brooks-Gunn, Duncan, and Rebello Britto suggest that disentangling the effect of income per se from the effects of other familial characteristics could help in understanding and preventing the negative effects of poverty. Pagani, Boulerice, and Tremblay (1997) fol-

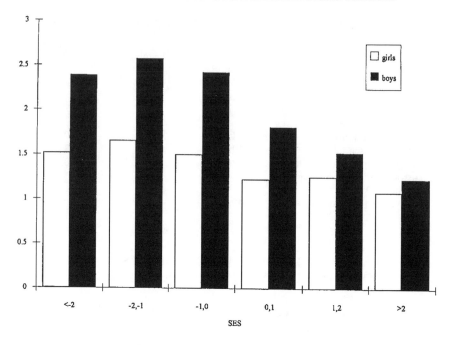

FIGURE 4.4. Physical aggression of boys and girls according to their families' socioeconomic status (SES).

lowed this suggestion by testing the effect of family income on the change in physical aggression between kindergarten and the end of elementary school for a random sample of boys and girls in French-speaking schools in the province of Québec ($N = 1,829$). Controlling for maternal education, mother's age at the child's birth, family status, sex of the child, and level of physical aggression during the kindergarten year, they showed that the children with the highest level of physical aggression at age 12 years (end of elementary school) were those living in a family that had always been poor. No significant effects were observed for having been poor at some point in time but not all of the time.

There are many reasons why individuals living in poverty would tend to commit more crimes and be more violent. Each of the relevant 20th-century sociological theories has focused on a restricted set of mechanisms. For example, cultural deviance theories such as differential association theory (Sutherland, 1939) suggest that youth living in low socioeconomic areas will have peer groups that positively reinforce involvement in crime; strain theory (Merton, 1938) suggests that living in a lower socioeconomic environment makes it more difficult to achieve one's "culturally induced" goals, thus creating frustration and fostering the use of antisocial means to

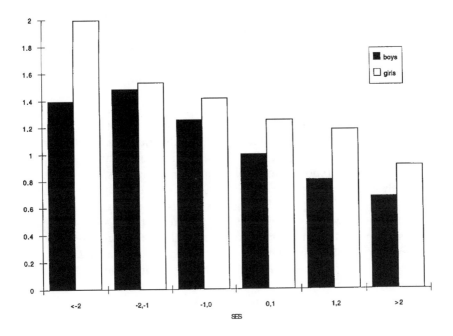

FIGURE 4.5. Indirect aggression of boys and girls according to their families' SES.

achieve one's aims; social disorganization (C. R. Shaw & McKay, 1942) or social ecological theories (Sampson, 1995) suggest that communities that are poor, densely populated, and have high population turnover are likely to shape routine activities of their youth in ways that lead to crime.

From these theoretical perspectives one would expect that all youth who live in low socioeconomic environments are equally at risk of criminal behavior. An obvious exception to this rule is gender differences; the intensity of the effects of socioeconomic environments are not the same for males and females, since they have different levels of physically aggressive and criminal behavior. It is also clear that not all male children from low socioeconomic environments become physically aggressive antisocial criminals. What are the protective factors?

Since the socioeconomic differences in physically aggressive behavior are present at 4 years of age, before school entry, one would expect that family environments play an important role in learning to control aggressive and antisocial behavior. It would indeed be surprising that the differences observed at age 4 could be attributed directly to the effect of deviant peers, the strain of not achieving "culturally induced" goals, or the disorganized physical environment of the community. One would expect that some families, although poor, would create a relatively well-organized environment for children to learn the social skills needed to live without frequent use of physical aggression.

Surprisingly, most studies of children's socialization have not been able to study family effects because only one child per family has been studied. The design of the NLSCY provided the opportunity to study family effects by assessing all the children (up to four) of the 10,287 two-parent families in the study. The results are extremely interesting. Tremblay, Boulerice, et al. (1996) showed that there were important family effects on aggressive behavior. For the total sample, family effects explained 38% of the variance in physical aggression ratings. This means than when a given child in a family is reported to be physically aggressive, his/her siblings are also likely to be rated physically aggressive. On the other hand, when a given child is rated not physically aggressive, his/her siblings are also likely to be rated not physically aggressive. With reference to physical aggression, siblings are more similar to one another than they are to children of other families. Comparable findings were obtained for indirect aggression, emotional problems, and prosocial behavior. The family effects were much smaller for hyperactivity.

Yet, by pointing to the family as an important explanation of physically aggressive behavior and other behavior problems, these results could not reveal the part poverty played in this effect. To determine whether poverty was in some way associated with these family effects, we had to look at family effects within socieconomic categories. There were a number of possible outcomes to this analysis. It could be argued that, if an important cause of physical aggression is living in a poor environment, one would expect that most children of poor families would tend to be physically aggressive, independently of which family they were part of; correspondingly, most children of well-off families would tend not to be physically aggressive. Thus, the magnitude of family effects would not be related to socioeconomic status. Others could argue that family effects should be greater in well-off families, compared to poor families, because the former have a better control over family events that can have a general impact on all the children in the family. For example, well-off families have more liberty in choosing the day care center to which they will send their children, and more liberty in choosing with whom their preschool children will interact by driving them to friends of their choice. On the other hand, it could be argued that most well-off families may have the economic, intellectual, emotional, and social resources to help each of their children develop fully their individual characteristics, thus fostering variability among siblings, whereas a number of poor families who do not have the necessary intellectual, emotional, and social resources could impose on all of their children a family environment conducive to physical aggression and other behavior problems.

Results of the analysis showed that the physical aggression scores of siblings living in families with a high socioeconomic status were almost as different from each other as they were from the scores of children of other families from high socioeconomic status. In other words, for families with high socioeconomic status, the family effect was weak; it explained only 3% of the variance of the physical aggression scores. At the other extreme of the social class distribution, the physical aggression scores of siblings living in families of low socioeconomic status were much more similar to each other than they were similar to the scores of children from other families of low socioeconomic status. In other words, the family effect was strong, explaining 53% of the variance in the physical aggression scores.

Figure 4.6 represents these results for each social class groupings from the lower status to the higher status. We can clearly see a very strong socioeconomic gradient for the family effects on physical aggression. The effects are independent of age, gender, and number of children in the family. Thus, the level of physical aggression of a child from a family with high socioeconomic status is relatively independent of the family characteristics shared with his/her siblings, while the level of physical aggression of children becomes more and more dependent on shared family characteristics as the socioeconomic status gets worse. One can draw an analogy to horticulture. The differences among flowers that are growing in fertile ground will be

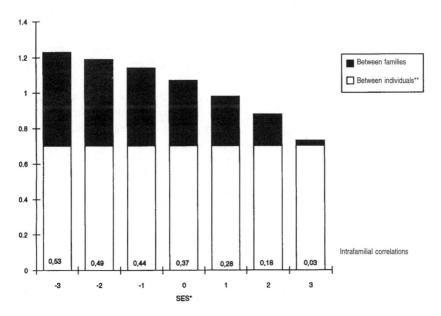

FIGURE 4.6. Family effects on physical aggression according to the SES of the family. *Standardized such that the total variance is 1 when SES = 0. **The interindividual variance varies across sex and age but does not depend on SES.

mainly due to genotype differences, whereas differences among flowers growing in less fertile ground will be due to the quality of the added care (e.g., water, fertilizer) given to these flowers.

An important conclusion from this study is that a major part of the poverty effect on physical aggression of children, delinquency of adolescents, and criminality of adults is probably mediated by the family before children enter the school system. The larger family effect on children from low socioeconomic status families tells us that the risk of chronic physical aggression and antisocial behavior is not evenly distributed among children from low socioeconomic status families. It is children from a restricted number of families who are most at risk. Thus, if poverty is a risk factor, the family can be a protective factor. Studies are needed to differentiate between the characteristics of the poor families that succeed and those that fail in socializing their children before they enter the school system. We also need to understand what mechanisms underlie the socioeconomic gradient in physical aggression and the gradient in family effects on physical aggression. Understanding these mechanisms is important for preventing the development of physical aggression and antisocial behavior. It is however clear that the majority of children from a poor community are not at high risk. Reaching the high-risk children within the poor community's families is an important challenge.

PHYSICAL AGGRESSION DURING EARLY CHILDHOOD

Most people believe that children learn to become aggressive as they grow older. This perception probably stems from the fact that as children grow older they become physically more powerful and thus an angry reaction at 12 years of age is more "dangerous" than an angry reaction at 2 years of age. But, as we have seen, from 4 years of age to late adolescence most children decrease the frequency of their physically aggressive behavior. Jean-Jacques Rousseau's conviction that children are born with "good" inclinations and learn "vice and error" from their environments has had much more influence on the way most people perceive children than has Thomas Hobbes's characterization of humans as selfish, reward-seeking machines who learn society rules through fear. It is thus difficult for most of us to acknowledge that young children can be physically aggressive, and accordingly few studies have attempted to describe the development of physical aggression during the first 3 years of life.

Cross-sectional data from the NLSCY suggest that the decline in physical aggression that was shown from 4 years of age to adolescence actually starts during the second year of life. Figure 4.7 shows that mothers perceive their 2-year-old children as "hitting, kicking and biting" others more often than at any other age. This picture fits the common expression "the terrible 2s." A longitudinal study in Belgium (Sand, 1966) provides evidence that

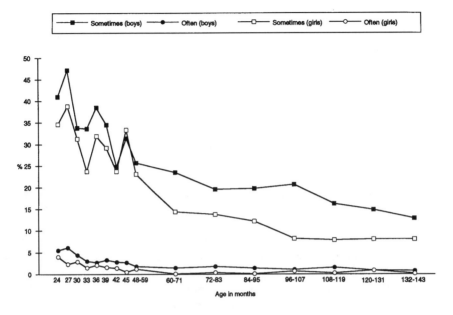

FIGURE 4.7. Frequency of hitting, biting, and kicking from 2 to 11 years of age.

the cross-sectional picture from the NLSCY may be an adequate representation of the true developmental path. From Figure 4.8 it can be seen that mothers report more temper tantrums around 18 to 24 months than at any other time between birth and school entry. We also can see that the frequency of tantrums increases from birth to age 18 months and then decreases constantly.

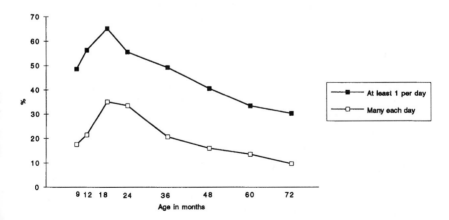

FIGURE 4.8. Frequency of temper tantrums from birth to 6 years of age. Based on Sand (1966).

This representation of the course of problem behaviors during early childhood could be an artifact of the mothers' perceptions. Fortunately, there are observational data available that confirm mothers' reports. Noël, Leclerc, and Strayer (1990) showed that the frequency of observed menaces and competition for toys in a Montréal day care center steadily decreased from 2 to 5 years of age. Restoin et al. (1985) showed that the relative frequency of aggressions in a French day care center increased from 6 to 24 months of age and then decreased from 24 to 36 months of age. Dunn and Munn (1985) showed that physical aggression of British children toward their siblings and expression of anger toward their mother increased from 14 to 24 months of age.

These curves are very similar to the delinquency curves during adolescence. How can an increase and decrease in physically aggressive and disruptive behavior during early childhood be explained? One would expect that physical, cognitive, and emotional development would be important variables. Within the first 24 months after birth babies grow in height by more than 70% and almost triple their weight. At birth babies can hardly lift their heads; 9 months later they can move on all fours; by 12 months they can walk; and by 24 months they can run and climb stairs.

The ability to grasp objects is an important development for social interactions. At birth babies do not control their arms, but at 6 months they can reach and grasp for objects. If they see an interesting toy in the hands of another 6-month-old, they will reach and grasp the toy. A struggle for the toy will occur if the other child does not let go. Note that at 6 months the child does not have the language ability to ask the other child for the toy—this ability will come much later—but the frequency and complexity of interactions between babies and other persons in their environment increase at least as rapidly as their physical growth. Infants' waking time is spent exploring their physical environments. Before 12 months of age they spend most of their playtime exploring one object at a time. Between 12 and 18 months they imitate real-life activities alone. By the end of the second year they are "pretend playing" with others (Rubin, Fein, & Vandenberg, 1983).

Thus, over the first 15 months after birth children are becoming more and more able to discover their environment by being more physically mobile and better equipped cognitively. The frequency of their interactions with peers increases with age, and playing with others increases dramatically from the end of the first year to the end of the second year (H. S. Ross & Goldman, 1977). This is the period when the rate of physical aggression increases to its maximum. At this age children are exploring social interactions with their newly acquired walking, talking, running, grasping, and throwing skills. Most of their interactions are positive, but conflicts become more frequent (Hay & Ross, 1982; Restoin et al., 1985). Most of these conflicts are over possession of objects. During these conflicts children learn that they can hurt others and be hurt. Most children will quickly learn that a physical attack will be responded to by a physical attack and that adults will not tolerate these behaviors. Most children will learn to wait for the toy to be free and learn that asking for toys rather than taking them away from someone will more likely prevent negative interactions.

Learning to wait for something you want (delay of gratification) (Mischel, Shoda, & Rodriguez, 1989) and learning to use language to convince others to satisfy your needs may be the most important protective factors for chronic physical aggression and antisocial behavior. Stattin and Klackenberg-Larsson (1993) showed that language skills between 18 and 24 months was a good predictor of adult criminality in a Swedish sample of males followed from birth to adulthood. Tremblay, Pihl, Vitaro, and Dobkin (1994) found that hyperactive–impulsive behavior was one of the best kindergarten predictors of early onset of delinquency. In fact, numerous studies have shown an inverse correlation of verbal skills with impulsivity and criminal behavior (Moffitt, 1993). We need to understand the mechanisms underlying these associations. They are clearly operating in the first few years of life. In a recent pilot study Landry (1996) showed that a high correlation between verbal skills and aggressive behavior was already present at 12 months of age.

By the age of 12 months children have the physical, cognitive, and emotional means of physically aggressing others. It appears that most children will at some point hit, bite, or kick another child or even an adult. Children's individual characteristics can explain part of the variance in the frequency and stability of this behavior, but the quality of the child's relations with his/her environment and the environment's reaction to his/her behavior should also be important factors. If the child is surrounded by adults and children who physically aggress each other, he/she will likely learn that physical aggression is part of everyday social interactions. On the other hand, if he/she lives in an environment that does not tolerate physical aggression and rewards prosocial behavior, it is unlikely that the child will acquire the habit of using physical aggression as a means of obtaining what he/she wants or of expressing his/her frustration. Keenan and Shaw (1994) have shown that physical aggression of boys at 2 years of age was predicted by a history of familial criminality. The same group (D. S. Shaw, Vondra, Hommerding, Keenan, & Dunn, 1994) showed that mothers' responsiveness to their sons at 12 months of age predicted externalizing behavior problems at 3 years of age.

CAN WE PREVENT THE DEVELOPMENT OF CHRONIC AGGRESSION AND ANTISOCIAL BEHAVIOR?

Most experiments to prevent antisocial behavior have been done with adolescents and preadolescent boys who were referred for behavior problems. Lipsey (1992) identified 443 such experiments. His meta-analysis of the treatment effects showed a mean effect size of .18; that is, the average treatment group scored .18 standard deviations higher than the average control group on the average outcome measure. He concluded that the average effect of these interventions was "perilously close to zero" (p. 126). The same conclusion had been reached almost 20 years earlier when Lipton, Martinson, and Wilks (1975) reviewed the adult and adolescent correctional treatment evaluation studies.

There have been very few intervention studies with children who have followed the subjects long enough to observe the effects on adolescent or adulthood antisocial behavior. However, the studies which have done long term follow-ups have shown long-term positive effects.

The Montréal Longitudinal–Experimental Study randomly allocated highly disruptive kindergarten boys to a treatment group and a control group. The treatment was based on the idea that the impact would be greater if both school and home environment were targeted. Parent training was selected to change the boys' home environment, while social skills training and teacher support were selected to change the school environment. The intervention lasted 2 years, starting at 7 years of age. Professionals made home visits for the parent-training program. The social skills program was implemented in the schools by the professionals. The disruptive boys were included in small groups of prosocial peers who met to learn self-control and prosocial skills. Follow-up of the treatment and control subjects showed that at the end of elementary school the treated subjects performed better in school, were less aggressive, had less aggressive friends, and were less delinquent (Tremblay et al., 1991; Vitaro & Tremblay, 1994). The last assessment at age 15 showed that the treated boys were reporting less delinquent behavior, less delinquent gang involvement, fewer police arrests, less alcohol abuse, and less drug use (Tremblay, Kurtz, Mâsse, Vitaro, & Pihl, 1995; Tremblay, Mâsse, et al., 1996).

The High/Scope Perry Preschool Study (Schweinhart et al., 1993) is famous for having shown that a preschool program for 3- and 4-year-old poor and low-IQ African-American children had very-long-term positive effects on school achievement, delinquency, unemployment, and use of social services up to age 27. Children attended the preschool daily for 2½ hours on weekday mornings, and teachers visited each mother and child for 1½ hours a week in the afternoon. The program lasted 30 weeks a year and was aimed at stimulating cognitive development by active learning, with systematic assessment of individual needs and interests.

Chronic physically aggressive and antisocial behavior appears to generally start in early childhood. This would indicate that prevention of the life course of miseries that follows should start by helping infants and toddlers learn alternatives to physical aggression. To our knowledge, no experiments have been conducted to test if this aim can be achieved. However, a number of experiments have tried to enrich the quality of care that children receive during the perinatal period and up to toddlerhood. Long-term follow-ups after the interventions indicate positive effects on the quality of family environments and children's behavior (Tremblay & Craig, 1995). For example,

Olds, Henderson, Chamberlin, and Talelbaum (1986) showed that a program of prenatal and postnatal home visits for at-risk first-time parents (young, single, poor) reduced the parent's child abuse and children's behavior problems. Other intervention experiments with newborns have shown that support to at-risk families and enriched day care programs have long-term positive effects on the children's cognitive development and behavior problems (Achenbach, Phares, & Howell, 1990; Infant Health Program & Development, 1990; D. L. Johnson, 1990; Wasik et al., 1990).

CONCLUSION

Longitudinal studies with repeated measurements from birth to adulthood clearly show that most seriously antisocial adolescents and adults had behavior problems during childhood. The origin of these behavior problems can be traced back to fetal development and infancy. Preventive interventions over the first 3 years of life for at risk families clearly reduce the prevalence and the seriousness of behavior problems. It appears clear that money invested in well-planned early prevention efforts with at-risk families will give greater payoffs than money invested in later preventive efforts with the same at-risk families. This policy is difficult to apply because criminal adults and aggressive adolescents attract much more public attention than do at-risk infants. It is difficult for politicians and policy planners to decide to invest less resources in these social "cancers"; however, it is clear that the prevention strategy will, within a 20-year period, reduce substantially the relative amount of resources needed for corrective interventions in the education, health, and justice systems. The idea that societies need to make early childhood development a priority has been recognized at least since Plato wrote *The Republic*. Twentieth-century science has simply demonstrated the validity of this statement. The challenge is now to transform it into policy.

ACKNOWLEDGMENTS

The research results presented in this chapter are from studies supported by grants from Canada's Social Sciences and Humanities Research Council and National Health Research Development Program, the Ministry of Human Resource Development of Canada, Québec's Conseil Québécois pour la Recherche Sociale, and Fonds pour la formation de chercheurs et l'aide à la recherche (Fonds FCAR). The author also received generous support from the Molson Foundation and the Canadian Institute for Advanced Research. A large number of collaborators have been involved in the research program described in this chapter. The names of the major collaborators can be found in the papers cited in the text. Lyse Desmarais-Gervais, Hélène Beauchesne, and Lucille David coordinated over the past 20 years the huge infrastructure needed to carry on the longitudinal studies.

5

Quality and Inequality in Children's Literacy

THE EFFECTS OF FAMILIES, SCHOOLS, AND COMMUNITIES

J. Douglas Willms

Two important indicators of the success of a society are the level of literacy of its children and youth, and the extent of disparities in literacy skills among children and youth with differing characteristics and family backgrounds. These indicators are markers of how investments of material, social, and cultural resources made during the past decade have been translated into skills and competencies in the present generation: they denote the success of families, schools, and communities in producing a literate society. The distribution of literacy skills also provides some indication of the pool of economic and cultural capital available to sustain the labor market over the next three or four decades, and to the extent that there is a relationship between education and health (Borjas, 1995; Britton, Fox, Goldblatt, Jones, & Rosato, 1990; Hertzman, 1994; C. E. Ross & Wu, 1995) it foretells the future health of our society. Indicators of the level of literacy skills and of inequalities in literacy skills are therefore "postmeasures" of returns on past investments and "premeasures" of future success.

The indicators most commonly used to gauge the success of a society are elemental economic statistics, such as unemployment rates, average annual income, and gross domestic product. But these are insufficient because they do not portray subjective aspects of social life or characterize the processes that generate social and economic outcomes. They also fail to describe the extent of inequalities in these outcomes among high- and low-status groups (Land, 1983; Murnane & Pauly, 1988; Willms & Kerckhoff,

1995). Literacy is a key social indicator because it is itself a defining characteristic of social class. People use language to engage in social relations that increase their knowledge and develop their potential. They become a part of a culture by learning to interpret and use its particular signs and symbols (Langer, 1991). Reduction of inequalities in literacy is therefore crucial for achieving tolerance, social cohesion, and equality of opportunity in a modern society.

This chapter examines levels and gradients in children's and youth's literacy skills in Canada. The term "gradient" is being used increasingly to refer to the relationship between individuals' educational or health outcomes and their social status. In most analyses, educational outcomes include academic achievement or high school dropout rates; health outcomes pertain to mortality and disease rates; and social status is represented by socioeconomic factors such as family income or the prestige of a person's occupation. The term "gradient" can be used also to refer to gaps in educational or health outcomes between minority and majority groups or between males and females. The interest in gradients often concerns whether people's outcomes are related to the educational and occupational success of their parents, as this relationship indicates the degree of social mobility in a society. In "open" societies, gradients are shallow: a person's success depends mainly on his or her own ability and effort, and relatively little on family background; the opposite is the case for "closed" societies (Bielby, 1981; T. N. Clark & Lipset, 1991).

The ability to characterize the distribution of literacy skills in Canada and to understand some of the processes generating literacy has been greatly improved because of a concerted effort by the federal and provincial governments to collect data describing the literacy skills of the Canadian population. Canada took a lead role in the International Adult Literacy Survey (IALS) (Organization for Economic Cooperation & Development [OECD] & Statistics Canada, 1995), which was conducted jointly by seven countries with support from the OECD, the European Union Task Force for Human Resources, and UNESCO. In 1989 the Council of Ministers of Education, Canada (CMEC) initiated the School Achievement Indicators Program (SAIP), and in 1994 it conducted a large-scale assessment of the reading and writing skills of 13- and 16-year old children. In 1994 Human Resources Development Canada launched the National Longitudinal Study of Children and Youth (NLSCY), which included a representative sample of more than 20,000 children ranging in age from newborn to 11 years. Children in the age 4–5 cohort were administered the Peabody Picture Vocabulary Test (PPVT), a measure of early language skills that is a relatively good predictor of later school success. Some of the provinces conduct their own assessments of children's literacy skills. New Brunswick, for example, has developed a comprehensive testing program to evaluate children's skills in reading and writing at the end of grades 3, 6, 8, and 11, and there are discussions among the four Atlantic provinces to collaborate on assessment.

These efforts have been enhanced considerably because of important advances in the measurement of cognitive skills, in sampling techniques, and in statistical methods. Early attempts to define literacy were based on a limited set of reading skills and were typically measured with multiple-choice tests. In the IALS, literacy was defined broadly as "using printed and written information to function in society, to achieve one's goals, and to develop one's knowledge and potential" (Organization for Economic Co-operation & Development [OECD] & Statistics Canada, 1995, p. 14). The tests used in the IALS reflect that broad definition: they assess an individual's ability to read and comprehend written materials (including reports, documents, and mathematical charts and displays); to use that information to solve problems, evaluate circumstances, and make decisions; and to communicate that information verbally and in writing. In other recent studies, literacy skills have been assessed using a variety of techniques, including questions that solicit open-ended responses or require lengthy written compositions. Similarly, school-based assessments have begun to place greater emphasis on "authentic" forms of evaluation, including appraisals of in-depth projects, journals, recitals, debates, and oral presentations. Advances in measurement theory and sampling techniques, particularly item response theory (Suen, 1990; Lord, 1980) and matrix sampling techniques (Bock & Mislevy, 1988), have enabled researchers to accurately characterize the performance of test items and tasks such that they can estimate a person's skill levels in several domains of literacy without having to administer unreasonably long tests. Because of these theoretical advances, it is now possible to conduct more valid comprehensive assessments of a society's literacy skills.

One of the problems that has plagued researchers in this area is that until recently there have not been appropriate methods for analyzing multilevel data. Data in the social sciences are usually nested in a multilevel hierarchy, such as data describing students, classrooms, and schools; patients, wards, and hospitals; or, more generally, people and communities. Conventional statistical techniques can only handle variables describing units at one level of a hierarchy. However, recent advances in statistics and computing have provided appropriate methods for analyzing multilevel data (Bryk & Raudenbush, 1992; Goldstein, 1995). The new techniques are powerful in that they estimate a set of statistics (e.g., regression coefficients) for each group of a hierarchical structure using data for that group while borrowing strength from the information available on all groups. These sets of statistics can then be used as outcome measures in models that posit relationships among group-level variables. Four advantages of these new techniques over conventional approaches, relevant to the work reported in this chapter, are that they allow the researcher to (1) discern the extent to which schools or communities differ in their levels of literacy after controlling statistically for respondents' social-class background and other characteristics, (2) provide estimates of social-class gradients (or of gaps between high- and low-status groups) for all schools or communities, (3) ascertain whether particular policies or practices are associated with differences among schools or communities in their levels of literacy or gradients, and (4) take account of how accurately the statistics for each group have been estimated (Raudenbush & Willms, 1995).

INTERNATIONAL AND INTERPROVINCIAL COMPARISONS OF LITERACY SKILLS

The models commonly used by sociologists to describe social mobility presume that individuals' academic attainment and ultimately their occupational attainment are largely determined by their family origins and educational experiences (e.g., Bielby, 1981; Sewell, Hauser, & Featherman, 1976; Kerckhoff, 1996). Family origins are assumed to have a direct effect on attainment through a wide variety of mechanisms that begin at birth, or even prenatally, and an indirect effect, through education. For example, children from more advantaged backgrounds are more likely to have better access to quality education, and greater financial and cultural capital to support educational activities during the elementary and secondary school years. Children with these resources are then more likely to have the high school grades and financial resources to pursue further education. These experiences contribute cumulatively to their level of literacy. Literacy is also considered to be affected by experiences at work, and through other experiences related to one's economic, cultural, and social capital. At this point, however, the models become complicated because levels of literacy affect the type of job and income an individual acquires, and these in turn affect levels of literacy. The models discussed in this chapter simply describe the relationship between literacy scores and parents' education and gender for children and youth. More extensive models of the IALS data, which include factors such as ethnicity, income, employment experiences, high school completion, and type of community, are presented elsewhere (Raudenbush & Kasim, 1998; Willms, 1997).

International Differences in Youth Literacy Skills

Figure 5.1 shows the relationship between literacy scores and parents' education for youth aged 16–25 in seven OECD countries, based on data from the IALS. The literacy score is the average score on the three tests (prose, document, and quantitative), standardized on the full IALS sample. Parents' education is the average of the number of years of education completed by the mother and father of the respondents. The lines for each country are drawn such that approximately 90% of a country's respondents had average parental education within the range covered by the line.

Two findings revealed by the analysis are particularly striking. First,

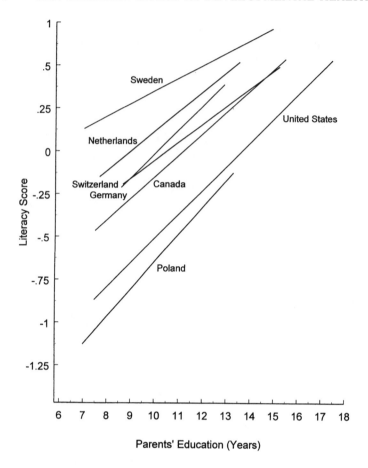

FIGURE 5.1. Socioeconomic gradients for youth in seven OECD countries. Data from 1994 International Adult Literacy Study (OECD & Statistics Canada, 1995).

countries vary substantially in their literacy scores, even after account is taken of parents' levels of education. Youth in Poland and the United States, for example, whose parents had both completed 12 years of education, on average scored approximately 30 to 40% of a standard deviation lower than comparable Canadian youth. This is a very large difference: on average, youth increase their literacy scores on this test by about 12–13% of a standard deviation for each additional year they remain in school (Willms, 1997). Thus, the literacy scores of youth in Poland or the United States who had completed 2 years of postsecondary schooling were similar to those of Canadian youth who had completed the 11th grade. However, Canadian youth lag behind the top-scoring country, Sweden, by nearly the same amount—about one-third of a standard deviation. Youth in Germany and Switzerland had scores comparable to those of Canadian youth, and youth in the Netherlands scored about 17% of a standard deviation above Canadian youth. The second striking finding is that countries with high scores tend to have shallow gradients. The correlation between the overall levels of achievement and the steepness of the gradients in this analysis was –.79. In Sweden, for example, youth whose parents had completed only the 8th grade, on average scored 13% of a standard deviation above the international average, whereas in the United States, the country with the steepest gradient, youth with similar family backgrounds scored 60% of a standard deviation below the international mean. In contrast, the variation among countries is relatively small for youth whose parents had both completed college.[1]

For all seven countries combined, there were no statistically significant differences between males and females in their average literacy scores. This was also the case for five of the countries. Poland and Germany were the exception: in Germany males scored about 12% of a standard deviation higher than females, and in Poland females outperformed males by about 16% of a standard deviation. For Canada, there was a significant sex-by-parental-education interaction, indicating that the parental education gradients for females were somewhat steeper for females than for males (a slope of .12 for females compared with .08 for males). However, the province-by-province analyses for Canada reported below suggest that the picture is more complicated, because females outperform males in some provinces whereas the reverse is true in other provinces.

Interprovincial Differences in Youth Literacy Skills

Figure 5.2 displays the relationship between literacy skills and socioeconomic status (SES) for each province.[2] The measure of SES is a statistical composite of the education level of the respondent's mother and father, and the occupation of the respondent's father. The national literacy–SES gradient in this analysis is .282. However, the analysis reveals that there is substantial variation among the Canadian provinces in their gradients. The provinces are clustered into two very distinct groups: Québec and the three prairie provinces have relatively shallow gradients; British Columbia, Ontario, and the four Atlantic provinces have relatively steep gradients. As was the case with the above international data, the provinces that have high adjusted average scores tend to have shallow gradients: the correlation between average levels of literacy and gradients is –.72. Two conclusions are immediately apparent: provinces that do well overall have high levels of performance among their youth from lower socioeconomic backgrounds; differences among provinces are relatively small if one considers youth from average or above-average socioeconomic backgrounds, but there are large differences among provinces in the performance of youth from lower socioeconomic backgrounds.

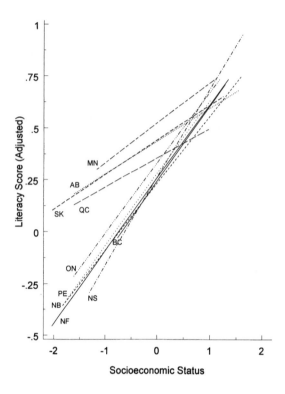

FIGURE 5.2. Socioeconomic gradients for youth by Canadian province. Data from 1994 International Adult Literacy Study (OECD & Statistics Canada, 1995).

These stark interprovincial differences raise a number of questions concerning their likely cause.[3] Are these differences evident during the preschool years? If so, they would raise further questions concerning interprovincial differences in the provision of prenatal and perinatal care, the quality of day care and preschool programs, and the early effects of parenting. Or do the differences arise mainly during the elementary and secondary years? If so, the findings would have important implications for teachers, principals, and district and provincial administrators concerning the quality and equality of educational provision. The differences could also arise at the end of secondary schooling, during the transition from high school to postsecondary education, or from formal schooling to the labor force. For example, it could be that youth from lower socioeconomic backgrounds are more likely to remain in school longer in some provinces than in others, leading to differences in levels of literacy. A more general question, relevant to each of the above questions, concerns the distribution of literacy skills among communities within provinces. For example, are the steep gradients observed in the Atlantic provinces and in British Columbia and Ontario, relatively consistent across schools, districts, and geographically defined communities within each province? Or are there some communities within each of these provinces with particularly low levels of literacy and others with particularly high levels? The answers to these questions have important implications for national and provincial policies aimed at reducing inequalities.

The remainder of this chapter will examine some of the evidence pertaining to these questions, based on findings from the NLSCY, a study of elementary schooling in New Brunswick, and a number of small-scale studies. The overarching question is whether levels of literacy and social-class gradients are immutable; that is, could Canada's (or other "steep gradient" nations') distribution of literacy skills look more like that of Sweden? Or are the mechanisms that lead to low levels of literacy and steep gradients embedded in historical, economic, and cultural relationships that defy interventions by governments and the efforts of citizens?

FAMILIES MAKE A DIFFERENCE

Beginning at birth, most children are immersed in the language and literacy of their immediate family. As infants watch and listen to their parents and siblings, speech emerges naturally. Their first incoherent utterances produce reactions in their parents, who attempt to perceive their needs and respond to them. Children learn that certain cries and sounds result in particular reactions from family members, and gradually they begin to copy the speech and language sounds of adults in an effort to communicate. Usually at age 12–18 months children begin establishing a recognizable vocabulary, which takes off and grows exponentially over the next few years. Language structures emerge as children try to communicate in a variety of contexts. Speech and language continues to develop as children experiment with it and learn how to manipulate it to achieve their goals (Courts, 1991; Ollia & Mayfield, 1991). These infant and toddler years are critical for establishing a foundation for future literacy development.

Children do not develop language and literacy at the same rate, and there are many factors that influence children's rate of development. Even within the same families, children display a wide range of literacy skills. Much of the research has been concerned with whether the observed variation in early literacy skills is attributable mainly to differences in children's innate capacity or to differences in their exposure to speech and language. Evidence for heredity effects are weak: only about 10–12% of the variation in children's vocabulary scores is attributable to parents' vocabulary scores (Scarr & Weisberg, 1978; F. Williams, 1975), and the correlation between children's and mothers' vocabulary scores are equally strong for children reared in adoptive and biological families (Scarr & Weisberg, 1978). Huttenlocher and her colleagues used multilevel growth models to examine children's vocabulary growth between 14 and 26 months, using data collected from several time points (Huttenlocher, Haight, Bryk, & Seltzer, 1988; Bryk & Raudenbush, 1992). They found that children vary considerably in the rate at which they acquire vocabulary and that about 20% of this variation is associated with the quantity of mothers' speech. They also found that the frequency with which mothers use particular words is strongly related to the age at which children acquire those words, thereby providing strong evidence of the importance of both *quantity* and *quality* of parental speech.

Preliminary Findings from the NLSCY

The NLSCY is the first study to assess the early language skills for a nationally representative sample of Canadian preschoolers. The PPVT was administered to more than 3,000 children in their homes on the same occasion as the parent interviews. Figure 5.3 displays the relationship between PPVT scores and SES for each of the 10 provinces. As with the analysis of international literacy scores, the PPVT scores were standardized to have a mean of 0 and a standard deviation of 1 for the full sample of Canadian 4- and 5-year-old children.[4] The SES measure is a composite measure comprising the prestige of the mother's and father's occupation, the mother's and father's level of education, and household income,[5] and for this analysis, like the PPVT, SES was standardized on the full sample of 4- and 5-year-old children. The regression estimate for SES, which can be considered the average within-province "SES gradient," is .287. This suggests that for each 1 standard deviation increase in SES, PPVT scores are on average about 27% of a standard deviation higher.

Figure 5.3 illustrates that the gradients are remarkably similar across the 10 provinces. (The observed variation in gradients was not statistically significant.) The provinces did differ, however, in their SES-adjusted average PPVT scores: Ontario and British Columbia had SES-adjusted scores that were about 10% of a standard deviation below the national average; Newfoundland and Nova Scotia had SES-adjusted scores that were about 10% of a standard deviation above the national average; the other provinces were between these extremes. These differences are not trivial: they suggest that a child with nationally average background characteristics would score at about the 46th percentile in Ontario and British Columbia, and at about the 54th percentile in Newfoundland and Nova Scotia. The results raise the question of whether children in different provinces vary in their exposure to adult language in the places where they spend the majority of their time during the toddler years. For example, are there disproportionately more children in Ontario and British Columbia in preschool or day care settings and, if so, to what extent do these settings vary in the

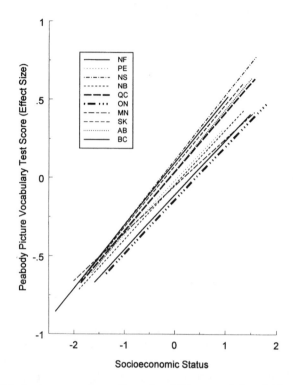

FIGURE 5.3. Socioeconomic gradients for children aged 4 and 5 by Canadian province. Data from National Longitudinal Study of Children and Youth, 1994–1995 (Statistics Canada & Human Resources Development Canada, 1995).

quality and quantity of language exposure? The amount of time children spend in day care and preschool settings, the adult-to-child ratio in these settings, and the average levels of education of the caregivers would give some indication of these effects. When data for successive waves of the NLSCY become publicly available, researchers will be able to test hypotheses relevant to these questions.

Table 5.1 shows the relationships between PPVT and a set of family background variables. The estimates are regression coefficients derived from multiple regression analyses. In each case the coefficient denotes the expected change in the outcome measure for a 1-unit change in the explanatory variable (i.e., the child background variable), given that all other explanatory variables are held constant. Coefficients marked with an asterisk are statistically significant at the .05 level; that is, it is unlikely (less than 5 times in 100) that the observed relationships occurred by chance alone.

The first column shows the relationships for the PPVT scores. The coefficient for female is .040 and is not statistically significant. Thus we can

TABLE 5.1. Relationship between Children's PPVT Scores and Their Family Background Characteristics

	Model 1	Model 2
Constant	−.004	.019
Girls	.040	.045
Socioeconomic status		.343*
Education: mother	.065*	
Education: father	.017*	
Occupation: mother	−.007	
Occupation: father	.091*	
Household income	.002*	
Single parent	−.197*	
Number of siblings	−.092*	

*Statistically significant at the .05 level.

conclude that males and females scored equally well on the test. The effect of years of education of the mother[6] is .065, which is statistically significant. This indicates that, on average, PPVT scores increase about 6.5% of a standard deviation for each additional year of education of the mother, with all other variables in the model held constant. The effect of the father's level of education was also statistically significant, but only about one-quarter as large. On the other hand, the prestige of the father's occupation had a strong and statistically significant relationship with PPVT scores. Household income was also significantly related, but the effect was relatively small (.002). This indicates that with other factors held constant, each additional Can. $1000 in annual household income was associated with an increase of one-fifth of 1% of a standard deviation. PPVT scores were negatively related to the number of brothers and sisters a child had. On average, each additional sibling was associated with a decrease in PPVT scores of 9.2% of a standard deviation. Finally, the PPVT scores for children living in single-parent families were on average about 19.7% of a standard deviation lower than the scores of children in two-parent families.

The second column of Table 5.1 shows the overall socioeconomic gradient for Canada, which is .343. This indicates that PPVT scores increase about one-third of a standard deviation for each 1 standard deviation increase in SES.

Taken together, these national-level findings support the conclusions of the small-scale, detailed studies of family interactions that have emphasized the importance of the quality and quantity of maternal language: the most important predictor of the early literacy skills measured by the PPVT is the mother's level of education. This is the case even after the prestige of the father's occupation and the household income are taken into account. Moreover, the results pertaining to family size and structure suggest that children have more frequent interactions with adults in smaller, two-parent families.

Goelman and Pence (1988) conducted a study of 126 young (3- and 4-year-old) children who attended three different types of day care settings in Victoria, British Columbia. Their study entailed collection of extensive data on children's cognitive and behavioral outcomes, program quality, and parents' and caregivers' characteristics. They found that children's expressive and receptive language scores at preschool age were related to the level of their mothers' education, program quality, and experience of the caregiver. Ten years later the same authors were able to capture follow-up data for 60 children who had participated in the 1987 study; they found that the early differences among children in the programs had persisted to age 13 (Goelman & Pence, 1996). The follow-up data suggested that the qualities of the caregiver may be more important than the type of day care setting. Their correlational study does not provide strong evidence that the quality of care in day care settings has a significant effect on children's early literacy skills, because it could be that parents with higher levels of education tend to choose better settings. However, the findings do indicate that the quality of day care provision varies significantly, even among settings in a relatively affluent city.

SCHOOLS MAKE A DIFFERENCE

Researchers studying school effectiveness have used multilevel models to determine whether schools have an effect on children's outcomes, over and above the effects of family background. Thus the same techniques used above to examine variation in literacy scores among countries and provinces can be used to examine variation among school districts or schools within provinces. The models used to examine the effects of schools presume that children's academic achievement is determined mainly by their ability upon entry to school, their family background, and their experiences at school (Raudenbush & Willms, 1995). Research in a number of countries has shown that there are large and significant differences among schools in their outcomes, even after students' family background characteristics and their ability upon entry to school are taken into account (Gray, 1989; Willms, 1992). Thus schools differ in their "added value."

For example, Willms and Jacobsen (1990) examined children's rate of growth in mathematics skills between grades 3 and 7 for an entire cohort of students attending 31 elementary schools in one British Columbia school district. The analysis was particularly powerful because the data included a measure of cognitive ability at the end of grade 3 (a more global measure of ability than the PPVT) and a longitudinal record of children's achievement derived from annual testing. The multilevel modeling examined each child's growth trajectory over the 5-year period and estimated the average rate of growth in each school, taking into account children's initial level of cognitive ability. The study found that in the three best-performing schools in the district, children with average cognitive ability grew in mathematical skills at a rate of at least 11 months of schooling per (10-month) school year, whereas in the four worst-performing schools the average growth rate was less than 9 months per school year. After 5 years of schooling, therefore, a student with average ability attending one of the three best-performing schools was more than a full year of schooling ahead of comparable children attending one of the four worst performing schools.

Figure 5.4 displays average reading scores plotted against average family SES for 119 elementary schools in New Brunswick. In this study, SES is a composite measure of family structure (single- vs. two-parent family and number of children), home possessions (an indicator of financial capital), and cultural capital. As we would expect from the discussion above, there is a relationship between reading scores and SES. However, at each level of school mean SES, there is a difference of more than one-half of a standard deviation between the best and worst-performing schools. This is equivalent to about 6–8 months of schooling at this grade level. Thus, schools differ substantially in their reading results, even after students' family background characteristics are taken into account.

Researchers are now attempting to determine whether differences in school effects such as these are attributable to measurable aspects of "school climate" that can be altered by teachers' and principals' practices (Bryk, Lee, & Smith, 1990; Pallas, 1988; Raudenbush & Willms, 1991, 1995). The studies include factors that portray the inner workings of school life: how students are organized for instruction; the formal and informal rules governing the operation of the school; the nature of interactions between participants; and teachers' and students' attitudes, values,

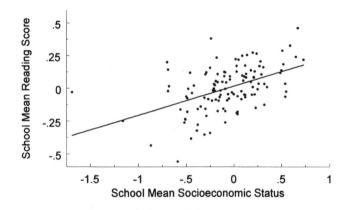

FIGURE 5.4. School mean reading scores by socioeconomic status. Data from 1996 New Brunswick Assessment Program (Willms, 1998).

and expectations. For example, in a study of U.S. middle school students and their parents, Ho and Willms (1996) found that schools with higher levels of parental involvement, on average, had higher levels of reading achievement and shallower gradients, even after controlling for the effects of students' family background. Ma and Willms (1995) found similar effects associated with the disciplinary climate of the school. A number of studies have suggested that successful schools are those where the principal and teachers project the belief that all students can master the curriculum. Their high expectations are manifest in a number of teaching practices and school routines, such as the content and pace of the curriculum, the type and amount of homework, and the way that time and resources are used in the classroom and school (Anderson, 1985; Dreeben & Gamoran, 1986; Plewis, 1991). In schools with such high academic press, students are more likely to engage in challenging activities and establish high norms for their own academic success.

In the New Brunswick study, academic press associated with peer expectations was a strong predictor of academic achievement, particularly for mathematics. An increase of 1-point on the 5-point scale was associated with an increase of nearly 40% of a standard deviation (or about 4 months of schooling). Classroom discipline was positively related, with an estimated effect of about 10% of a standard deviation for a 1-point increase on the 5-point scale, but was not statistically significant. The variables pertaining to parental involvement at home were negatively related to student achievement, indicating that parents who met more often with the teacher or worked more regularly with their children tended to be parents of children who scored lower on the achievement tests. Parents had relatively little involvement in the schools as volunteers at this grade level, and the effect of volunteering was negligible.

An important aspect of school reform, including its likely effect on levels of achievement and gradients, concerns the manner in which students are allocated to schools, classrooms, and instructional groups. The extent to which students are segregated is important because a child's reference group can have a substantial effect on his or her outcomes, over and above the effects associated with the child's own ability and social class.[7] Schools or classrooms with high social-class or high ability intakes tend to have several advantages associated with their context. On average they are more likely to have greater support from parents, fewer disciplinary problems, and an atmosphere conducive to learning. They are more likely to attract and retain talented and motivated teachers. Usually there are peer effects that occur when bright and motivated students work together. Consequently, when students are segregated, either between classes or tracks within schools or between schools within a community, students from advantaged backgrounds do better whereas those from disadvantaged backgrounds do worse. Thus levels of segregation are an important contributing factor of socioeconomic gradients.

Segregation between schools along social-class lines arises in many jurisdictions through residential segregation. In most school districts, children are assigned to particular schools on the basis of school "catchment areas" and the geographic boundaries of these areas are not necessarily drawn to achieve a heterogeneous mix of students across schools. Some districts have "open enrollment" policies, which allow parents to choose schools outside their designated catchment area. However, research in the United States and the United Kingdom suggests that these policies actually increase segregation, because parents with more resources are more likely to exercise this right (Lee, Groninger, & Smith, 1994; Echols & Willms, 1995; Willms & Echols, 1992). Thus some segregation can be reduced simply by redrawing catchment boundaries in townships and cities where there are two or more schools. This would likely result in higher achievement for students from lower social-class backgrounds, thereby flattening gradients.

Other school, district, and provincial policies can also contribute to between-school segregation. Private schools contribute to between-school segregation, because parents of middle class backgrounds are more likely to send their children to a private school. Therefore, policies such as tuition tax credits that support private schooling are likely to increase segregation. Denominational schooling may also contribute to between-school segregation, but data on this issue are not available for Canada. Many educators believe French immersion programs or programs for "gifted" children contribute to both between- and within-school segregation, depending on where they are situated and the nature of the selection mechanisms. Recently, some school districts have allowed—and, in some cases, encouraged—the development of charter schools or magnet schools. These schools usually offer special curricula (e.g., the Langley Fine Arts School in British Columbia) or have a particular mission set out in a parents' charter. The problem is that these schools attract students who are predominantly from middle class backgrounds. Sometimes the schools have selective criteria that contribute to the segregation of students over and above the segregation stemming from choice of residence, and often children with special needs are excluded because charter schools do not typically have adequate services. The existence of charter schools contradicts the principle of "equal access and opportunity for all students" served by a public system.

The research on school climate and segregation has had considerable influence on efforts to "restructure" schools in ways that make schools a more supportive environment, especially for children from disadvantaged backgrounds. Three prominent models for restructuring—*Accelerated Schools* (Levin, 1987), *Success for All Schools* (Madden, Slavin, Karweit, & Livermon, 1989), and the *School Development Program* (Comer, 1980, 1988)—have been adopted by schools throughout the United States and to some extent worldwide. All three models emphasize prevention over remediation, a highly contextualized curriculum with strong components in reading and language, parental participation, and site-based governance structures (King, 1994). More general efforts to restructure schools have attempted to provide learning activities that integrate different aspects of the curriculum, are longer term, and are more relevant to students' everyday lives. They aim to provide students with instruction in heterogeneous groups, with more team-teaching and student-based learning approaches (Lee & Smith, 1993). In Canada, a number of schools have embarked on restructuring efforts, and generally the philosophy of "middle schools" (which serve children in grades 6–8) is consistent with the restructuring movement. However, there is no widely accepted Canadian model for restructuring schools or for supporting disadvantaged children.

COMMUNITIES MAKE A DIFFERENCE

The research on the effects of families and schools has been fruitful in that it has identified many of the important factors that contribute to a child's development. However, the effects of school policy and practice are circumscribed by the social, economic, and political context of the community and state. These larger forces have not been accommodated by the "input–process–output" models, in which schools are "treatments" in a quasi-experimental design without regard to their surrounding communities. The term "community" is difficult to define, both theoretically and operationally, which perhaps causes many researchers to steer clear of community-level analyses. "Community" usually refers to a group of people living in the same locality and organized through some political or municipal body. But it is also used to refer to a group of individuals that share certain beliefs, values, or goals, such as a religious community or a community of scholars. A simple definition suffices for the purpose of studying children's educational and health outcomes: "a community is a group of individuals who share responsibility for the education and care of their children." With this definition, there are multiple overlapping communities that warrant consideration, such as municipalities (defined geographically with attention to local government structures), school districts and schools, health regions, neighborhoods, religious groups, and families.

   Research on the Scottish educational system, conducted by the Centre for Educational Sociology (University of Edinburgh) between 1985 and 1995, provides some insight into the effects of community that are relevant to the Canadian system. McPherson and Willms (1986) examined levels of academic attainment and socioeconomic gradients for 50 Scottish communities that had two or more schools. The definition of community was based on geographic boundaries and on the historical relationships between primary "feeder" schools and secondary schools. They found that communities varied substantially in both levels of attainment and socioeconomic gradients. They also observed that single-school communities on average had steeper socioeconomic gradients within schools than did schools in larger communities. Some communities had relatively shallow gradients, particularly the Scottish "new towns"—five communities established after World War II to accommodate overspill from the large cities. They noted that there was a stability of student intake and schooling outcomes that spanned nearly a century: schools founded during the Victorian and Edwardian eras were on average more effective in 1980 than schools founded after 1945. McPherson and Raab (1988) noted that after 1945 the Scottish teachers who served on the national curriculum and examination committees and on Her Majesty's Inspectorate had been disproportionately recruited from the small set of Victorian and Edwardian schools that McPherson and Willms (1986) had identified as being more effective.

When parental choice of schools was introduced by the Thatcher government in 1980, parents could elect to enroll their child in a school outside of their designated catchment area. However, analyses of patterns of enrollment revealed that middle class parents were more likely to exercise choice and disproportionately chose schools with above-average social-class intakes, particularly the Victorian and Edwardian schools (Echols, McPherson, & Willms, 1990). By 1995, some 15 years after parental choice had been introduced, the level of segregation along social class lines had increased dramatically in most Scottish communities (Willms, 1996).

Raffe and Willms (1989) hypothesized that some of the variation within and between Scottish communities in their educational attainment was associated with variation in local opportunity structure. They were able to link data describing the employment rates of males and females in local "travel-to-work" areas with data describing pupils' academic attainment. They found that in communities where there were few opportunities for employment, pupils achieved better grades on national examinations and were more likely to remain in school beyond the compulsory period. The effect of "local opportunity structure" provided a plausible explanation for the exceptional performance of females in rural communities (Willms & Kerr, 1987) and of Catholics in the West of Scotland (Willms, 1992).

Social Capital

The foregoing Scottish work shows that the effectiveness of schools is affected by far-reaching social and economic factors and is entrenched in schooling systems through historical and political relationships between schools and their local communities. Coleman (1988) maintained that the success of many Catholic schools in the United States was due to the strong sense of community shared by the parents and school staff. He distinguished between "human capital," as used by Schultz (1963) and Becker (1964) to embody the skills and capabilities that enable people to act in new ways, and "social capital," which "comes about through changes in the relations among persons that facilitate action" (Coleman, 1988, p.

S100). Coleman elaborated the concept of social capital by identifying three forms in which social relations become assets that bring about action.

The first form—obligations, expectations, and trustworthiness of structures—relies on the notion of social exchange: when one individual does something for another, it establishes an expectation in the giver and an obligation in the receiver. The number of these expectation–obligation relationships present in a social structure varies, depending on how trustworthy the environment is. Trustworthiness might be low, for example, in an environment where the population is relatively transient. It may also be low if members of the social structure are relatively independent, such that there are few outstanding expectation–obligation relationships. This could be the case in areas where people are affluent and where there is strong provision of social services. The extent of expectation–obligation relationships can also vary among ethnic or religious groups.

Social capital also entails information channels. People use social relations to keep informed. For example, when parents have the opportunity to choose a school for their child, they consider information from friends, neighbors, and acquaintances as one of the most important sources of information about available schools (Echols & Willms, 1995). The networks that parents establish through social clubs, sports activities, church groups, or other institutions are an important form of social capital.

Norms and effective sanctions are the third form of social capital. Coleman (1988) argues that when these are effective, they constitute an especially potent form of social capital. He suggests that the safety of neighborhoods depends largely on effective norms that inhibit crime, and that these norms are more important than the presence of a police force. Similarly, norms for high academic achievement established by rewards from the community outside the school reinforces and strengthens the mission of the school. More generally, effective norms lead people to work for the public good.

SUMMARY AND DISCUSSION

The data on literacy from the 1994 IALS suggest that Canada's youth outperformed youth in the United States but scored well below Swedish youth. The differences were most pronounced for youth whose parents had low levels of education. Within Canada, the literacy scores of youth in Québec and the three prairie provinces more closely resembled those of Swedish youth, whereas the scores of youth in British Columbia, Ontario, and the four Atlantic provinces were closer to those of American youth. The results of both the international and national analyses indicate that successful societies have shallow gradients: the countries and provinces with high overall literacy scores have relatively high scores for youth from less advantaged backgrounds. Two questions immediately arise: (1) Are gradients immutable; that is, could Canada look more like Sweden? (2) If so, what policies and practices might bring about that change?

One line of research on social action emphasizes the independent actions of individuals (Coleman, 1988). Parents make independent decisions to achieve what they perceive to be best for their family—what economists call "maximizing utility." Gradients persist because parents with more economic and social capital do things differently: on average, they are likely to talk more with their children, read to them more often, buy them more educational toys—generally provide them with a richer environment—than parents with fewer resources. Differences in individuals' behaviors that affect developmental outcomes begin during pregnancy with choices regarding nutrition, smoking, and the use of alcohol and drugs. For example, breast-feeding is a protective factor against infectious diseases (L. A. Hanson, Lindquist, Hofvander, & Zetterstrom, 1985). Just over one-half of Canadian babies are breast-fed, and of these about two-thirds are breast-ed longer than 3 months (McIntyre, 1996). Moreover, the effects of protective factors, or factors that place children at risk during the period their brain and nervous system are being developed, appear to be cumulative. Thus differences in individuals' actions might account for the social-class gradients in children's early literacy that are observed at age 5 in the NLSCY.

But it seems unlikely that differences in individual behavior could account for the differences among provinces in children's early literacy scores or the large variation among provinces in both levels and gradients in the literacy skills of young adults. Another line of research, more characteristic of sociologists, stresses the importance of social context in shaping, constraining, and redirecting individuals' actions (Coleman, 1988). In this line of research, mothers' choices regarding the use of alcohol or drugs during pregnancy, or whether to breast-feed their babies, depend heavily on the norms of their immediate community and the social support available to them. Research in a number of countries has provided convincing evidence that schools and schooling systems can vary considerably in their effects on children's outcomes and that their effectiveness depends on their social context. Three of the most important features of school context concern the norms and expectations established by school staff, the disciplinary climate of the school, and the support of parents and the wider community. The steepness of gradients, therefore, depends on the extent to which children from differing socioeconomic backgrounds have equal access to supportive school contexts.

An essential link between gradients and context is the effect of segregating low-status groups from mainstream society. Ethnic minorities, people with low incomes, and the unemployed are segregated by their place of residence in most cities worldwide (London & Flanagan, 1976). This segregation limits their access to certain labor markets, exposes them to more crime and health risks, and restricts their access to the best schools, hospitals, and other social services. It affects their health and their general economic and social well-being (Massey, Condron, & Denton, 1987). The effects of residential segregation can be either reduced or exacerbated by structural features of the community that determine where certain programs are located and what rules govern access. The development of a "charter school" in a high social-class area, with selective admission criteria, would be a good example. The segregation of low- and high-status groups can also be occur within institutions, for example, by streaming children with differing academic abilities. A plausible explanation for differences among provinces in their social-class gradients is that some school systems may have greater segregation between schools within communities and between classrooms or school programs within schools.

Thus, any explanation of why some provinces have particularly steep social-class gradients, like any discussion of policies that might increase equality of opportunity and outcomes, necessarily requires an understanding of the competing individual interests of those with differing social status and how these affect access and opportunity within communities. If we consider geographically defined communities, for example, as was done in the Scottish research, a province could have steep gradients if there were a number of communities with very low levels of economic and social capital, resulting in low levels of educational attainment. If this were the case, socioeconomic gradients within communities would be relatively shallow but the gradient for the province would be steep. This kind of distribution would call for policies that aimed to strengthen the social capital of deprived communities in conjunction with compensatory policies that increased resources for schools in those communities. Alternatively, a province's gradient could be steep if within most communities students were allocated to schools or school programs, through either formal or informal selective mechanisms, in ways that segregated children along social-class lines. If this were the case, social class gradients would be steep for most communities and for the province as a whole. This would call for policies that aimed to increase the heterogeneity of schools and classrooms, and provide greater opportunities for children from lower social-class backgrounds.

We return to the questions—could Canada look more like Sweden, and if so, what policies and practices might effect that change? A. Heath (1990), a prominent British sociologist, offered a pessimistic view that social-class gradients are immutable, which he supported with analyses that suggested class inequalities in educational attainment in England and Wales had been relatively constant since the turn of the century. My conjecture is that socioeconomic gradients are indeed relatively stable, because societies establish some tolerable equilibria, which are maintained by powerful economic and political forces. But there is ample evidence that these can be altered through policy, practice, and reform. Canada is an ideal setting for studying questions about gradients for several reasons. One is that it is that is possible to study variation across provinces in children's outcomes and in the policies and practices aimed to support children. Second, cross-sectional data describing large samples of Canadian children and youth have recently become available and longitudinal data will soon be available. Third, and perhaps most important, is that there is an optimistic spirit prevailing among many Canadians that change is possible, even during a time of dwindling government funding. Better support for children is high on the policy agendas at both federal and provincial levels.

ACKNOWLEDGMENTS

I am grateful to Human Resources Development Canada and Statistics Canada for providing the data for this study, to the U.S. Spencer Foundation for its funding of the study, "School and Community Effects on Children's Education and Health Outcomes," and to the Social Sciences and Humanities Research Council for its funding of "The Elementary School Climate Study." I am also grateful to the Canadian Institute for Advanced Research (where I am the New Brunswick–CIBC Fellow), which provides the primary funding for the Atlantic Centre for Policy Research in Education. Opinions reflect those of the author and do not necessarily reflect those of the granting agencies. I am thankful to Sandy Harris for help in preparing the manuscript.

NOTES

1. It is unlikely that the observed relationships stemmed from "ceiling effects" on the test. In every country, there was a relatively small proportion of respondents scoring at level 5—the top level on the literacy test.
2. The analyses are presented in detail in Willms (1997). The model includes a statistical control for whether the respondent spoke the language of the test (either French or English) since birth, and if not, the length of time he or she had been speaking the language of the test.
3. One hypothesis is that the observed differences among provinces are simply an artifact of sampling and measurement error. However, the levels of reading and writing skills of 16-year old children, collected by the CMEC as part of the SAIP, correlate highly with the IALS results (Willms, 1997). The SAIP data do not include measures of students' family background, so it is not possible to use them to examine social-class gradients. Human Resources Development Canada and Statistics Canada are currently supporting research to discern whether these interprovincial differences in levels and gradients in literacy are evident in other large databases and whether these findings are consistent across a range of children's educational and health outcomes. The U.S. Spencer Foundation is supporting research to examine the distribution of children's outcomes across Canadian communities and to determine whether some of the variation in children's outcomes can be explained by the social capital available to families, schools, and communities.

4. The scores for the *Échelle de vocabulaire en images Peabody* (EVIP), the Francophone version of the PPVT, were standardized separately, whereas the scores for the Anglophone version were based on the standardization provided by the developers of the test. Therefore, the average score and standard deviation for the sample from Québec, which comprised 89.5% Francophone children, is close to the Canadian average, as are the mean and standard deviation for New Brunswick, which comprised 29.1% Francophone children.

5. See Willms and Shields (1996) for details.

6. The data identify the "person most knowledgeable" (PMK) about the child, which in more than 90% of the families was the mother or stepmother. Similarly, the "spouse of the primary care giver" was nearly always the father or stepfather. For ease of presentation, I refer to the PMK and the spouse of the PMK simply as the mother and father.

7. See Brookover et al. (1978), Henderson, Mieszkowski, and Sauvageau (1978), Rumberger and Willms (1992), Shavit and Williams (1985), Summers and Wolfe (1977), and Willms (1985, 1986), regarding between-school segregation. See Gamoran (1991, 1992) and Kerckhoff (1986, 1993) regarding tracking and streaming. See Dar and Resh (1986), Dreeben and Gamoran (1986), Rowan and Miracle (1983), Slavin (1987), Sorensen and Hallinan (1984), and Willms and Chen (1989) regarding within-classroom segregation.

6

Are Socioeconomic Gradients for Children Similar to Those for Adults?

ACHIEVEMENT AND HEALTH OF CHILDREN IN THE UNITED STATES

Jeanne Brooks-Gunn
Greg J. Duncan
Pia Rebello Britto

Socioeconomic (SES) gradients have been observed for a broad range of adult outcomes, with the bulk of the work focusing on the United States, United Kingdom, and Canada. Individuals lower in SES have poorer physical and emotional health, across diseases and conditions, and for morbidity and mortality outcomes (Adler et al., 1994; Illsley & Baker, 1991; Seeman & McEwen, 1996). These gradients for health indicators are not totally accounted for by differentials in educational attainment (Adler et al., 1994; Hertzman & Wiens, 1996). SES differentials also are not accounted for by access to and use of health care (Marmot et al., 1984, 1991; Marmot & Shipley, 1996).

The SES gradients are not just seen between those at the bottom and the top of the distribution but across the socioeconomic distribution (Marmot et al., 1991). However, it is important to focus on the differences between those individuals or families at the bottom and those close to the bottom of the distribution (i.e., in comparisons between poor and near-poor individuals), since economic policies are likely to target the poor (and at best raise poor individuals' incomes only modestly above the poverty threshold; Brooks-Gunn & Duncan, 1997; Duncan & Brooks-Gunn, 1997a; Duncan, Yeung, Brooks-Gunn, & Smith, 1998).

Typically, SES is defined by several indicators within a particular country. Education, occupation, and income are the three most frequently used SES indicators. Sometimes individual indicators are the focus; more frequently, comparisons involve a number of SES indicators. The grouping of SES indicators renders it difficult to make comparisons across studies within a particular country, since researchers often use different categorization strategies in defining SES. Problems also arise when researchers are examining SES gradients in different countries (even though across-country comparisons are made vis-à-vis the *relative* ranking of individuals in different deciles, e.g., of each country). The steepness of the SES gradient represents the response of the health outcome to SES.

With respect to SES gradients for child outcomes, most work has focused on family income and parental education as indicators of SES. In this chapter, data are presented separately for these two indicators. Our rationale is that the associations between income and children's development, on the one hand, and between education and children's development, on the other, may be somewhat different. Parental decisions and constraints regarding investments in their children may vary by both parental income and education (Becker, 1991). Furthermore, the pathways through which income and education might influence children may vary. As an example, maternal education is strongly associated with reading and literacy activities in the home, two variables that are linked to school achievement and verbal ability (see Willms, Chapter 5, this volume; R. H. Bradley et al., 1989; A. W. Gottfried, 1984; Hart & Risley, 1995; Klebanov, Brooks-Gunn, & Duncan, 1994; Klebanov, Brooks-Gunn, McCarton, & McCormick, 1998; Phillips, Brooks-Gunn, Duncan, Klebanov, & Jencks, 1998; Snow, 1993; Wachs & Gruen, 1982). While income also is linked to reading, the association is weaker than between education and reading. In contrast, the purchase of learning materials in the home is constrained directly by family income (even though such purchase is also associated with maternal education). So while reading and the purchase of learning materials both may be associated with children's achievement, maternal education may be more important for the former and family income for the latter (Brooks-Gunn, Klebanov, & Duncan, 1996; Mayer, 1997a).[1]

In the literature on SES and adult health, the extensive knowledge about the existence of SES gradients is not matched by comparable understanding of the pathways through which SES influences physical and emotional health. Adler and her colleagues (1994) outline four major sets of pathways, the first having to do with physical environment, the second with social environment, the third with socialization and experiences, and the fourth with health behaviors. They summarize these classes of influences as follows: "(i) the physical environment in which one lives and works and associated exposure to pathogens, carcinogens, and other environmental hazards; (ii) the social environment and associated vulnerability to interpersonal aggression and violence as well as degree of access to social resources and supports; (iii) socialization and experiences that influence psychological development and ongoing mood, affect, and cognition; and (iv) health behaviors" (Adler et al., 1994, p. 18).[2] The pathways through which income or education might influence children have been organized somewhat differently, although the same types of pathways are believed to be operating. We shall return to these pathways later on.

We have organized this chapter around six questions having to do with the nature and existence of SES gradients upon health and developmental outcomes of U.S. children (see Brooks-Gunn, Britto, & Brady, 1998; Brooks-Gunn & Duncan, 1997):

1. Why the focus on children?
2. Are income gradients found for indicators of child health and development?
3. Are gradient effects similar across the income distribution?
4. Does the timing of low income influence child outcomes?
5. What are some of the pathways through which income operates during childhood?
6. How do current federal policies in the United States address the existence of income gradients during childhood?

WHY FOCUS ON CHILDREN?

Our focus on children is driven by the belief that children, who are dependent on others for their well-being, are a concern of all adults in a community or country, not just of their parents. Children enter or avoid poverty by their birth into a family, not by any actions of their own. Their ability to alter their SES status is limited until the late adolescent years. And if growing up poor has adverse effects on their development, then, at least for the vast majority of children, being born into poverty also restricts their chances of leaving poverty as adults.

Rates of Poverty in Children and Adults

Western nations have policies to provide some necessities of life to their poor citizens, or at least to some of their poor citizens. How well has the United States done for its youngest citizens? In the late 1990s, about 14 million children (more than one in five of all U.S. children) are living in families below the poverty threshold. In 1996, the poverty threshold was U.S.$12,516 for a family of three people and U.S.$16,036 for a family of four. Poverty thresholds in the United States take into account household size and are adjusted each year for the cost of living (based on the Consumer Price Index, CPI). The threshold was originally developed based on expected food expenditures (the thrifty food basket) for families of particular sizes; this number was then multiplied by a factor of 3 since, in 1959, food constituted about one-third of household expenses (Orshansky, 1988). Consequently, the U.S. poverty line is absolute, not relative.[3] For any given year, families whose incomes are above the threshold are considered "not poor," and families below the threshold are classified as "poor." Adjustments to income for family size are often accomplished by calculating income-to-needs ratios; when translated into a ratio based on the poverty threshold, poverty is defined as 1.0.[4] Is a poverty rate of 20% for our children high? In 1959, the first year for which official poverty rates were available, the percentage of children living in poverty was about 27%. The poverty rate for children was substantially higher than that for adults aged 18–64 but was less than the rate for the elderly. Over the next 30 years, the proportion of poor in each of the three age groups has declined, as is illustrated in Figure 6.1. In recent years, however, as the rate of poverty has climbed, the proportion of children below the poverty threshold has risen faster than the proportion of adults. It is now about twice as high as the rate for adults and about 70% higher than that for the elderly. The increase in Social Security benefits is the major cause of the drop in the poverty rates for elderly individuals over the past 20 years (Hernandez, 1993, 1997). In addition, if we were to look at the rates of persistent poverty (poverty that lasts more than 1 year), these age differences would be even more pronounced.

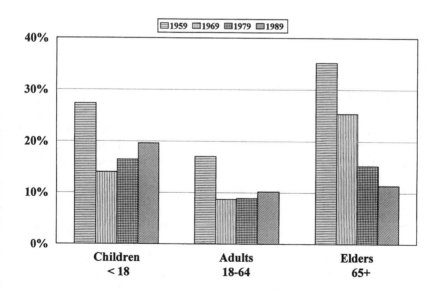

FIGURE 6.1. Percentage of children and adults who were poor from 1959 to 1989.

Causes of Increases in Children's Poverty Rates

The principal causes of the rise in children's poverty rates include changes in marriage and divorce patterns, in unemployment, and in falling infla-tion-adjusted wages for less-educated adults. Both the number of unmar-ried women having children and the number of divorces between couples with children are often cited as the most potent factors in the high rates of child poverty in the United States. By the mid-1990s, one in three births in the United States were to unwed couples. Two-thirds of black women and one-fifth of white women who become mothers have children outside of marriage (Ventura, 1995). While nonmarital childbearing is highest for ad-olescent mothers, the rates are also high for mothers in their 20s. Never-married mothers are often poor, as they are relying on one income (their own), they are young, and they have relatively low levels of education (Cherlin, 1992; Furstenberg, Brooks-Gunn, & Morgan, 1987; Hernandez, 1993; McLanahan & Sandefur, 1994). In 1990 there were over 1 million divorces in the United States (Divorces and Annulments Rates: United States, 1940–90, 1995). Of children born to married parents, approxi-mately 45% are expected to experience parental divorce before the age of 18 (Bumpass, 1984). Ever-married or divorced mothers also are more likely to be poor than are married mothers, as the incomes of divorced mothers drop by over a third after the marital disruption (Duncan, 1991; McLanahan & Sandefur, 1994; McLanahan, 1997).

The rise in children's poverty rates has also been attributed to the growing wage inequality. Research examining the association between U.S. trends in poverty and labor market opportunities indicates that even though economic expansion on the mid-1980s led to a drop in unemploy-ment by more than 4 points, it had very little effect on poverty rates (Blank, 1993; Blank & Card, 1993; Cutler & Katz, 1991). In one of the most thor-ough studies on this issue, Blank and Card (1993) present evidence suggest-ing that four factors—unemployment, wage level, wage dispersion, and family structure—each play an independent role in producing changes in poverty rates within regions. Unemployment itself has statistically signifi-cant but substantive modest effects, with a 1-point drop in unemployment associated with a .2 point drop in the poverty rate. Both the level and dis-persion of the labor market earnings played important independent roles in affecting the poverty rate.

The decline in manufacturing, relocation of jobs to the suburbs, and increasing polarization of the labor market into high- and low-wage sectors has lead to an increase in the level of unemployment and stagnation of wages among the semiskilled adults in the cities (Coulton, 1996; Danziger & Gottschalk, 1995; Sampson & Morenoff, 1997). These changes have lead to a concentration of extremely poor inner-city neighborhoods and middle- to upper-income suburban neighborhoods (Wilson, 1987, 1996). The effects of this geographic concentration of urban poverty and social isolation have been seen in individual-level outcomes, such as the degree of labor force attachment, and in family-level outcomes, such as higher levels of social and economic disadvantage (Sampson & Morenoff, 1997).

ARE INCOME GRADIENTS FOUND FOR CHILD OUTCOMES?

Domains of Child Health and Development

The consequences of low income (and the existence of an income gradient) upon children's health and development are being studied by a number of scholars. Research has focused on four general domains of health and development: physical health, cognitive and verbal abilities, emotional well-being, and school achievement (Brooks-Gunn & Duncan, 1997). Other childhood indicators have not received much attention (e.g., relationships, school engagement, self-efficacy, motivation; see Brooks-Gunn, 1995 and Hauser, Brown, & Prosser, 1997). The major outcomes within each domain are listed below (reviews of this literature may be found in Brooks-Gunn & Duncan, 1997, and Haveman & Wolfe, 1995):

1. *Physical health outcomes* include low birth weight, preterm delivery, perinatal complications, infant death, anemia, and lead exposure.
2. *Cognitive abilities outcomes* include scores on tests of intelligence, verbal ability, reasoning ability, and visual–spatial ability.
3. *School achievement outcomes* include grade failure, learning problems, attention problems, school completion, and achievement test scores.
4. *Emotional outcomes* include behavior problems, juvenile delinquency, depressive or anxious behavior, aggressive behavior, antisocial behavior.[5]

Use, access, and cost of service use or food patterns are not included in this list, as they are conceptualized as process rather than outcome variables in this chapter. Food consumption, food expenditures, receipt or recommended well-baby visits, up-to-date immunizations, cost of health care, and access to health care services are known to influence potential child outcomes. The same is true of parental behaviors such as smoking during pregnancy, drug use during pregnancy, postpartum parenting practices, and provision of learning experiences. That is, effects of income upon child outcomes may operate through the receipt of health, nutrition, or social services, as well as parental food choices and interactions with the child. The pathways through which poverty might operate are discussed in a later section.

Developmental Periods in the First 20 Years of Life

Income gradients vary both by domains of well-being (physical health, cognitive and verbal abilities, emotional well-being, and school achievement) and across various age periods that characterize the first two decades of life (Baydar, Brooks-Gunn, & Furstenberg, 1993; Brooks-Gunn, Guo, & Furstenberg, 1993; Brooks-Gunn, Klebanov, Liaw, & Spiker, 1993). Five age groups are often described: prenatal and infancy years (prenatal to 2 years); early childhood years (ages 3–6); late childhood (ages 7–10); early adolescence (ages 11–15); and late adolescence (ages 16–19). The boundaries are often blurred; for example, 11-year-olds could be considered in the late childhood or early adolescent period. Each of these age groupings covers one or two major transitions in the child's life, such as school entrances or exits, cognitive maturation, role changes, physiological changes—or a combination of these. These groupings are characterized by developmental challenges that are relatively universal, that are navigated more or less successfully, and that require new modes of adaptation to changes (Graber & Brooks-Gunn, 1996; Rutter, 1994).

Each of these age groupings are characterized by distinctive capacities and require different resources. Hence they include somewhat different indicators of well-being. So, for example, grade failure is relevant in the late childhood years but not later, since most schools no longer hold students back by the end of middle school (Guo, Brooks-Gunn, & Harris, 1996). Furthermore, poverty might influence each indicator somewhat differently. As an illustration, income effects are much stronger for cognitive and verbal ability test scores than for indices of emotional health in the childhood years (Duncan & Brooks-Gunn, 1997b).

Three Data Sets in the United States

Much of our knowledge about the effects of income poverty upon children and youth in the United States is gleaned from large national longitudinal studies, including the Panel Study of Income Dynamics (PSID), the National Longitudinal Study of Youth (NLSY) and the follow-up (Child Supplement) of the children born to the women in this study, High School and Beyond, and the National Educational Longitudinal Survey of 1988 (see Brooks-Gunn, Brown, Duncan & Moore, 1995, for a description of these data sets as well as other national data sets with multiple years of family income data). Scholars have also used smaller scale studies that are longitudinal, have family income and household size information collected yearly, assess child outcomes, and are multisite. Three notable studies of this genre are the Infant Health and Development Program (IHDP; Brooks-Gunn, Klebanov, et al., 1993; Brooks-Gunn, McCarton, et al., 1994); the Iowa Farm Family Study (Conger, Conger, & Elder, 1997; Conger et al., 1993; Conger, Ge, Elder, Lorenz, & Simons, 1994); and the Québec Longitudinal

Studies of Behavior (Pagani et al., 1997). Additionally, all of the studies cited here provide estimates of income poverty in regression equations that control for other family conditions, including maternal ethnicity, age at birth, education, and marital status. It is possible that family characteristics not included in this list might account for, at least in part, any associations between income and child outcome.

We are using three data sets, each of which is described below: the PDID; the Child Supplement of the NLSY; and the IHDP (Table 6.1).

1. The PSID is a nationally representative sample followed annually since 1968 (Duncan & Hill, 1989; Hill, 1992). All members of the original households are included in the sample, and family members leaving the household (i.e., due to divorce or offspring setting up their own households) are seen. About 7,000 households were interviewed in 1996. Black families were oversampled. Roughly 60% of individuals present in the study's first wave were still present 29 years later. Currently, child and youth data are restricted to high school completion rates, teenage motherhood, and limited work experience data (see Duncan & Brooks-Gunn, 1997b, and Haveman & Wolfe, 1995, for reviews of this work).

2. The NLSY, begun in 1979, was a nationally representative sample of youth aged 14–21 (black, poor white, and Hispanic youth were oversampled, as were low-income whites). The approximately 12,000 NLSY cohort members were seen yearly through 1994 (and are now seen every other year). In 1996, the respondents were 31–38 years of age. Attrition has been remarkably low (about 10% between 1979 and 1991). School, fertility, and work information is collected on the youth, as well as drug use, self-esteem, and verbal ability data. The National Longitudinal Study of Youth–Child Supplement (NLSY–CS) is drawn from those women in the original 1979 NLSY cohort who have become mothers (Chase-Lansdale, Mott, Brooks-Gunn, & Phillips, 1991). All children in the family are seen every other year (beginning in 1986). Thus, as children are born, they are added to the cohort. The sample of children is not nationally representative, since the 1979 NLSY women have not completed their childbearing years (i.e., in 1996, the women were still in their 30's). However, the sample becomes more representative with every passing year. For children aged 5 and older, assessments include a school achievement battery, a verbal ability test, a digit span test, and a behavior problem index (reported by the mother). The 3- and 4-year-olds also are given the verbal ability test. The youth also are asked questions about grade failure, school completion, work experience, and fertility, similar to the questions in the PSID and NLSY surveys. The home environment is also assessed every other year. The NLSY–CS is the only U.S. national data set available with child assessments across the first two decades of life and yearly information gathered on family characteristics.

3. The IHDP is a multisite demonstration testing the efficacy of early

TABLE 6.1. Three Data Sets: Panel Study of Income Dynamics (PSID), National Longitudinal Survey of Youth (NLSY), and Infant Health and Development Program (IHDP)

PSID Survey Research Center of the University of Michigan	NLSY Cohorts 1986, 1988, 1990, and 1992	IHDP Follow-up conducted by Brooks-Gunn and McCarton

Ongoing longitudinal survey of U.S. households
  Begun in 1968
  Representative sample of nonimmigrant U.S. population and of major subgroups in the population
	Ongoing longitudinal study of youth
	  Begun in 1979
	  National representative sample of youth aged 14–21 in 1979, oversampled poor whites and blacks
	  Children of NLSY women seen from 1986 onward
		985 low-birth-weight, preterm infants and their families
		  Consists of 8 sites across the country
		  Seen 11 times from birth to age 8

Subsample of interest
  1,323 youth
  Born between 1967 and 1973
  Seen yearly between birth and age 20
  Yearly family income data collected
	Subsample of interest
	  3,057 (5- to 6-year-olds)
	  3,517 (7- to 8-year-olds)
	  2,879 (9- to 10-year-olds)
		Two intervention groups (randomized)
		Control (pediatric follow-up and referral)
		Treatment (pediatric follow-up and referral)
		  Home visiting over first 3 years of life
		  Center-based child development—second 2 years of life
		  Parenting groups—second 2 years of life

Outcomes of interest
  Incidence of out-of-wedlock teenage births
  School leaving before high school graduation
	Outcomes of interest
	  Peabody Individual Achievement Test (PIAT)—Math
	  Peabody Individual Achievement Test (PIAT)—Reading
	  Peabody Picture Vocabulary Test (PPVT)
	  Behavior Problems Index (BPI)
		Outcomes of interest
		  Cognitive and language
		  Behavioral competence
		  Health
		  Parenting behavior
		  Home environment

intervention services for low-birth-weight premature infants and their families (Infant Health & Development Program, 1990; Brooks-Gunn, Klebanov, et al., 1993; Brooks-Gunn, McCarton, et al., 1994; C. T. Ramey & S. L. Ramey, 1992). Almost 1,000 families were seen 11 times from the time of the children's birth through their 8th birthday. The attrition rate has been remarkably low (i.e., 92% of the birth cohort was followed through age 8; McCarton et al., 1997). Extensive data were collected on cognitive, emotional, linguistic, health, and social functioning. Parenting behavior and home environment were assessed repeatedly. Additionally, family social and economic data were collected yearly.

While not a nationally representative sample, the IHDP has a richer set of child outcome data than the NLSY–CS. Together, the two data sets provide most of the information about the effects of family income upon children in the first 8 years of life (given our requirement for multiple years of family income data being available as well as other family characteristic data). In this chapter, we shall look at evidence for gradients in the preschool, childhood, and adolescent years. Our focus will be on cognitive outcomes and school achievement (limited data on emotional well-being will be presented as well) using the IHDP and NLSY–CS data sets. The PSID is used to estimate income effects upon high school completion rates.

Income Effects in the Three Developmental Periods

The data reported for the three age groupings are in part based on a 1995 conference entitled "Growing Up Poor," which was sponsored by the NICHD Research Network on Child and Family Well-being and the Russell Sage Foundation (Duncan & Brooks-Gunn, 1997a). Longitudinal data from almost a dozen developmental studies were examined to understand the extent to which childhood poverty influences life chances. All of the research teams were asked to conduct "replication" analyses in which the same set of measures were included in regression models. These measures were family income, maternal schooling, family structure, and—if multiple race/ethnic groups were included—race/ethnicity. Our goal was to provide an estimate of income effects independent of the most common poverty cofactors (parental education, marital structure). Almost all of the studies had at least three annual observations of family income; consequently, the estimates of income-to-needs ratios are based on multiple years (since family income is known to vary from year to year, multiple year estimates yield more stable estimates).

In the discussion that follows, a "large" effect is one in which the effect sizes are significant and are almost always one-third of a standard deviation or larger. A "moderate-to-small" effect is one in which the income coefficients, while significant at the .05 level, are less than one-third of a standard deviation. We use the term "no effect" for those coefficients that are not significant at the .05 level. Studies not included in our conference proceedings do not always include maternal education and family structure as control variables, and sometimes define income differently than we do (i.e., studies may not use 3-years worth of data and may not have calculated an income-to-needs ratio based on family income and family size, with the poverty threshold set to 1.0; see Duncan,

Brooks-Gunn, & Klebanov, 1994). Tables 6.2 and 6.3 present a summary of the findings.

Preschool Years

In the young childhood period, studies have examined intelligence test scores, verbal ability scores, and behavior problem scores as associated with income poverty (Brooks-Gunn, Klebanov, & Liaw, 1994; Chase-Lansdale, Gordon, Brooks-Gunn, & Klebanov, 1997; Korenman, Miller, & Sjaastad, 1995; J. R. Smith, Brooks-Gunn, & Klebanov, 1997). This research relies on two data sets primarily: the NLSY–CS and the IHDP.

Controlling for other family characteristics, these income effects are quite large—about one-third of a standard deviation or higher—for the intelligence and verbal test scores at ages 2, 3, and 5 years. Since intelligence and verbal ability tests are normed to have a mean of 100 and a standard deviation of 15 or 16, this means that a hypothetical child whose family's income was at the poverty threshold (1.0) would have an IQ score 5 to 6 points lower than a hypothetical child whose family's income was twice the poverty threshold (these hypothetical children being reared by mothers with the same marital status, education, and ethnicity as well as these children being the same gender, birth weight, and age). The effect sizes are comparable across the age range of 2–5 years (Duncan et al., 1994; J. R. Smith et al., 1997). That is, lower income-to-needs ratios are associated with lower Mental Development Index scores, controlling for maternal education and family structure, at 2 years of age, as well as at ages 3, 4, and 5. Interestingly, family income is not associated with Bayley Mental Development Index scores at 1 year of age (Klebanov et al., 1998). We hypothesize that family income is not a significant contributor to infant intelligence test scores because the skills measured in the first 18 months of life are different than those tapped thereafter (i.e., verbal and reasoning skills are not represented in the early months of infant intelligence tests; Brooks-Gunn, Liaw, & Klebanov, 1992; M. Lewis, 1983; McCall, 1983).

Some children live in poverty for a short time, whereas others spend a significant portion of their childhoods in poverty. The number of years in poverty is significantly associated with negative child outcomes. For example, using the IHDP data on 5-year-olds again, children who lived in poverty for 4 years had IQ scores 9 points lower than those of children who had never lived below the poverty line in the first 5 years. In contrast, children who had been poor for some but not all of the years had IQ scores that were, on average, 4 points lower than those of the nonpoor children (Duncan et al., 1994).

Behavior problems have also been studied during the early childhood years. This literature is based on maternal report of children's behavior problems. Behavior problems include aggression, tantrums, anxiety, mood-

TABLE 6.2. Effects of Income on Verbal Ability and School Achievement Childhood Outcomes

Magnitude of effect	Preschool	Elementary school	High school
Large	Bayley IQ (2)[a] PPVT-R (3)[a] Stanford–Binet (3)[a] PPVT-R (3–4)[b] PPVT-R (5)[a] PIAT—Math (5–6)[b] PIAT—Reading (5–6)[b]	PIAT—Math (7–8)[b] PIAT—Reading (7–8)[b]	
Small/ moderate		Behind in grade for age (6–12)[d]	Odds of completing high school[e] Completed schooling (23)[c] AFQT Score (16–18)[f] Completed schooling[f] Odds of college attendance[h] Status of first job[h] Job status (52)[h] Earnings (52)[h] Hourly earnings (26–27)[f]
None			Self-reported grades (14–17)[i] Odds of high-school graduation[g] Odds of college attendance[g] Completed schooling[g] Odds of family poverty (52)[h]

Note. Numbers in parentheses indicate the ages at which the outcomes are measured. Studies with fewer than three income measurements are omitted from the table. All results come from regression-based analyses that control for mother's education, family structure, and other demographic measures. A "large" effect is one in which all of the income coefficients from the various income-based models are significant at the .05 level or below and the effect sizes are almost always one-third of a standard deviation or larger. A "small/moderate" effect is one in which most of the income coefficients from the various income-based models are significant at the .05 level or below but the effect sizes are consistently less than one-third of a standard deviation. "No effect" means that few if any of the income coefficients from the various income-based models are significant at the .05 level. From Duncan and Brooks-Gunn (1997b). Copyright 1997 by Russell Sage Foundation Press. Reprinted by permission.
[a] J. R. Smith et al. (1997), data from the Infant Health and Development Program.
[b] J. R. Smith et al. (1997), data from the National Longitudinal Survey of Youth.
[c] Axinn et al. (1997), data from the Detroit Longitudinal Study of Mothers and Children, income measured five times, from birth to age 17.
[d] Pagani et al. (1997), data from the Québec Longitudinal Studies of Behavior.
[e] Haveman et al. (1997), data from the Panel Study of Income Dynamics, income measured between ages 6 and 18.
[f] E. Peters and Mullis (1997), data from the NLSY.
[g] Teachman et al. (1997), data from the NLS cohorts of Young Men and Women.
[h] Hauser and Sweeney (1997), data from the Wisconsin Longitudinal Survey.
[i] Conger et al. (1997), data from the Iowa Youth and Family Project.

TABLE 6.3. Table of Effects of Income on Physical and Emotional Outcomes

Magnitude of effect	Preschool	Elementary school	High school
Large			
Small/moderate		Stunting (5–8)[a] Fighting (12)[b]	
None	Motor and physical development (0–3)[a]	Wasting (5–8)[a] Obesity (5–8)[a] Anxiety (12)[b] Hyperactivity (12)[b]	Odds of out-of-wedlock childbearing[c]

Note. See Table 6.2. From Duncan and Brooks-Gunn (1997b). Copyright 1997 by Russell Sage Foundation Press. Reprinted by permission.
[a] Korenman and Miller (1997), data from the NLSY Mother–Child File.
[b] Pagani et al. (1997), data from the Québec Longitudinal Studies of Behavior.
[c] Haveman et al. (1997), data from the PSID, income measured between ages 6 and 18.

iness, and so forth. Income-to-needs ratios are associated with family income for 3- and 5-year-olds (Chase-Lansdale et al., 1997; J. R. Smith et al., 1997). The effect sizes are small to moderate (between .15 and .18 of a standard deviation).

Elementary School Years

With entrance of the child into school, measures of his/her well-being now include school achievement test scores, behavior problems as reported by teachers as well as parents, grade failure, and learning and attention problems. Work is currently being conducted on other domains of well-being, such as child reports of school disengagement, of self-efficacy and self-esteem, and of depressive and aggressive behavior (Cairns & Cairns, 1986; Connell, Spencer, & Aber, 1994; Harter, 1990; Nolen-Hoeksema, 1994). However, large-scale studies have often not included these other aspects of child competence, so little is known about their links with income poverty (see, as exceptions, Lipman & Offord, 1997, and Pagani et al., 1997).

School achievement scores are linked with low family income. For example, the PIAT (Peabody Individual Achievement Test) was given to all children aged 5 or older in NLSY-CS. Large income-to-needs effects were found for math and reading scores of children aged 5–6 years of age and 7–8 years of age (J. R. Smith et al., 1997).[6] School reports of behavior problems by teachers also are linked to family income (Klebanov, Brooks-Gunn, & McCormick, 1994). Effect sizes for school behavior problems are smaller than those for school achievement, paralleling the differences between intellectual ability and behavior problems found in the young childhood years.

High School Years

Many studies have examined income effects for teenage child bearing in girls and for high school dropout or completion in boys and girls (Brooks-Gunn, Guo, & Furstenberg, 1993; Graham, Beller, & Hernandez, 1994; Haveman & Wolfe, 1995; Haveman, Wolfe, & Spaulding, 1991). At our 1995 NICHD conference, small-to-moderate income-to-needs effects and effects of completed schooling were found in four data sets (Axinn, Duncan, & Thornton, 1997; Haveman, Wolf, & Wilson, 1997; Hauser & Sweeney, 1997; E. Peters & Mullis, 1997). The only exception was the study by Teachman, Paasch, Day, & Carver (1997), which did not find income effects on schooling outcomes. Interestingly, the effects sizes for school completion are somewhat smaller than what is seen for achievement scores in childhood years (Baydar et al., 1993; Duncan & Brooks-Gunn, 1997b).

Summary

Taken as a whole, the results suggest that family income has at times large but rather selective effects on children's attainments. Most noteworthy is the importance of the *type* of outcome being considered. Family income has large effects on some of the children's ability and achievement measures but large effects on *none* of the behavior, mental health, or physical health measures represented by the dozen developmental studies. Specifically, roughly half the measures of ability and achievement listed in Table 6.2 had "large" associations with family income; in contrast, none of the measures of behavior, mental health, and physical health listed in Table 6.3 have what we have deemed as large effects. Emotional and behavioral well-being may be linked to family income. The lack of findings, however, may be due to issues of measure reliability.

A second noteworthy point from the tables is the importance of the childhood stage in which income is measured. Family economic conditions in early and middle childhood appear to be far more linked to school outcomes than are economic conditions during adolescence. In fact, *none* of the achievement studies with exclusively adolescence-based income measurement during early childhood found large income effects. Left unanswered in these and all other analyses is the importance for adolescent outcomes of family economic conditions in the earliest stages of childhood.

ARE GRADIENT EFFECTS SIMILAR ACROSS THE INCOME DISTRIBUTION?

Even if income gradient effects are demonstrated, we still do not know if the effects are similar across the income distribution. That is, any effects seen in our analyses to date might be due to the effects being concentrated in the low-income part of the distribution, such that large differences are found between the poor and the near poor, for example. Alternatively, the effects might be due to differences between low-income and middle-income families, such that comparisons between the poor and the nonpoor yield the largest effect sizes. In the adult literature on health outcomes, differences between the poor and the near poor have been demonstrated (Haan, Kaplan, & Syme, 1989). At the same time, gradations among individuals higher on the income distribution also exist (Marmot et al., 1984, 1991; also Chapters 2–5, this volume).

Are similar results found for child and adolescent outcomes? Three sets of findings are relevant—the first having to do with comparisons among poor, near-poor, middle-income, and affluent families; the second having to do with comparisons among families in deep poverty, just under the poverty threshold, just above the poverty threshold, and just under two times the poverty threshold; and the third having to do with comparisons of income effects on lower and higher income groups:

1. Our samples are divided into four family income groups—those below the poverty threshold (i.e., income-to-needs ratios below 1.0), those with income-to-needs ratios between 1.0 and 2.0, those with income-to-needs ratios between 2.0 and 3.0, and those with income-to-needs ratios above 3.0. The omitted category for these analyses is those with income-to-needs ratios between 1.0 and 2.0 (see J. R. Smith et al., 1997, for data using the IHDP and the NLSY–CS samples). Control variables include maternal education, age, ethnicity, and marital status, as well as child gender and birth weight. Income effects are found across the income categories for IQ and for math achievement. The effects are less striking for behavior problems, with significant differences only being seen between the poor and the near poor (Brooks-Gunn, Klebanov, Liaw, & Duncan, 1995).

2. We have divided the income categories more finely in order to explore the potential effects of deep poverty (i.e., income-to-needs ratios of less than one-half of the poverty threshold), as well as the effects of being very close to the poverty threshold (i.e., 1.0–1.5 of the threshold). Findings are presented for children aged 5–6 from the IHDP and Children aged 5 to 9 from the NLSY–CS (Figure 6.2 presents age 5 IQ data from the IHDP; and Figure 6.3 presents math achievement data from the NLSY–CS for three age groups: 5- to 6-year-olds, 7- to 8-year-olds, and 9- to 10-year-olds). It is clear that children in deep poverty (50% or less of the poverty threshold) fare less well than do those children near the poverty threshold (J. R. Smith et al., 1997). Furthermore, children just above the poverty threshold are doing better than children just below it (when we control for other family characteristics—maternal age, marital status, education, and ethnicity). The slopes are quite similar for math achievement and IQ. However the slopes are a bit steeper for the 9- to 10-year-olds than for the 5- to 6-year-olds on the PIAT mathematics test.

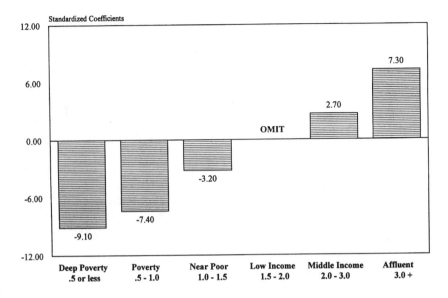

FIGURE 6.2. Income-to-needs ratios and child cognitive ability: Deep poverty and IQ scores, age 5 IHDP data set.

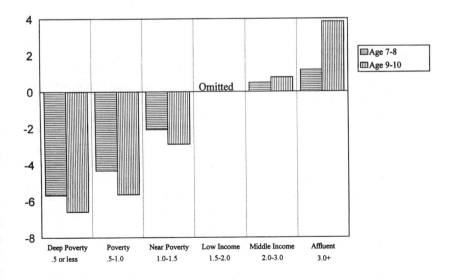

FIGURE 6.3. Income-to-needs and child cognitive ability: Deep poverty and math ability (PIAT—Math), NLSY–CS data set.

3. We have recently examined the income-to-needs effects upon high school completion using the PSID (Duncan et al., 1998). A little more than 1,300 youth born between 1967 and 1973 and seen yearly between birth and age 20 were included in these analyses. Yearly family income data were available from birth through age 15. Overall, U.S.$10,000 increments in family income were associated with a 34% increase in the probability of completing high school (with family income per year averaged across the 15-year period; Duncan et al., 1998). However, the income effect was also estimated for those individuals in the bottom half of the income distribution (the low-income group) and those in the top half of the income distribution (the high-income group). A U.S.$10,000 increment in family income was associated with a sixfold increase in high school completion for those children in the low-income group but only a 16% increase in high school completion for children with family incomes above U.S.$20,000.

DOES INCOME ACCOUNT FOR SES GRADIENTS IN CHILD OUTCOMES?

Earlier in this chapter, we acknowledged the fact that income is highly correlated with parental education and occupation as well as with family structure. Consequently, before we can say with certainty that SES gradients exist for child outcomes, links with other family characteristics must be examined. In the studies just reviewed, maternal education, age at birth of the child, ethnicity, and marital status were entered as covariates. Therefore, the estimated effects of income just presented in our brief review for the most part cannot be attributed to these characteristics.

However, it is important to consider the size of the associations between child outcomes and family characteristics other than income. After all, the research on SES gradients in adult health often includes education as part of the SES definition. In order to illustrate the associations between family characteristics other than family income and child outcomes, Tables 6.4 and 6.5 present a summary of regressions conducted using the IHDP and the NLSY–CS data. Child IQ and behavior problem scores at age 5 are the outcomes from the IHDP, and child math achievement and behavior problem scores at ages 5–6 are the outcomes from the NLSY–CS (see Brooks-Gunn, Klebanov, et al., 1993; Duncan et al., 1994; J. R. Smith et al., 1997). The unstandardized regression coefficients as well as the standardized coefficients and the standard error are presented for the following predictors: age of mother at birth of child (teenage vs. older); maternal education (three categories—less than high school, high school graduate, or some college); ethnicity (black vs. white); and single-parent household. Gender and birth weight are also entered (the coefficients are not presented here; complete results are available from the authors).

Three sets of regressions are presented (1) in the first, the income-to-

TABLE 6.4. Family Characteristics of Predictors of Behavior Problems and Math Achievement at Ages 5–6 and Ages 7–8: NLSY-CS

	Behavior problems[a]						Math achievement[b]					
	Ages 5 to 6			Ages 7 to 8			Ages 5 to 6			Ages 7 to 8		
	Model 1	Model 2	Model 3	Model 1	Model 2	Model 3	Model 1	Model 2	Model 3	Model 1	Model 2	Model 3
Family income-to-needs ratio	-.91*** (.09) [-.19]		-.69*** (.12) [-.14]	-1.07*** (.13) [-.18]		-.94*** (.16) [-.16]	2.95*** (.19) [.28]		1.41*** (.24) [.13]	3.08*** (.20) [.29]		1.65*** (.25) [.16]
Maternal education		-.45*** (.06) [-.14]	-.28*** (.07) [-.09]		-.45*** (.08) [-.13]	-.25** (.09) [-.07]		1.60*** (.13) [.23]	1.25*** (.14) [.18]		1.38*** (.12) [.22]	1.02*** (.13) [.16]
Teenage mother		-.20 (.38) [-.01]	-.32 (.37) [-.02]		-.34 (.45) [-.13]	-.46 (.45) [-.02]		-.11 (.79) [.00]	.12 (.79) [.00]		.60 (.58) [.02]	.95+ (.58) [.03]
Female head, some of the time		1.09*** (.31) [.08]	.54+ (.33) [.04]		1.07** (.39) [.07]	.40 (.41) [.03]		-.94 (.62) [-.03]	.14 (.65) [.00]		-.63 (.57) [-.02]	.36 (.59) [.01]
Female head, all of the time		.69* (.26) [.05]	.49+ (.26) [.04]		1.51*** (.43) [.08]	1.18** (.43) [.06]		.30 (.54) [.01]	.70 (.54) [.02]		-.96 (.64) [-.03]	-.43 (.64) [-.01]
Ethnicity, black		-.05 (.29) [-.00]	-.43 (.29) [-.03]		-.24 (.35) [-.02]	-.70+ (.36) [-.05]		-6.05*** (.56) [-.22]	-5.24*** (.57) [-.19]		-6.01*** (.51) [-.25]	-5.08*** (.53) [-.21]
Adj. R²	.04	.04	.05	.04	.03	.05	.08	.12	.13	.09	.13	.14

Note. Results from multiple linear regressions representing unstandardized coefficients, standard errors in parentheses, and standardized betas in brackets. All regressions control for gender of child and birth weight (1 = low birth weight, less than 2,500 grams). Family income-to-needs ratio averaged across first 3 years. Maternal education: three categories—less than high school, high school graduate, some college. Age of mother at birth of child: teenage = 1. Female headship: omitted category "female head none of the time." Ethnicity: black = 1. N = 2,845 for ages 5–6, math achievement (1,131 blacks, 1,714 whites); N = 2,474 for ages 7–8, math achievement (1,054 blacks, 1,420 whites); N = 2,742 for ages 5–6, behavior problems (934 blacks, 1,808 whites); N = 2,038 for ages 7–8, behavior problems (852 blacks, 1,186 whites).

[a]Higher scores = more behavior problems.
[b]Higher scores = higher math achievement test scores.

TABLE 6.5. Family Characteristics of Predictors of Externalizing Behavior Problems and Intelligence Test Scores at Age 5: The IHDP

	Externalizing behavior problems			Full-scale IQ score		
	Model 1	Model 2	Model 3	Model 1	Model 2	Model 3
Family income-to-needs ratio (ages 1–3)	−1.04*** (.28) [−.20]		−.67+ (.37) [−.13]	5.85*** (.49) [.58]		3.44*** (.60) [.34]
Maternal education at birth (years)		−.73*** (.22) [−.19]	−.53* (.25) [−.14]		2.93*** (.38) [.39]	1.92*** (.40) [.26]
Teenage mother		−.21 (1.27) [−.01]	−.08 (1.27) [−.00]		3.27 (2.15) [.07]	2.60 (2.06) [.06]
Female head, some of the time (ages 2–3)		.96 (1.35) [.04]	.55 (1.37) [.02]		−.88 (2.28) [−.02]	1.21 (2.21) [.02]
Female head, all of the time (ages 2–3)		.71 (1.13) [.04]	.28 (1.16) [.01]		−1.12 (1.92) [−.03]	1.08 (1.87) [.03]
Ethnicity, black		.33 (1.16) [.02]	−.43 (1.23) [−.02]		−14.15*** (1.96) [−.39]	−10.23*** (1.99) [−.28]
Adj. R^2	.11	.10	.11	.38	.40	.45

Note. Results from multiple linear regressions representing unstandardized coefficients, standard errors in parentheses, and standardized betas in brackets. All regressions control for gender of child and birth weight (grams), neonatal health, and site. Female headship: omitted category "female head none of the time." Only follow-up group, blacks and whites, and infants with birth weight greater than 1,000 grams were included in the analyses. N limited to geocoded only subjects. N = 348 for IQ (210 blacks, 138 whites); N = 377 for behavior problems (221 blacks, 156 whites).

needs ratio is entered alone (column 1); (2) in the second, the family characteristics are entered without the income-to-needs ratio being entered (column 2); (3) in the third, the income-to-needs ratio and the family characteristics are both entered (column 3). Of particular importance for SES gradients is the fact that income effects on child outcomes do not disappear when maternal education, age, and family headship are included as controls.

Interestingly, maternal education is associated with all of the child outcomes considered, even after the income-to-needs ratio is entered into the equation. We interpret these findings to mean that maternal education and family income have independent and significant effects on child outcomes. Therefore, if we had included both in one measure of the SES gradient, the gradients would be steeper than they are for either separately.

Residing in a female-headed household is significant when the income-to-needs ratio is omitted from the equation for behavior problem outcomes. However, it becomes insignificant or is reduced after income is entered. Similar findings are reported by Pagani et al. (1997) for aggression over the elementary and middle school years in the Québec Longitudinal Studies of Behavior. Others (e.g., Conger et al., 1997; T. L. Hanson, McLanahan, & Thomson, 1997; Lipman & Offord, 1997; McLanahan & Sandefur, 1994; Pagani et al., 1997) report that family structure (specifically, residing in a female-headed household) is associated with lower emotional health and adjustment in teenagers, over and above family income variables.

Effect sizes are in the range of .10 to .20 in these studies. These effects are due in part to divorce and family disruption, not just to single parenthood per se (Hetherington & Clingempeel, 1992; Cherlin et al., 1990; McLanahan & Sandefur, 1994). For example, family structure changes such as divorce and remarriage are known to cause short-term perturbations in relationships among all family members. Children and adults have to renegotiate roles and relationships, one result of which is often an increase in behavior problems (Hetherington, 1993). In our analyses of the IHDP and NLSY–CS data sets, a change from a two-parent to a one-parent structure was more strongly associated with children's behavior problems than living in a one-parent family in the preschool years (Duncan et al., 1994; J. R. Smith et al., 1997).

However, the question still remains as to whether or not we have controlled for every family characteristic that might account for family income effects. We have only included a relatively small set of potential covariates in our regressions (even though those selected are clearly relevant to child outcome). Low-income families may still differ from middle-income families in as yet unknown ways. If so, then the income effects really might be due to other, unmeasured differences (commonly referred to as selection effects due to "as yet unknown" omitted variables). Several approaches to estimating selection bias for income effects on child outcomes are considered here.

One approach has examined income effects based on the different components of income. Income has been differentiated based on the degree of influence of parental behavior. For instance, welfare use and earnings are more influenced by parental behavior than are asset income or net worth. According to Mayer (1997a, 1997b), welfare use and earnings are more strongly associated with child outcomes and more likely to be influenced by unmeasured characteristics of family than is asset income. However, since low-income families do not have many assets, this test tells us little about unmeasured bias in poor and near-poor families.

Yet another line of research estimating effects of income has looked at siblings within families. Besides the fact that siblings being reared in the same family share many of the same unmeasured characteristics, this method enables us to compare children at the same age within families while allowing us to look at the income of the family at different time points (e.g., if a firstborn was 5 years old in 1985 and the second child was 5 years old in 1988, we can look at their achievement levels at this age and the family income in 1985 and in 1988). In our work estimating income effects on completed schooling, we used this method with 328 sibling pairs from the 1,323 children from the PSID (Duncan et al., 1998). The income coefficient was very similar to that for the individual-based model. Our interpretation is that income effects are seen when controlling for unmeasured family characteristics.

Finally, the most convincing demonstration of income effects is witnessing a change in child outcomes as a result of providing low-income families with cash. The Income Maintenance Studies of 25 years ago provided partial support for the premise that income matters (Salkind & Haskins, 1982). Currently, another such demonstration is underway in two provinces in Canada. In this demonstration mothers receiving public assistance have their incomes supplemented if they enter the workforce (a comparison group does not get the income supplement). Thus far, preliminary results suggest that the supplement is associated with greater entry and stability in the workforce; however, child and family outcome data are not as yet available.

DOES THE TIMING OF LOW INCOME INFLUENCE CHILD OUTCOMES?

Our brief review suggests that the income gradient is operating throughout the first two decades of life (Duncan & Brooks-Gunn, 1997b). However, the effects of income are very strong during the preschool and childhood years; the size of these effects is illustrated in the data presented for cognitive and school achievement outcomes in this chapter. Relatively large effect sizes are also reported for physical health outcomes (see Tables 6.2 and 6.3, above; J. E. Miller & Korenman, 1994; Korenman & Miller, 1997). Interestingly, more modest income associations (effect sizes ranging from small to medium) are reported in the adolescent literature, which has focused on out-of-wedlock teenage childbearing, high school completion, and completed years of schooling (Brooks-Gunn & Duncan, 1997; Haveman & Wolfe, 1995; Haveman et al., 1991). It is not known why these differences exist.

One possible explanation is that the variability in effect sizes is because the childhood and adolescent outcomes are not the same; that is, if we had measures of math and reading achievement for the teenage samples paralleling those for the childhood samples, then comparable effect sizes would be seen. We eagerly await the "aging" of the NLSY–CS cohorts in the United States to test this hypothesis (Chase-Lansdale et al., 1991). The National Longitudinal Study of Children and Youth (NLSCY) cohort in Canada is also available (Statistics Canada, 1996).

Another possibility is that the timing of low income is critical. So, for example, the coefficients for family income–developmental outcome links are smaller for high school completion than for earlier school achievement measures because the adolescent-based studies, in general, have not included measures of family income during the early childhood years. And perhaps income in these years is influencing later schooling outcomes. In support of this premise, a longitudinal study of more than 300 children of young black urban mothers in Baltimore reports that welfare receipt in the preschool years is more highly associated with adolescent outcomes (literacy, high school completion, and school failure) than is family welfare receipt in the childhood or early adolescent years (Baydar et al., 1993; Brooks-Gunn, Guo, & Furstenberg, 1993; Furstenberg et al., 1987).

More direct evidence showing the importance of early childhood income comes from Axinn et al.'s (1997) study of completed schooling. Using a PSID-based sample of children observed between birth and at least age 20, we found much more powerful effects of income between birth and age 5 than at other points in childhood. For example, when we controlled for family size, mother's education, her age at the birth of the child, and other demographic characteristics, having an average income above U.S.$10,000 between birth and age 5 as opposed to an average income of less than U.S.$10,000 was associated with .14 more years of schooling. Comparable income differences in middle childhood (age 6–10) or early adolescence (age 11–15) produced much smaller and statistically insignificant effects.

Our current thinking about these timing effects has to do with the importance of school readiness in determining the course of schooling for children. Income poverty is highly associated with preschool readiness and verbal scores. And the level of school readiness sets the stage for children's transition into the formal school system. Children who have not learned skills such as color naming, sorting, counting, letters, and the names of everyday objects are at a disadvantage compared to children who have mastered these skills (see, e.g., Case, Griffin, & Kelly, Chapter 7, this volume). Schools tend to classify children very early, such that language arts groups are often formed in kindergarten or first grade. And teachers tend to identify children as having potential school problems in the first years of school as well, with these ratings being as predictive as readiness test scores in the early elementary school years (Alexander & Entwisle, 1988; Alexander, Entwisle, & Horsey, 1997). Skills such as the inability to inhibit behavior may be associated with teachers' ratings of readiness as well as difficulties in letter recognition and verbal ability (Lee, Brooks-Gunn, & Shnur, 1988). Low readiness test scores are associated with grade failure, school disengagement, and school dropout (Barnett, 1995; Brooks-Gunn, Guo, & Furstenberg, 1993; Guo et al., 1996; S. L. Ramey & C. T. Ramey, 1994; Schweinhart & Weikart, 1997).[7]

WHAT ARE THE PATHWAYS
THROUGH WHICH SES GRADIENTS OPERATE?

How does income (or how do SES indicators more generally) influence children's outcomes? As indicated in the introductory remarks to this chapter, the literature on the existence of SES gradients on adults and child outcomes far outstrips current knowledge about the ways in which SES gradients actually work. Adler and her colleagues (1994) outlined four major classes of pathways: physical environment, social environment, socialization and life experiences, and health behavior. We have considered two major types of pathways for children—family-based and community-based pathways (Brooks-Gunn & Duncan, 1997; see also Table 6.6). Under each, physical environment, social environment, socialization factors, and health behavior factors are included. Health behaviors such as access to and use of appropriate health care (both preventative and acute) are typically controlled by parents, at least until the high school years. Examples from our work will be presented for two family-based pathways and for one neighborhood-based pathway.

Family Mediators of Income Effects in the Childhood Years

During the childhood years, we know the most about potential pathways that involve the family. Perhaps the most well-developed literature is that which focuses on parent–child interactions and parental mood. Another set of studies has targeted learning experiences in the home as a major path-

---

TABLE 6.6. Pathways through Which Poverty Operates

Family

Nutrition and health behavior
Provision of learning experiences
Parental interactions with children
Parental emotional and physical health
Use of health care services
Choice of schools and child care
Household stability

Community and neighborhood

Exposure to violence in safety of neighborhoods
Environmental toxins
Neighborhood spirit and connectedness
Peer groups
School characteristics
Existence of parks, playgrounds, libraries, community center,
    organized child-oriented activities
Access to health care

---

way through which income influences preschool and elementary school children. For example, addition of the HOME scale (a commonly used measure of the home environment; R. H. Bradley, Caldwell, & Rock, 1988; R. H. Bradley, 1995) into a regression reduces the effect of income upon children's achievement and the ability scores by more than one-half (Klebanov, Brooks-Gunn, Chase-Lansdale, & Gordon, 1997; J. R. Smith et al., 1997). We do not know if these effects (seen over age groups and over data sets in the childhood years) are due to the purchase of materials (e.g., educational toys, computers, books, concerts) or to the use of such materials. The HOME scale does not allow for a differentiation of these possibilities (i.e., it is difficult, in a 2-hour home visit to observe a mother's use of materials). The effects are accounted for by activities in the home, not outside the home (Klebanov et al., 1998). However, studies of maternal interactions, especially reading and literacy activities, reveal high correlations between maternal language use and child outcomes (Brooks-Gunn, Denner, & Klebanov, 1995). A few studies have included observational measures of maternal interaction as well as the HOME scale; in these studies, maternal interaction and provision of learning experiences as measured on the HOME are associated with young children's developmental outcomes (Berlin, Brooks-Gunn, Spiker, & Zaslow, 1995). Studies have not compared the ability of parental interactions and provision of learning experiences to mediate income effects, however.

Often income loss, through unemployment, underemployment, and unstable work conditions, rather than poverty per se, is the focus of the family mediators literature. This work is exemplified by the Family Stress Model, as developed by Conger and his colleagues (1992, 1993, 1997) and McLoyd (1990). According to their model, income loss and uncertainty influence parenting behavior and parent–child interactions through parental depressed and/or irritable moods associated with marital and family conflict, which in turn is caused by family economic pressure. Conger and colleagues have suggested that parent–child interaction (especially conflictual interactions) are the proximal cause of child and youth emotional problems and school disengagement. Several studies, including the study of children of the Great Depression and children of the farm recession in the Midwest during the 1980s, have yielded confirmatory findings. However, it is unclear whether similar processes operate in single-parent families where child outcomes and parenting behavior may be influenced either by low income or by the effects of conflict other than marital conflict (e.g., conflict in single-parent households or in multigenerational households). McLoyd (1990; also McLoyd, Jayaratne, Ceballo, & Borquez, 1994) has reported complementary work on single-parent families, focusing more on low income than on income loss (see also, Jackson, Brooks-Gunn, Huang, & Glassman, in press). However, her models postulate parent–child interaction as just one of a number of pathways through which poverty might influence children. It is difficult to compare findings across these studies, as family structure and family race are confounded (the work of Elder, 1979, and Conger et al., 1992, 1993, 1997, has focused on white families; the work of McLoyd et al., 1994 on black families; and Jackson et al., in press, on primarily single parents). Consequently, little is known about the similarity in the processes operating in different groups of families (Brooks-Gunn & Duncan, 1997).

Our research on preschool children is combining elements of the Family Stress Model and the Learning Experiences Model. Two sets of outcomes are examined: behavior problems and cognitive functioning at age 3. Using the IHDP data set, we have examined links between low income and three sets of potential mediators: maternal depression, provision of learning experiences in the home, and maternal parenting behavior (in this case, harsh, punitive behavior and responsive, sensitive behavior). Following McLoyd, our expectation was that low-income effects on child outcomes would in part be mediated by maternal emotional health and interaction with the child, both of which could have direct effects on child outcomes. Additionally, in line with Conger's work on adolescents, we explored whether or not the mother's emotional health operated upon child outcomes through her interaction with the child. Figure 6.4 presents a schematic of our results for IQ scores when the children were 3 years of age (Linver, Brooks-Gunn, & Kohen, 1999). Parenting behavior—specifically provision of learning experiences and absence of harsh, punitive interactions—was highly associated with IQ. Additionally, about one-half of the family income effects was mediated through parenting behavior. The pathways are somewhat different for child behavior problems. Mothers with poorer emotional health rated their children as having more behavior problems. However, low income was not associated with low scores on emotional health. Parenting interactions and provision of learning experiences were associated with children's behavior problems, but not as strongly as these parenting measures were for children's IQ scores (Figure 6.5).

Neighborhood Mediators of Income Effects during Childhood

The influence of neighborhood contexts on individuals has been cogently argued and demonstrated by several researchers. Concentration of poverty, female-headed families, absence of the middle class, and joblessness have often been cited as factors influencing child and adolescent development (Crane, 1991; Hogan & Kitigawa, 1985; Wilson, 1991). Several key economic and demographic indices have been used to define neighborhoods. In keeping with the underlying theme of this chapter, we are characterizing neighborhoods based on the extent of neighborhood poverty or income gradients (i.e., percentage of nonelderly poor neighbors). Neighborhoods with poverty rates of 30–40% or more have been termed high-poverty concentration neighborhoods (Jargowsky & Bane, 1991; Wilson, 1991, 1996). Poor neighborhoods are often characterized by high crime and overcrowd-

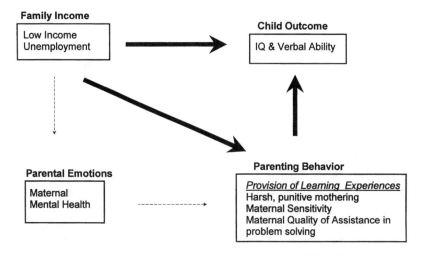

FIGURE 6.4. Theoretical model predicting verbal ability during preschool years.

ing, as well as higher levels of male joblessness, public assistance use, and female-headed families (Ricketts & Sawhill, 1988). Neighborhood-level geocoded data from the PSID show that approximately 17% of all children lived in very poor neighborhoods (i.e., poverty rates in excess of 30%), 16% of the children lived in neighborhoods with few (i.e., less than 10%) poor neighbors, approximately 33% of the children lived in neighborhoods

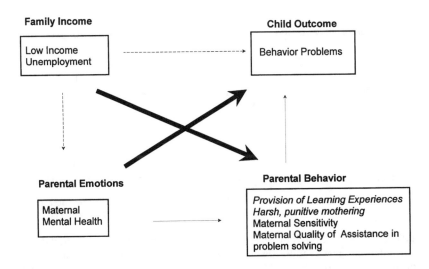

FIGURE 6.5. Theoretical model predicting behavior problems during preschool years.

with 10–20% poor neighbors, and approximately 27% of the children lived in neighborhoods with 20–30% poor neighbors (Duncan et al., 1994). Thus, based on the PSID sample estimates, nearly 1 child in 10 lives in a very poor neighborhood and another 2 children in 10 live in a moderately poor neighborhood.

Neighborhoods may influence the lives and development of children both directly (e.g., organization of the neighborhood) and indirectly (i.e., through the family). In our research we have looked at the indirect effects of neighborhoods being mediated through the family both for the IHDP and the NLSY–CS. Within the IHDP, an examination of neighborhood effects on the family indicated that living in poor neighborhoods and residing in ethnically diverse neighborhoods were each associated with poorer physical home environments and less cognitive stimulating homes (as measured by the HOME scale). For the NLSY–CS data set comparable findings were not obtained. However, male joblessness in the neighborhood was associated with lower cognitive stimulation HOME scores for preschool-aged children (3- to 4-year-olds). For school-aged children presence of high SES neighbors was associated with better home environments (Klebanov, Brooks-Gunn, & Duncan, 1994; Klebanov et al., 1997, 1998).

We have also looked at whether or not neighborhood effects on child outcomes are mediated by family level characteristics (see Figure 6.6). Within the IHDP, the mediating effect of the family was associated with the economic and social composition of the neighborhood. For instance, the learning environment in the home did not mediate the association between affluent neighbors and children's' intelligence test scores. However, residing in an ethnically diverse neighborhood was associated with worse learn-

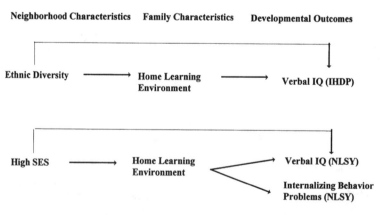

FIGURE 6.6. Two models of neighborhood and family influences on child development outcomes ages 5 and 6. From Klebanov, Brooks-Gunn, Chase-Lansdale, and Gordon (1997). Copyright 1997 by Russell Sage Foundation Press. Reprinted by permission.

ing environments in the home, which in turn was associated with children's' lowered verbal ability. For the NLSY–CS, the quality of the home environment mediated the association between high SES neighborhoods and better reading scores and verbal ability. The home environment also mediated the association between residing in a high SES neighborhood and more internalizing behavior problems (Klebanov et al., 1997; Leventhel & Brooks-Gunn, in press).

CONCLUSION

While our interest is in SES gradients more generally, this chapter has focused on the consequences of low income. Income, though important, is not the only determinant of children's developmental health. Additionally, income is only one component of SES. However, it is the component that determines the parental ability to provide basic needs to children (food, shelter, clothing, the ability to purchase goods necessary for parents to work). In the United States, qualification for programs to help families provide these basic needs is based on the income-to-needs ratio, based in turn on the poverty threshold. Nutrition programs include food stamps, Women, Infants, and Children (WIC, a food supplement program for pregnant women and young children), and school lunch subsidies. Shelter programs include public housing, Section 8 vouchers (which provide vouchers for renting private housing), and heating subsidies. Welfare payments (Aid for Dependent Children, Social Security Insurance) are actual income transfers for children's basic needs, unlike the programs mentioned earlier. Other programs target health and schooling, which also may be considered necessities. Some of the programs are also means tested, including Medicaid and child care vouchers. Our point is that low family income is recognized as the major barrier to ensuring that children's basic needs are met (Currie, 1997).

Our data demonstrate the existence of income gradients during childhood. These gradients are seen in the earliest years of life—starting with low birth weight (and other complications at birth), including physical growth and exposure to lead and other toxins in the first few years of life), and moving to cognitive ability by the end of the toddler stage of development (Brooks-Gunn & Duncan, 1997). The gradients do not seem to be reduced by the advent of school. We suspect that schools tend to reinforce existing disparities in children's outcomes rather than reducing them, although some recent data suggest that the primary reason for continuing disparities has to do with stimulating experiences in the home rather than school (Gamoran, Mane, & Bethke, 1998). And the gradients continue through the adolescent years. Interestingly, the gradients are much more pronounced for school achievement and growth than for behavior problems.

The gradients exist along the entire income distribution, not just at the high or low ends. Children in deep poverty fare more poorly than children just at or above the poverty threshold. The federal programs in place in the United States do not raise all children out of deep poverty (defined as 50% or less of the poverty threshold). And more children in the United States than in other Western countries are in deep poverty, in part because supports to families with children are less generous in the United States than in nations such as Canada, France, Sweden, Italy, and Germany.

Comparing across chapters in this volume suggests that income gradients during childhood are steeper in the United States than in Canada or the United Kingdom. This difference is due to at least two factors. First, as we just stated, more U.S. children are in deep poverty than in the two comparison nations. Second, the income disparities between the rich and the poor and near-poor are much larger in the United States than in Canada or the United Kingdom. Unless policies address these inequities (via more generous transfer payments, change in tax policies such as Earned Income Tax Credit, or change in minimum wages), it is likely that the SES gradient will remain steeper for U.S. children than for Canadian or British children, with the consequent risks for the developmental health of the American population that we have identified.

ACKNOWLEDGMENTS

The research reported in this chapter was supported by the National Institute of Child Health and Human Development (NICHD) Research Network on Child and Family Well-Being and the MacArthur Foundation Network on Family and Work. In addition, analyses of the Infant Health and Development Program (IHDP) data set were funded by grants from the March of Dimes Foundation, the Bureau of Maternal and Child Health and the Russell Sage Foundation. We also wish to thank the Robert Wood Johnson Foundation, NICHD, and the Pew Charitable Trusts for their support of the IHDP. The participating universities and site directors were Patrick H. Casey, University of Arkansas for Medical Sciences (Little Rock, AR); Cecelia M. McCarton, Albert Einstein College of Medicine (Bronx, NY); Marie McCormick, Harvard Medical School (Boston); Charles R. Bauer, University of Miami School of Medicine (Miami); Judith Bernbaum, University of Pennsylvania School of Medicine (Philadelphia); Jon E. Tyson, and Mark Swanson, University of Texas Health Science Center at Dallas; Clifford J. Sells, and Forrest C. Bennett, University of Washington School of Medicine (Seattle); and David T. Scott, Yale University School of Medicine (New Haven, CT). The Longitudinal Study Office is directed by Cecelia McCarton and Jeanne Brooks-Gunn. The Data Coordinating Center is directed by James Tonascia and Curtis Meinert at the Johns Hopkins University, School of Hygiene and Public Health. We would like to thank Judith Smith, Pamela Klebanov, Kyunghee Lee, and Wei-Jun Yeung for their collaboration on the studies reported here. We are also thankful for the ongoing discussions about SES gradients across countries with our colleagues in the Canadian Institute for Advanced Research; special thanks go to Clyde Hertzman, Daniel P. Keating, J. Douglas Wilms, Robbie Case, and Richard E. Tremblay. Portions of this chapter also appear in Brooks-Gunn and Duncan (1997). Copyright 1997 by *The Future of Children*. Reprinted by permission.

NOTES

1. The developmental literature generally has not included measures of family income; when such data have been collected, they often are not gathered yearly, making it difficult to calculate stable estimates of the effects of family income or family size or adjusted family income. Three or more years of family income data are needed for such estimates because yearly incomes fluctuate widely (Duncan, 1988; Duncan et al., 1994). Therefore, much of our knowledge about SES gradients comes from studies using maternal educational status (and sometimes paternal education status). Occupational status also has been used in some studies (Brooks-Gunn, Phelps, & Elder, 1991; Hauser, Sewell, & Warren, 1994; A. E. Gottfried, Gottfried, & Bathurst, 1995). The data presented in this chapter are representative of those studies that have maternal education as well as family income data, the latter collected for at least 3 years (see analyses in Duncan & Brooks-Gunn, 1997b).

2. Several investigative teams have been using the term "allostatic load" to denote the ways in which such environmental conditions, health behaviors, and experiences might translate into physiological stress (McEwen & Stellar, 1993; Seeman & McEwen, 1996). Allostatic load has been described as the "cumulative strain on the body produced by repeated ups and downs of the physiologic response, as well as by the elevated activity of physiologic systems under challenge" (McEwen & Stellar, 1993, p. 2094). The physical environment, social environment, socialization experiences, and health behaviors all contribute to allostatic load (Adler et al., 1994). See also Chapters 2, 3, and 10 in this volume.

3. Other countries have employed a relative rather than an absolute poverty threshold. For example, in Canada, the poverty threshold is sometimes estimated on a percentage of the median income of all Canadian households. Consequently, the poverty threshold changes (in real dollars) as the median income of the nation's households is altered. Recently, the National Academy of Sciences has proposed altering the way that the U.S. poverty threshold is calculated to take into account expenditures on basic necessities, based on a percentage of the median income (Citro & Michael, 1995). Others have looked at poverty rates using relative measures (see, e.g., the excellent work by Hernandez, 1993, 1997).

4. Sometimes more fine-grained distinctions are made; for example, families living in deep poverty (50% or less than the poverty line) may be compared to families who live closer to the poverty threshold (between 50 and 100%). Likewise, comparisons are often made between families who are below the poverty threshold and those who are just above it (often called the near poor, defined as either between 100 and 150% of the poverty line or between 100 and 200% of the line; Duncan & Brooks-Gunn, 1997a; J. R. Smith et al., 1997).

5. Teenage parenthood is sometimes considered an emotional or physical health outcome. Additionally, it could be included in a separate domain entitled fertility. Since we are looking at the first two decades of life in this chapter, a separate domain of fertility is not included (Brooks-Gunn & Duncan, 1997).

6. However the size of this effect is reduced by about half when a measure of maternal cognitive ability is added to the equation for the NLSY–CS sample (Phillips et al., 1998).

7. The same may not be true for behavior problems. The correlations between preschool behavior problems and elementary school behavior problems are not as strong as those found for achievement and verbal ability scores over the same time period (J. Stevenson, Richman, & Graham, 1985). Additionally, behavior problems seem to be more strongly associated with family events such as residential moves and marital and partner changes of parent, over and above family income, than are school achievement measures (McLanahan, 1997; McLanahan & Sandefur, 1994).

7

Socioeconomic Gradients in Mathematical Ability and Their Responsiveness to Intervention during Early Childhood

Robbie Case
Sharon Griffin
Wendy M. Kelly

As was demonstrated in the three previous chapters socioeconomic gradients in health, education, and social well-being are ubiquitous. No matter what country one looks at, no matter what aspect of well-being one selects, and no matter what form of measure one uses, one finds that groups with higher socioeconomic status (SES) have an advantage over their lower-SES peers. They arrive at school better prepared for the sort of learning that is required there, both cognitively and affectively (Griffin & Case, 1996; see also Chapters 4 and 6, this volume). They exhibit better social adjustment, attain higher test scores, and maintain better health throughout the school years (Chapters 4 and 5, this volume). After school is over they carry these early advantages into their adult lives, showing superior achievement, higher income, better social adjustment, and greater resistance to disease at all ages (Chapter 3, this volume). Finally, even if one controls for SES in adulthood, one finds that children whose childhood was spent in high-SES homes do better in retirement, showing fewer degenerative ailments and living to an older age (Chapter 3, this volume).

Although effects such as these are present in all countries, their magnitude varies considerably from one country to the next. Moreover, within any country, the size of these effects varies considerably from one region to the next. Regions with steep gradients in income and low levels of social cohesion tend also to show the following: (1) the steepest gradients and lowest means in regard to infant mortality, early childhood disease, and readiness for learning; (2) the steepest gradients and lowest means in educational achievement; (3) the steepest gradients and lowest means in measures of adult health and well being; and (4) the steepest gradients and lowest means in longevity (see Chapters 3 and 5, this volume; also Fuchs & Reklis, 1997; Kaplan et al., 1986; Kawachi, Kennedy, Lochner, & Prothrow-Stith, 1996).

The question that we now need to address is one of mechanism. How are these SES gradients produced in the first place, and how are they sustained? In Chapters 8 and 9 of this volume, a link is established between the early experience to which an organism is exposed and its subsequent neurological and behavioral functioning. As Cynader and Frost (Chapter 8) point out, the capability for early biological "tuning" confers a great evolutionary advantage. Infants of all species are born into a wide variety of different local circumstances. If their biological hardware can be tuned to these circumstances at an early point in their lives, their likelihood of survival is increased while the amount of genetic preprogramming that is required is decreased. What makes sense in terms of evolutionary theory has also been demonstrated to hold true in experimental studies. Depending on the visual experience that a kitten is exposed to during its first few days of life, its visual cortex will develop along one of two quite different pathways. By altering the early rearing conditions that a rhesus monkey is exposed to, one can also alter the corticosteroid response to stress that it exhibits throughout its lifespan (Chapter 9). Many other examples of such early biobehavioral effects are provided in Chapters 8, 9, and 10.

THE BIOLOGICAL SUBSTRATE OF HIGHER-ORDER COGNITIVE PROCESSES IN HUMANS

If early experiential influences of the sort just discussed are demonstrable throughout the animal kingdom—and if they are particularly strong in our closest primate cousins—one might expect them to be present in human beings as well, and to be implicated in some way in the socioeconomic gradients mentioned above. In fact, many of the indices used by S. J. Suomi in his research with primates have also been used in research with young children. Although the early experiential variation that has been studied in research with young children has been naturally rather than experimentally produced, the results have been very similar (see Chapter 4, this volume). The possibility therefore exists that the different sorts of early life events to which low-SES children are exposed—and particularly the different forms of stressors and/or opportunities that they encounter—may also set them on different biobehavioral pathways.

What about higher-order cognitive functioning? Is it possible that this sort of functioning, too, might have a biological and/or neurological component to it that could be shaped by children's early experience? At first glance, this possibility might appear to be a rather remote one. Still, it is one that is worthwhile keeping in mind, particularly in view of recent research in primatology and neuropsychology. As the reader may be aware, recent research with primates has revealed that many of the higher cognitive capabilities that we exhibit as humans are also present—albeit in less developed form—in other primates. Although the work is not uncontroversial, there is considerable evidence that chimpanzees can learn an artificial sign-based language and use it in a fashion that bears a striking resemblance to the way in which children use their natural language (R. A. Gardner & B. T. Gardner, 1984). Chimpanzees can also learn to understand human language (Savage-Rumbaugh et al., 1993), and to use human tools in a sophisticated fashion (Boysen & Bernston, 1995; Gibson, 1990; Russon, 1995). In short, many of the high-level cognitive capabilities that were once presumed to be unique to humans have recently been shown to be present, albeit in a considerably less developed form, in other members of the animal kingdom. Since work with other species suggests that these same higher-order intellectual capabilities and the neurological substrate on which they depend can be affected by early experience (Diamond, Krech, & Rosenzweig, 1964; see also Chapter 9, this volume), this gives further weight to the suggestion that SES gradients might have their origin in early childhood and be maintained, at least partially, by factors that become biologically embedded.

Of course, the history of science is full of examples where hypotheses that were eminently reasonable on theoretical grounds turned out to be false when they were subjected to close empirical scrutiny. Thus, it is important to look at the evidence concerning the neurological substrate of higher cognitive functioning in humans and the extent to which this substrate can be impacted by the sort of differential early experience that different social environments offer.

The particular form of higher cognitive activity with which we have been concerned in our own research is mathematical reasoning. Although it was once thought that the ability to understand and manipulate numbers was unique to humans, recent work has shown that this ability, too, is present in our primate cousins. Although it can take several years to train them, common chimpanzees can learn to differentiate sets of different numerical magnitude and to associate each with a different numerical symbol (Boysen & Berntson, 1989, 1995). They can also learn to answer questions regarding the relative magnitude that these symbols represent (Boysen & Berntson, 1995). Finally, they can learn to solve numerically presented problems involving the addition of small numbers (Boysen & Berntson, 1995; Boysen, Berntson, Shayer, & Hannan, 1995).

Interestingly, the sort of training to which chimpanzees are responsive and the sort of strategies that they appear to use in executing these numerical tasks appear to be very similar to those observed in human children who range in age from 2½ to 3½ years. Our own work has been done with human children who are just a bit older than this (4–6 years of age). One of the most interesting capabilities that children develop during this later age range is the ability to respond to a purely verbal question about quantity ("Is 4 bigger than 5 or smaller than 5?"). Another capability that they develop at this later age is mental addition. Six-year-olds can solve simple addition problems where the answer is not obvious on perceptual grounds but must be computed via mental counting. These two tasks are of special interest not just because they appear to be just beyond the range of chimpanzees and younger children but because the cortical areas and circuits on which they depend are the most recent in evolutionary terms and undergo a period of particularly rapid development during the preschool era.

The numeral comparison task is of particular interest, since Stanislas Dehaene and his colleagues (Dehaene & Changeux, 1993; Dehaene & Cohen, 1995) have developed a neurological model to explain the cortical responses of adult humans to the simple question "Is the number on the screen bigger or smaller than 5?" In their studies, subjects are expected to press one key if the number on the screen is bigger than 5 and to press another if it is smaller. In the learning phase of this task (and most other mathematical tasks as well), a region of the brain that appears to play an important role is the frontal lobe. As the reader may be aware, one function that the lobes at the front of the brain perform is that of acting as an "executive" and orchestrating the response of the posterior lobes to novel and potentially misleading stimuli. It has also been suggested that in humans, these lobes play a role in integrating linguistic and nonlinguistic inputs, and that this is the reason these lobes are so extensively developed in *homo sapiens* (Jerison, 1997).

Once a task such as that mentioned above becomes relatively automatic, neurological processing is no longer so strongly localized in the frontal lobes. Instead, it is taken over by the posterior regions of the brain. On each trial, there is a rapid activation of the areas of the brain that are responsible for dealing with three different kinds of material. The following are the areas in question: (1) an area at the base of the occipital lobes, which is important for recognizing visual patterns such as those presented by written words or numerals and which becomes active approximately 100 milliseconds after the stimuli are presented; (2) an area in the left temporal lobe, which is known to be important for the rapid serial processing of verbal material and which becomes active during the next 50 milliseconds or so—particularly if the stimulus is a written word rather than a numeral; and (3) an area at the juncture of the right (and, to a lesser extent, the left) occipital and parietal lobes, which appears to be responsible for making judgments of relative size. This latter area reaches its maximum activation shortly after the previous two areas, and about 200 milliseconds before a response is made, and is more strongly active if the number presented is close to the target in magnitude (e.g., 5 vs. 4) than if it is distant (5 vs. 10). Finally, on trials where the subject slips up and makes an error, an area of frontal cortex lights up again about 120 milliseconds later—and a correction is made.

The top panel of Figure 7.1 illustrates these three areas and the tracts that connect them, and Dehaene's description of the processing for which they are responsible. Note once again that many of the areas indicated (especially the left temporal area) are considerably more developed in humans than in other higher primates. Note also that these areas and the connections among them are known to undergo a substantial process of development during the period in which the response in question is acquired (see Case, 1992; A. Diamond, 1991; Fischer & Rose, 1994; Thatcher, 1992; Zelazo, Carter, Reznick, & Frye, 1997). Once again, then, it seems reasonable to suggest that this system might be particularly open to experiential effects during the preschool years and that some of these effects might be long lasting ones.

EARLY SOCIOECONOMIC INFLUENCES ON HIGHER-ORDER COGNITIVE PROCESSES

Such behavioral evidence as is available appears to be broadly compatible with this suggestion. Gradients in mathematical achievement do not have

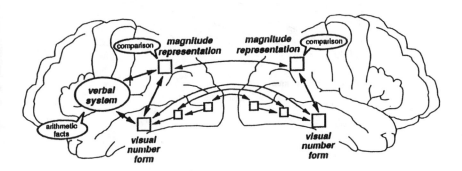

FIGURE 7.1. Dehaene's model of the neural centers and pathways that are involved in making comparisons of magnitude. The model assumes that numerals are stored in the ventral occipital lobes, which are labeled *visual number form* in the diagram. Number words are stored in the left temporal lobe, which is labeled *verbal system* in the diagram. The magnitude of each number is presumed to be represented analogically and stored in the parieto-occipital-temporal junctions, which are indicated as *magnitude representation* in the diagram.

exactly the same pattern across countries as those in reading that Willms discussed in Chapter 5 of this volume. However, they are just as ubiquitous. Figure 7.2 presents the scores received by 13-year-olds from several different countries on the Third International Mathematics Study. As may be seen, for all countries there is a linear increase in score with SES. As may also be seen, the gradient in the United States is relatively steep compared to countries such as Germany and Canada, whose general level of achievement is in the same general range.

The U.S. case is a particularly interesting one, not just because it exhibits such steep SES gradients but because such good data have been gathered on the range of social conditions that are found and the influence that they have on young children's early cognitive growth. As Brooks-Gunn and her colleagues point out in Chapter 6 of this volume, SES gradients are present in American children's cognitive performance before they ever reach the school years. Even with other factors such as mothers' IQ controlled, preschool cognitive performance is a function of (1) the income of the mother and (2) the home environment that she provides for her child. Indeed, with

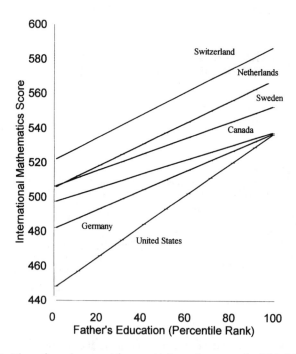

FIGURE 7.2. Plot of math scores for grade 8 students on the Third International Mathematics and Science Study. Note that the mean score for the total population tested is 500; the standard deviation is 100. Note further that father's education level has been expressed as percentile, that is, relative to others in the same country. The countries selected for comparison are the same as those discussed by Willms in Chapter 5.

these variables controlled, SES gradients in cognition are no longer apparent (Duncan et al., 1994).

The sort of abilities that Brooks-Gunn and her colleagues have studied are those that are tapped by preschool intelligence tests, such as picture–vocabulary and block design. Until recently, good measures of children's numerical abilities in this age range were not available. In recent years, however, several different teams of investigators have investigated children's mathematical abilities in this early age range. Their results converge on the following general conclusions: (1) human children are born with an innate sensitivity to number and an ability to predict the result of certain elementary perceptual transformations of a numerical nature (Starkey, 1992; Wynn, 1992); (2) socioeconomic differences in these capabilities are not evident at birth and indeed do not emerge until about 2½–3 years of age (Saxe, Guberman, & Gearhart, 1987; Starkey, 1992); and (3) beginning at about this age, socioeconomic differences begin to become apparent (Ginsburg & Russell, 1981; Starkey & Klein, 1992). In one set of studies that we conducted, for example, we found that 75% of the children in an upper middle class kindergarten were capable of executing the elementary tasks mentioned above, that is, the task of judging the relative magnitude of two different numbers and the task of performing simple mental additions (Griffin, Case, & Siegler, 1994). By contrast, the corresponding percentage in a school with lower-income students in the same community was only 7%. When we calibrated the difference in terms of age equivalents, it turned out that the high-SES students were a full year and half ahead of their lower-income peers. Very similar results have been found by Herbert P. Ginsburg at Columbia University and by Sharon Griffin at Clark University (Ginsburg, Choi, Loez, Netley, & Chao-Yuan, 1992; Ginsburg & Russell, 1981; Griffin, Case, & Siegler, 1994), using much large samples.

Before proceeding, it is important to enter a series of caveats. First, the evidence on the maturation of the neurological systems that control early numerical processing, although it is suggestive, is by no means definitive. Second, even if this evidence were stronger, it would not imply that the different experiences that the different SES groups encounter during this age range actually *produce* a difference in the underlying neurological systems. Third, even if a causal connection of this sort were established, it would not imply that the effect on the underlying neurological systems was a permanent one. To the contrary, everything we know about the nervous system suggests that it retains a great deal of plasticity well through adolescence and into adulthood.

Still, the fact that SES differences in numerical competence do emerge at such an early age, during the very period in which so much of the basic circuitry on which numerical processing depends is still being laid down, is clearly a cause for concern. Moreover, one could argue that, biological considerations aside, if one wishes to prevent too broad a divergence in the functioning of different SES groups, the best time to do so is either just before or just after this divergence first begins to become apparent. Regardless of whether one's perspective is biological or behavioral, the same general conclusion follows: it is important to understand what sorts of experience early mathematical competence depends on and to see if a more level playing field can be provided for different SES groups by systematically manipulating that experience in some fashion.

EARLY CHILDHOOD EDUCATION AS AN INSTRUMENT FOR FLATTENING SOCIOECONOMIC GRADIENTS

Early childhood education and the compensatory effect that it can have on SES gradients have been of particular interest in the United States, where steep gradients in school achievement often co-occur with an equally strong commitment to equity. Project Head Start was a massive federally funded project that was specifically designed for the purpose of providing children from low-SES homes with a high-quality preschool experience so that they would be on a more equal footing with their high-SES peers when they entered school and thus better able to take advantage of the opportunities which schooling offers. A good deal of controversy surrounded the initial evaluation of the Head Start project (Cicerelli, 1969; M. S. Smith & Bissell, 1970). However, a consensus now appears to be emerging (Currie & Thomas, 1994; Zigler & Muenchow, 1992). Although Head Start programs tended to produce an initial elevation in measures of general cognitive ability, these gains showed an equally rapid attrition. Long-term effects did remain, however, especially those relating to social and/or attitudinal factors. In one study it was shown that children who participated in Head Start stayed in school an average of 2 years longer than siblings reared in the same family who did not attend Head Start—even though the Head Start group did not achieve higher scores on IQ tests (Currie & Thomas, 1994). Other studies showed that Head Start graduates had a lower incidence of teenage pregnancy and delinquency than control populations, higher general feelings of empowerment, and a more positive attitude toward the education of their own children (Zigler & Muenchow, 1992).

The foregoing results are by no means trivial. Still, they would be stronger if they were joined by results showing an improvement in cognitive functioning. In this regard, it is important to note that early compensatory programs tended to target characteristics that were either very general and stable, such as IQ, or very specific and easily influenced, such as the ability to recognize letters and numerals (see Wiekart, Kamii, & Radin, 1994; Bereiter & Engleman, 1966). A possibility that has recently begun to receive some attention is that a greater impact may possibly be made by targeting conceptual competencies that are intermediate, both in their generality and in their susceptibility to short-term environmental influence. As it turns out, most elementary school subjects cannot be learned with any real insight unless certain general conceptual understandings are already in place. For example, learning the rules for visual–phonic mapping depends on understanding that words have sounds as well as meanings, that these sounds may be broken up into sequences of more primitive sounds. Children who come to school with this "phonemic awareness" in place respond very well to early reading instruction, regardless of whether it is phonically based or based on more holistic techniques, and tend to end up with higher reading scores (Adams, 1990). A similar point can be made with regard to writing. Learning to write depends on certain very general understandings regarding the form and content of what one writes, that is, concerning the basics of narrative structure (McKeough, 1992). Once again, children who come to school with these insights in place tend to take to early instruction in writing very naturally, whereas those who come without them do not.

A similar analysis obtains in the domain of mathematics. Learning the rules for elementary arithmetic depends on being able to assign some sort of quantitative meanings to numbers, recognizing that the problem of computing small sums or differences can be solved by counting, and so on (Fuson, 1982; Siegler, 1996). Children who come to school with these general insights in place respond very well to their first instruction in arithmetic, whereas children who come to school without them do not (Griffin & Case, 1996; Griffin et al., 1994). In the early years of the Head Start movement, little guidance was available regarding instruction in such general competencies, since their existence was only dimly understood at best. In recent years, however, advances in cognitive science have made it possible to understand these competencies in great detail and to make equally detailed suggestions regarding how they might be taught. In order to get a better sense of these recommendations and the rationale on which they are based, it is worthwhile to consider a specific example.

RECENT DEVELOPMENTS IN OUR UNDERSTANDING OF PRESCHOOLERS' MATHEMATICAL COMPETENCE

In the late 1960s and early 1970s a new field was born from the integration of cognitive psychology, computer science, linguistics, and neurology. Dubbed "the mind's new science" (H. Gardner, 1985), this field permitted a much more detailed mapping of mental structures and processes than had previously been possible.

Early Knowledge of Counting and Addition/Subtraction

Rochel Gelman at UCLA was one of the first to apply the new tools of cognitive science to the analysis of preschool children's thought. One of her most widely cited studies (Gelman, 1978) had to do with preschoolers' intuitive understanding of counting. By the age of 4–5, most preschoolers' can count a small set of objects without error. By designing novel counting tasks and watching how children respond to them, Gelman came to the conclusion that preschoolers have an extensive set of understandings about number, which include the following intuitive concepts: (1) that each number word occurs in a fixed and necessary sequence; (2) that each number word must be assigned to one and only one object in an array; (3) that the order in which objects are counted is not significant; and (4) that when each object has been assigned a number word in an ordered fashion, the last number word mentioned indicates the total number of objects in the array (Gelman, 1978). The mental "blueprint" or "schema" that children possess at this stage may be illustrated graphically in the manner shown in the top panel of Figure 7.3.

Prentice Starkey at Berkeley is another researcher who has conducted extensive research on preschoolers' quantitative thinking, using the tools that cognitive science has made available. One of his most widely cited dis-

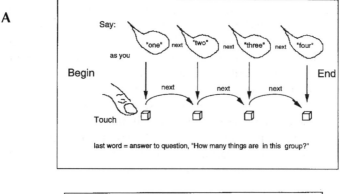

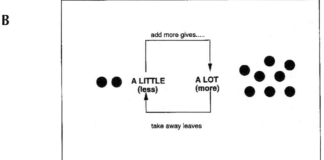

FIGURE 7.3. *A:* Preschoolers' counting schema. *B:* Global quantity schema (add/subtract compare).

coveries is that infants are born with a natural sensitivity to number and can distinguish actions that preserve the numerical value of small arrays from those that change it (Starkey, 1992, see also Wynn, 1992). Equally important is his finding that, by the age of 4 years, most children appear to understand all the relationships indicated in the bottom panel of Figure 7.3. As may be seen, the core understandings in their global quantity schema concern relative quantity (more, less, same), and the transformations that change this variable (adding objects or taking some away).

Differentiation and Elaboration of the Counting Schema

Several changes take place in children's knowledge of counting as they enter the elementary school years. The most obvious change is that they learn more words in the number sequence: typically, they learn to count from 1 to 20 instead of just 1 to 5. A less obvious change—and one that is a great help to them when they encounter subtraction problems in first grade—is that they learn to count backward, at least for small numbers. This new counting knowledge is indicated in Figure 7.4.

At first glance, Figure 7.4 may appear to be an overly complex way to illustrate the improvement in such a simple skill as counting. One of the main points of the diagram, however, is that the knowledge that appears to be so simple from the adult's point of view is in fact quite complex from the point of view of the child. For example, for adults there is a single sequence of number words that remains invariant across all number tasks. Although an adult may choose to recite the sequence backward or forward, the sequence itself remains the same in his/her eyes. For the young child who is just learning to count, however, counting forward and counting backward

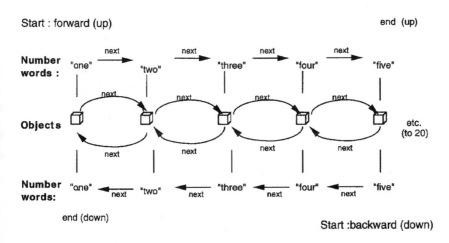

FIGURE 7.4. Elaborated counting schema.

are two separate skills. Moreover, the second one (counting backward) is a good deal harder to master not just because it is encountered less frequently but because the associations learned in forward counting keep intruding when the child is trying to learn to count backward. Thus, it takes a good deal of time before backward counting assumes the same ease and efficiency as does forward counting (Fuson, 1982).

Differentiation and Elaboration of the Add/Subtract Schema

Robert S. Siegler is a researcher at Carnegie–Mellon University who has made a detailed study of children's early understanding of addition and subtraction. He has also built elaborate computer models that behave in the same fashion that young children do when they are solving addition and subtraction problems (Siegler, 1996). One of the findings that has emerged from his research is that, as children make the transition to the school years, their global quantity schema becomes a good deal more differentiated and elaborated. For a 4-year-old, the numbers 4 and 5 are both "big" numbers: that is, numbers—that signal one has "a lot." If asked which one is bigger, most preschoolers are unsure and have to guess. By contrast, by the time they have reached the end of kindergarten, these two numbers have become clearly differentiated in their minds, as each is associated with a different perceptual configuration (Siegler & Robinson, 1982).

Another change that takes place as children make the transition to formal schooling is that they begin to distinguish between adding and taking away—as global operations—and additions and subtractions that have a particular magnitude associated with them. Now 4 and 5 not only become numbers that are associated with particular perceptual appearances, but they also become "set sizes" that can be derived from each other: 5 can be derived from 4 by adding 1, while 4 can be derived from 5 by taking 1 away. Once again, these two simple insights, each so obvious to an adult, are normally constructed quite gradually by young children because they entail such an elaborate network of concepts, associations, and linguistic terms. Figure 7.5 is intended to illustrate the complexity of the new knowledge that children acquire in this area in the same fashion as Figure 7.4 indicated the increased complexity of their knowledge about counting.

Integration of the Counting Schema with the Add/Subtract Schema

Probably the most famous scientist to study children's early understanding of number was the Swiss psychologist Jean Piaget, whose work predated the birth of cognitive science but anticipated many of its core postulates (Piaget, 1970). Piaget stressed that, as children develop, their later number

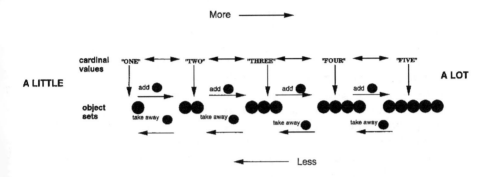

FIGURE 7.5. Elaborated quantity schema.

knowledge always develops out of their earlier knowledge in an organic fashion. As children assimilate new experience and relate it to their existing mental representations, these representations inevitably become more differentiated and elaborated. As children reflect on their mental representations, their representations are also reorganized and in the process become more integrated. In our own work, we have studied this process in some detail. Our research indicates that, as children's knowledge of counting and their knowledge of quantity become more elaborate and differentiated, it gradually merges into the single knowledge network indicated in Figure 7.6. We call this network a *central conceptual structure* because of the central role it assumes in children's scientific and mathematical thought.

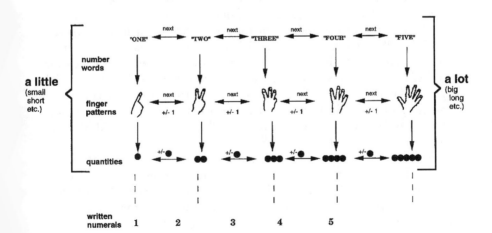

FIGURE 7.6. Mental counting line.

As may be seen, most of the elements in Figure 7.6 are just more so-phisticated versions of the knowledge that was diagrammed in earlier fig-ures. The first row of the figure (labeled "number words") is very similar to the elaborated counting schema that was illustrated in Figure 7.4. The main difference is that the forward and backward counting words have now been merged into a single set of entries that can be "read off," as it were, in either direction, whether or not a specific set of objects is present. The row one line from the bottom (labeled "quantities") is the same as the elabo-rated quantity schema that children constructed earlier and that was illus-trated in Figure 7.5. It has simply been diagrammed in a more economical fashion. In the second row of Figure 7.6 is a representation of the standard pattern in which quantities are represented with one's fingers. The advan-tage of fingers over other forms of representation is not just that they are portable. They can also be used for two distinct purposes: (1) counting (by moving one finger at a time, in sequence), and (2) indicating a set size (by forming the standard "cardinal number pattern" directly). As a result, they can serve as a transitional integrating device, which serves to link children's two earlier schemata.

As children merge their previous structures into a single and more uni-fied structure, they gradually come to realize that a question about addition or subtraction (bottom row) can be answered, in the absence of any con-crete set of objects, simply by counting forward or backward along the string of counting words (top row). They also come to realize that a simple verbal statement about a transformation such as "I have 4 things, then I get 1 more" has an automatic entailment with regard to quantity. One does not need to see the objects that are involved or know anything else about them. This simple understanding actually betokens a major revolution in children's understanding—a revolution which changes the world of quanti-tative transformations from something that can only occur "out there" to something that can be modeled in their own heads via mental counting (Resnick, 1983; Riley, Greeno, & Heller, 1983). As this revolution takes place, children gradually begin to use their counting skills in a wide range of other contexts. This broadened usage is indicated at the left and right edges of Figure 7.6. In effect, children come to realize that counting is something one can do in order to make a determination of the relative value of two objects on a wide variety of dimensions (e.g., width, height, weight, musical tonality) (Case, 1992).

A final change that takes place during this time period is that children begin to learn the (Arabic) system of notation that is used for representing numbers on paper. This new understanding is indicated at the bottom of Figure 7.6 with dashed vertical lines. Note that the numerals stand as sym-bols for both uses of numbers simultaneously (i.e., their use as array sizes and their use as counting operators). They thus further serve to bind the el-ements of the new cognitive structure together.

HARNESSING THE NEW UNDERSTANDING TO IMPROVE EARLY PROGRAMS IN MATHEMATICS EDUCATION

Assessing Children's Mathematical Knowledge before They Enter School

The cognitive structure described in Figure 7.6 is very similar to the one that Stanislas Dehaene has studied in adults in his electroencephalographic (EEG) studies. Thus, it is worthy of note that the component concepts and skills outlined in Figure 7.6 bear a close resemblance to those his studies have revealed. The written numerals in the bottom row correspond to Dehaene's visual/symbolic representations of number, which appear to be localized in the occipital cortex. The representations of quantity that appear in the third row correspond to Dehaene's analogical representations of magnitude, which appear to be localized at the juncture of parietal and occipital lobes, with some lateralization on the right side of the cortex. The number words in the first row correspond to Dehaene's verbal/numerical system, which appears to be localized in the inferior region of the left temporal lobes. The one set of entries that does not appear in Dehaene's model are those for manual representation of numbers. However, it must be remembered that adults have had a long time to detach their judgments of quantity from this sort of digital representation, and the present model is designed to capture children's mental representations.

What we see, then, is an increasing convergence of the data and models from several different fields of inquiry. There is increasing agreement among primatologists and developmentalists with regard to the fundamental building blocks on which numerical cognition depends and on the advantage that human children demonstrate—by about the third or fourth year of life—in their ability to assemble these building blocks into sophisticated and uniquely human forms of cognitive structures. At the same time, there is increasing agreement among cognitive psychologists and neuropsychologists on the details of what numerical thinking entails: what its basic components are, how they are connected, and what sorts of neurological circuitry they depend on.

It is in the light of this converging evidence, then, that the SES gradients in mathematical cognition must be considered. As mentioned earlier, if one uses tests that are especially designed to assess the presence of the structure in Figure 7.6, one finds that social-class gradients of the same general magnitude as those indicated in Figure 7.2 are already present before children ever enter the first grade. Of course, the presence of these gradients does not mean that children from low-SES homes have some sort of neurological handicap. It does not even mean that they have some sort of psychological handicap. It simply means that their early home environment has not had such a strong numerical emphasis as has been present in middle class homes, and that they come to school with a knowledge base and a set of numerical capabilities that are less well developed.

On the other hand, however, it seems clear that children from low-SES homes are at considerable risk that these early differences will be reified and that they will *develop into* a handicap. At the present moment, schools are not equipped to diagnose the subtle differences in knowledge with which children arrive at school. Nor are they equipped to do anything about them, even if they were so diagnosed. There is great danger, therefore, that what starts out as a mere difference in knowledge may be misidentified as a difference in native ability and eventually converted into a difference of a much deeper nature—perhaps even one that includes some sort of biological component. In short, children from low-SES homes are at risk for much more serious outcomes, if nothing is done to address their early differences.

It is in this regard that the importance of the analysis in Figure 7.6 becomes apparent, for it permits something to be done about the early differences that children from different backgrounds exhibit, in a principled manner. In particular, it permits one to (1) specify what knowledge is most crucial for early success in mathematics, (2) assess where any given population stands with regard to this knowledge, and (3) provide children who do not have all this knowledge with the experience that they need in order to construct it. In short, it permits a better bridge to be built between the implicit curriculum of the home and the explicit curriculum of the public school system (Strodtbeck, 1965).

Designing Preschool Programs Tailored to Children's Knowledge at School Entry

This is what we have attempted to do, in the context of a math-readiness program that we have labeled "Rightstart." At the time that we designed our curriculum, several math-readiness programs already existed that were intended to teach children all the prerequisite skills and concepts that they need in order to succeed in first grade. The program that we designed differed from these existing programs in the following respects:

• *Presence of additional elements in curriculum.* First, our program included elements that these other programs were missing, since it was based on a more detailed analysis of what the cognitive requirements for early mathematics success actually are. For example, most programs that were already in existence taught children the string of number words in the forward direction and to use them in a one-to-one fashion when counting sets of objects (the top row in Figure 7.6). They also gave children worksheets where they had to match different numerals with different cardinal values (the top and bottom rows). If children possessed these skills, they were deemed "ready" for formal training in addition and subtraction. The problem, of course, is that they were often *not* ready, but no one knew quite what to make of this fact. By contrast to existing programs, our program made provision for children to acquire the entire network of elements and relations indicated in Figure 7.6, which meant a much stronger emphasis on (1) learning to count backward as well as forward (top row); (2) learning the "increment" and "decrement rules" (third row); (3) learning that movement forward and backward in the number string could be treated as a reliable guide to movement forward and backward in the sequence of cardinal values (top row to third row mapping); (4) learning that the entire sequence could be used as a basis for making dimensional judgments (see the outside brackets of Figure 7.6), and (5) learning the conventional labels for referring to the relations in each row (next, up, etc.) as well as the elements themselves.

• *Stronger and more explicit developmental emphasis.* A second way in which our program differed from programs that were already in existence was that it had a much stronger developmental emphasis—both in the sense that activities were sequenced in a developmental fashion and in the sense that teachers were provided with "benchmark" assessment devices for determining where any individual student was situated in their general developmental journey. This permitted an intervention that could be adapted much more easily to the existing knowledge possessed by the students in any particular school, neighborhood, or community, at their current level of development.

• *Mix of didactic and nondidactic methods.* A third difference between our program and others was in the pedagogical methods that we employed. At the time, most kindergarten and/or grade 1 math programs were of two varieties: those that used classical didactic methods (exposition, followed by drill and practice), and those that concentrated on providing hands-on activities which encouraged children to construct their own mathematical meanings and insights. The program that we designed drew on both these general approaches. The materials were always ones that children could manipulate on their own. Moreover, the children were always given the time and opportunity to do so. At the same time, however, teachers were encouraged to ask children carefully targeted questions as they participated in these activities, and to reformulate and reinforce the insights that they created for others to share. In effect, then, our program was both child centered and teacher centered.

• *Emphasis on board games and language.* A final way in which our program differed from programs that were already in existence was that it included a heavy emphasis on affectively involving games and the mathematical language that such games elicit. Figure 7.7 presents a game of the sort that was presented. The object of this game is to progress down the line of boxes to the end in order to put out the fire of a dragon who lives in the box at the end and is terrorizing a city. Children roll a die and count the

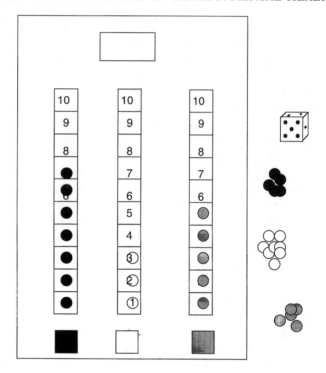

FIGURE 7.7. Board game played in Rightstart math-readiness program. (See the text for an explanation.)

number of dots that it displays. They then count out the corresponding number of chips and place them one by one along the line. As they do, the teacher asks questions about who is closest to the dragon, how many more chips they need to reach the dragon, and so on. The general idea is to embody, in a spatial context, as many as possible of the nodes and relations in Figure 7.7, thereby encouraging children to move backward and forward among them with ease.

EVALUATING THE SUCCESS
OF THE NEW MATH PROGRAMS

The math program that we created has now been tried out in several different communities in Canada and the United States. Several different forms of evaluation have also been conducted. In the first, children who participated in the program were simply compared with matched controls, who had received a readiness program of a different sort. On tests of mathematical knowledge, on a set of more general developmental measures, and on a set of experimental measures of learning potential, children in the experimental program were consistently superior to those in the control groups (Case & Sandieson, 1988; Griffin, Case, & Sandieson, 1992; Griffin et al., 1994). In a second type of study, children who had had the experimental program were followed up 1 year later, and evaluated on a variety of mathematical and scientific tests using a double-blind procedure. Once again, those who had had the program were found to be superior on virtually all measures, including teacher evaluations of "general number sense" (Griffin & Case, 1996). In a third type of study, graduates of the program were compared with graduates of programs designed to improve children's readiness in the area of language arts. In this case, the graduates of the experimental program showed the same degree of superiority in the area of first grade mathematical concepts as they had in other studies, while those who had had the linguistic training showed a parallel advance in the language arts area (Case, Okamoto, Henderson, & McKeough, 1993; Griffin et al., 1994).

Although all these studies were encouraging, the most dramatic results were obtained from a longitudinal study by Griffin in which graduates of the Rightstart program were tracked over a 3-year period and given a follow-up program that was based on the same general principles described above. At the beginning of the study and at the end of each year, the treatment children were compared with two other groups: (1) a second low-SES group who were originally tested as having superior achievement in mathematics, and (2) a mixed (largely middle class) SES group who also showed a higher level of performance at the outset and who then attended a magnate school with a special mathematics coordinator and an enriched mathematics program. As may be seen from Figure 7.8, what happened was that the low-SES group who received the Rightstart program gradually outstripped both other groups. They also compared very favorably with high-SES groups from China and Japan that were tested on the same measures (Griffin & Case, 1997).

PLACING COMPENSATORY MATH EDUCATION IN A BROADER EDUCATIONAL CONTEXT

The results in Figure 7.8 are stronger than any others that have been reported in the literature to date. While they are extremely encouraging, they naturally raise several further questions.

Fostering Readiness for Other Kinds of Learning

One obvious question has to do with the possibility of improving the preschool curriculum for low-SES students in other subject areas such as reading and writing. Although mathematics is a school subject that is of

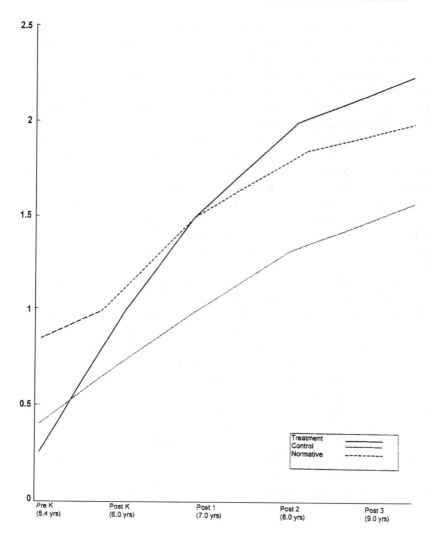

FIGURE 7.8. Mean developmental level scores on number knowledge test at five time periods.

increasing importance in the modern world, it is not the only subject that is important. As mentioned above, the amount of work that has gone into analyzing the cognitive prerequisites for success in reading and writing is at least as great as the amount of work that has been done in mathematics (see Adams, 1990, and Bereiter & Scardamalia, 1987, for reviews). Parallel compensatory programs have also recently been developed in these other areas, which have led to results of equal promise (Bereiter & Scardamalia,

1987; L. Bradley & Bryant, 1985; Case, Stephenson, Bleiker, & Okamoto, 1996; McKeough, 1992). To the best of our knowledge, no data exist in these other areas that are as strong as those illustrated in Figure 7.8. However, that is not because the effects in kindergarten have not been as great. It is simply because no follow-up programs have been devised of equivalent efficiency. As programs such as these are devised, there is reason to be optimistic about our ability to deliver high-quality education across the full socioeconomic spectrum.

Moving to Scale

Since the results of the math program have already been replicated in more than a dozen small projects, another question that needs to be raised concerns the feasibility and cost of implementing such projects on a broader scale. A new preschool program is much like any other invention in that its first version requires a great deal of time and money to develop. Implementing the program on a wider scale or across a broader array of subject areas may be difficult at first due to the requirement for training the teachers who will be using the new methods. Such training may be costly. Still, as is the case with any technology, the unit costs for implementation normally go down as further experience is gathered and improvements made. Ultimately, the cost may prove to be little more than that of (1) purchasing one math kit per preschool classroom, (2) investing modest sums for in-service workshops, and (3) supporting participating teachers or day care workers with two or three peer visits during the first year of program usage.

Problems Posed by Fixed or Declining Resources

A third question has to do with the cost of increasing the emphasis on preschool intervention, whether in one or in several different school subjects. If the total financial resources available to the system are fixed or declining, where should the resources for this sort of compensatory effort come from? Are the costs likely to jeopardize programs that are already in place, either for older age groups or for higher-SES groups or for other (noneducational) efforts? Can we afford to add a cognitive emphasis to our existing preschool programs at this time? Our belief about these questions is that they cannot be answered independent of political considerations. Each community, each region, or each country must make its own determination on these questions and come to a decision that is consonant with its own values. All that educators, social scientists, and economists can do is to offer guidance as to what actions will have what consequences and costs, not which set of consequences are most desirable or what trade-offs are to be preferred.

As such deliberations take place, it may be worthwhile to take into account the long-term costs of *inaction*, as well as those of action. There is good evidence that, as we make the transition to an era of high technology, the economic penalty for not completing high school is increasing, while the reward of university or postuniversity education is increasing. This is a trend that is at work across all advanced industrial economies, and it is leading to an increasing slope in income distribution in all countries as well (Atkinson, Rainwater, & Smeeding, 1995; Smeeding & Gottschalk, 1996). If we do *not* put additional effort into compensatory education, then we may well run the risk of increasing the educational gap between rich and poor even further and thus jeopardizing (1) our sense of common purpose and/or (2) our ability to maximize our international competitiveness. In any full calculation of costs these factors also have to be taken into consideration.

Indirect Consequences of Altering the Slope of Achievement Gradients

One final factor to consider is the effect that compensatory education is likely to have on the tail rather than the center of the educational distribution. The gradients that were illustrated in Figure 7.2 were gradients in mean scores. It is a statistical fact of life, however, that any difference between the mean score of two populations is accompanied by a difference in the tails as well. Moreover, for every small difference in mean scores, there is a much bigger difference in the tails. As an example (Figure 7.9), a difference of 1.2 standard deviations (which is roughly what one finds in the case

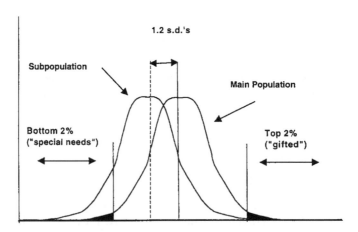

FIGURE 7.9. Idealized representation depicting displacement of subgroup with regard to main population on any variable that is normally distributed, such as academic achievement. Note that relatively small displacement in mean produces much larger change in the proportion of children at the extremes because definition of "extreme" depends on tests formed for general population.

of the British, U.S., or New Zealand populations) will be accompanied by a difference on the order of 5 to 1 in the percentage of children who are at the extreme upper end of the academic distribution (and thus judged to be "gifted"), and a corresponding difference of the same size but opposite direction in the percentage of children who are at the lower end of the distribution (and thus judged as learning disabled, or mildly retarded). This means that the incidence of "giftedness" may be five times higher in high-SES populations than in low-SES populations, while the incidence of mild retardation and learning disabilities may be five times higher in low- than in high-SES populations.

If the only way of flattening SES gradients was to increase the performance of low-SES children at the expense of high-SES children, then this fact would perhaps need to be taken into account in computing the overall costs and benefits. What was gained by one group would simply be lost by another. However, that does not appear to be the case. Special preschool programs move the low-SES distribution up but have no negative effect on the high-SES distribution. What this suggests is that—in addition to any other effects—any widely implemented early intervention program is likely to have two secondary consequences if it is successful: an increase in the pool of highly talented individuals, and a decrease in the expense that must be devoted to special and remedial services.

CHANGING ACHIEVEMENT GRADIENTS IN A CHANGING WORLD ECONOMY

Before we conclude, it seems worthwhile to set the issues that have been raised in the present chapter in a broader social and historical context. Social-class gradients in educational achievement are a universal phenomenon in the modern world. Indeed, it would be surprising if they were not. All modern societies offer differential rewards of some sort to different occupational groups. Since the desire to provide for one's children is a universal one, it would be surprising if such gradients were *not* present. That is to say, it would be surprising if groups who have access to more material resources did not find some way to parlay these resources into an educational advantage for their offspring. It would also be surprising if the SES gradients in educational achievement were not part of a broader picture: one which includes a broad range of other social and economic variables.

What *is* surprising, however, or at least worthy of note, is that the slope of these SES gradients varies so much from one country or locality to the next. As we move in the direction of a global economy, these gradients are likely to become an increasing source of attention, both because of the external effect that they may have on economic competitiveness and because of the internal effects that they may have on social stability (Goldstone, 1991). Attention to these gradients may also increase as the slope of the income distribution becomes more steep. The increase in the slope of income distributions across different SES groups is a trend that appears to be taking place across all modern industrial economies regardless of their political ideology (Atkinson et al., 1995; Smeeding & Gottschalk, 1996). Although it is too early to determine what effects the increased income gradient will have on cognitive and educational gradients, it seems quite reasonable to assume that it may be substantial. The interesting situation that may possibly arise, then, is this: at the same time as our potential to exert a leveling influence on educational gradients increases, the gradients themselves may actually become steeper. To the extent that a situation such as this does develop, we can expect that pressure for improved compensatory programs will build and that programs such as those discussed in the present chapter will be perceived as being of increasing economic and social relevance. In Parts III and IV of this volume the issues that arise when communities decide to implement early childhood education programs such as these will be considered. Attention will also be given to the changing requirements that young children from *all* SES groups are likely to face in the future, as well as new ways that they can be prepared for these challenges.

CONCLUSION

Since the argument that has been advanced in the present chapter is a rather lengthy one, it is perhaps worthwhile to recapitulate it, by way of conclusion. Recent research on children's early mathematical abilities has gone a long way toward identifying the early cognitive prerequisites on which later mathematical learning depends and the neurological circuitry on which these capabilities are dependent. Recent research has also shown that, like most other high-level cognitive capabilities, children's early mathematical capabilities show a considerable degree of differentiation by social class during the years when the neurological circuitry on which they depend is showing its most rapid development. This differentiation may or may not result in biologically embedded changes analogous to those discussed in other chapters. We do not need to await the answer to this question, however, to determine whether or not something can be done to make the SES gradient less severe and to put children from all SES groups on a more equal footing. Drawing on recent developments in cognitive science, we have shown that a well-designed early intervention program can have powerful effects, providing it is targeted at the central conceptual structures that children will need for their subsequent learning and development. The practical questions that arise now that we have such data in hand have to do with the best way to make such interventions available on a broader scale, to minimize their costs, and to tailor them to the needs of different local communities. These and other issues related to the changing needs of young children in an increasingly global economy are taken up in subsequent chapters in this volume.

ACKNOWLEDGMENTS

The work that is reported in the present chapter was supported by grants from the McDonnell Foundation and Spencer Foundation, whose assistance is gratefully acknowledged. We are also endebted to Richard Wolfe and Tahany Gadalla for their help in analyzing the data that are reported in Figure 7.2.

Part II

Fundamental Processes: Biology and Development

Based on the evidence reviewed in Part I, we take up in Part II the notion that biological embedding is a potential explanation for the gradient effects in developmental health. We examine the development of the central nervous system, the neuroendocrine system, and the neuroimmune system, and the connections between these aspects of brain development and identified cognitive, social, and behavioral functioning in animals, nonhuman primates, and human infants and young children. Of particular importance is the recognition that the various systems of brain development are interconnected through mutual influences, which provides a strong basis for the inference that the large effects in developmental health may have a common origin in development, especially early development.

In Chapter 8, Max S. Cynader and Barrie Frost review the powerful evidence emerging from a variety of animal species that critical periods exist in brain development such that the analyzing and processing capabilities of the cortex are shaped by the input received during these times. The interaction between the genetic history of the individual and the stimulation received at these times will be an important determinant of lifelong skills in competence and aging. Systematic differences in opportunities for stimulation during early childhood likely correlate with systematic differences in appropriate stimulation during critical periods in brain development and may help explain the observed gradients in cognitive and behavioral development over time.

In Chapter 9, Stephen J. Suomi describes the primate models of the life cycle that demonstrate the powerful effects of nature–nurture interactions in early life on circumstances throughout life. In particular, manipulating the early socioemotional environment of vulnerable monkeys can change their life chances from the poorest to the best. These changes in life chances are accompanied by changes in the developing monkey's biological response to stressful circumstances, which helps to define the basis of biological embedding. These nonhuman primate models are particularly valuable in that they can also reveal the stress–physiology–behavior connections in the context of group functioning, offering a vivid and comparable perspective for human behavior in society.

In Chapter 10, Christopher L. Coe notes that research can provide a more detailed model of biological embedding. Over the last two decades there has been growing interest in the interaction between psychosocial factors and a different dimension of health that involves immunological well-being and disease. The principal axes are the "psychoneuroimmunological" and "psychoneuroendocrinological," which link perception of circumstances to the function of organ systems and also to behavior.

In Chapter 11, Daniel P. Keating and Fiona K. Miller review studies of the determinants of competence and coping that show that early opportunities in the socioemotional sphere, particularly responsive relationships with significant others and the development of regulatory systems, may be more important than early cognitive competence per se. This reinforces Suomi's findings (Chapter 9), in that it shows the development of cognitive competence to be inescapably a social process. This, in turn, creates a significant challenge for societies that strive to be cognitively sophisticated but at the same time lag behind when it comes to creating the social and emotional conditions for success in the cognitive realm.

8

Mechanisms of Brain Development

NEURONAL SCULPTING BY THE PHYSICAL AND SOCIAL ENVIRONMENT

Max S. Cynader
Barrie J. Frost

Although gradients appear ubiquitous in many spheres of the human condition and endeavor, it is of considerable importance to attempt to understand how the underlying neural mechanisms that result in these individual differences in abilities and coping strategies are built over a lifetime. Since antiquity humankind has intuitively understood that both nature and nurture interact to produce competent adult behavior. In fact the writings of Plato and Aristotle are often contrasted as early examples of nativism and empiricism, respectively, but some modern scholars (Baumrin, 1975) have argued that Aristotelian writings reveal a more sophisticated interactionism that lies quite close to contemporary views. In this chapter we will take an interactionist or *epigenetic* approach (see Table 8.1) and argue

---

TABLE 8.1. Epigenetic Sources of Information

1. Genetic information
2. Chemical and physical information (*microscale*) residing in the nature of matter
3. Ecological environmental information (*macroscale*) derived from—
   a. layout of world, plant, animate, and inanimate objects
   b. social information obtained through behavioral interactions with conspecifics

---

that during development, information from genetic sources, the material environment, and biological and social environments *all* contribute in complementary ways and at critical times during neural differentiation to forge competencies for the current ecology of the individual.

The explosion of scientific research in the 20th century has yielded knowledge not only about the nature of the inanimate universe and its fundamental laws and dynamic processes but also about the evolution of life itself. With J. D. Watson and F. H. C. Crick's discovery of the structure of DNA and subsequent elucidation of the "central dogma" of molecular biology, we have now in our possession the "Rosetta stone" for understanding the genetic code and the genome of individual species. (The central dogma is as follows: All DNA is copied from other DNA—replication. All RNA is copied from DNA—transcription. All proteins are copied from RNA using three nucleotide bases to specify one amino acid in a protein chain—employing a code that is the same for nearly all organisms; some viruses are different.) In fact, in many instances molecular geneticists have sequenced the entire genome of species such as the nematode worm *Caenorhabditis elegans,* the fruitfly *Drosophila,* and even the mouse. Work on the human genome project is proceeding at an accelerating pace.

However, with the wonderful repertoire of techniques at the disposal of molecular geneticists and the precision with which they can describe the sequence of specific genes, one often loses sight of what information "the code" really contains, or (put another way) where "meaning" resides in genetics. As Hofstadter (1979) has eloquently explained in his book *Gödel, Escher, Bach: An Eternal Golden Braid,* the total information content of a coded message always involves much more than is explicitly specified. Thus, the self-organizing principles of physics and chemistry need not be specified in the genetic code because they already reside in the material building blocks of matter itself. What is not generally appreciated is that high-probability events such as what young organisms typically see, hear, touch, smell, taste, and experience, through interactions with their particular physical and social environments (their ecological niche in other words), also contain critically important information *that is presumed and required* to sculpt and mold their brain and nervous system in very lawful and specific ways. These sources of information may be as essential as the self-organizing principles of matter itself for building members of a species that can successfully and competently cope with all aspects of their physical and social environments, and therefore provide selective advantage for their particular set of genes.

We now understood that the successful development of an embryo from a single fertilized ovum requires the critical sequencing and expression of the appropriate genetic information at the appropriate time during development. Likewise, there appear to be "critical periods" when *specific high-probability information from the physical or social environment* is required, in addition to genetic information, to build adult brain structures and processors to produce and control adult behavior. In this chapter we will describe how these "critical periods" for neural development exist in a number of different species, for a number of different brain areas that are specifically responsible for a number of different aspects of adult behavior. They will range from critical periods for sculpting and wiring the visual, auditory, and somatosensory areas of the brain, as well as critical periods for laying down neural templates for social recognition, bonding, and affiliation.

NEURONAL DEATH AND SYNAPTIC PRUNING

When we think about the development of the brain, a representation that is useful and evocative is that of Michelangelo's unfinished "Atlas," which is illustrated in Figure 8.1. The organism begins as a single cell, and there is then an extraordinarily complicated process of development in which cells divide repeatedly, migrate to their appropriate positions within the embryo,

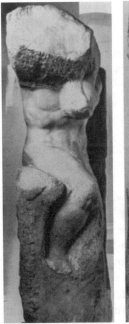
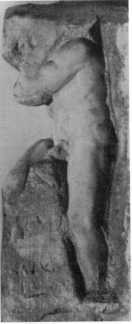

FIGURE 8.1. Michelangelo's unfinished "Atlas." From *Michelangelo, the Sculptor* by Martin Weinberger. Copyright 1967 by Columbia University Press. Reprinted with permission of the publisher.

differentiate, and eventually produce the large volume of tissue that becomes the organism. Yet, in parallel with this addition of neurons, neural pathways, and synapses (representing connections between cells) in the developing brain, there is an important process of elimination, or sculpting away, which occurs in parallel with these generative programs. An appropriate metaphor is that of an expanding ball that is being sculpted at the same time as it expands. Cell death plays a crucial and necessary role in neural development. Elimination of cells, connections between cells, and even of entire neural pathways is an important feature of brain development. For example, more than half of the cells in the retina die before a child is 1 year of age. Over one-third of the neurons in the cerebral cortex are eliminated in the first 3 years of postnatal life (Meinecke & Rakic, 1992). In addition to a major expansion in synaptic connections that occurs during the first few years of postnatal life in the developing human cortex, there is also massive elimination of synapses, connections, and even entire pathways. For instance, early in postnatal life there is a substantial pathway connecting the visual and auditory cortex, this pathway largely disappears later in postnatal life.

What are the rules that govern the sculpting process? Stated in most general terms, neural development proceeds by overproducing neurons, connections, and pathways. Thereafter, development recapitulates evolution and only the fittest and most useful of these neurons, synapses, and pathways are retained in the mature organism. It is important to understand that the needs of an individual neuron may not always coincide with the needs of the entire organism. Some neurons must die in order for the organism to survive. At a metaphorical level, one can think of each neuron as an individual striving to grow, prosper, and accumulate as much synaptic territory and other neurons willing to listen to him/her as possible. This type of biological aggression is valuable to neurons, because it enables them to survive in spite of the difficult developmental challenges that they face, and it seems intuitively reasonable that such a process should occur in a situation where many neurons will have to be eliminated.

As mentioned above, the dynamic interaction between genetic and environmental information to forge an adult organism that is optimally matched to its ecological niche is driven in part by mechanisms of redundancy reduction; there is no need to specify in the genetic code information that exists in the physical and social environment itself. Also operating on this complex system is selection for adaptive tuning of neural mechanisms so that slight variations in the "expected" (by the genetic predispositions) high-probability environmental information can be accommodated or compensated for. The following examples show how the visual system, although genetically predisposed or biased to extract certain features of patterns from visual images, can be modified profoundly by experiences that occur in sensitive or critical periods early in an animal's life by the selective survival of neurons and synapses previously described.

EARLY VISUAL EXPERIENCE
SCULPTS THE VISUAL SYSTEM

Figure 8.2 tries to make some of the somewhat abstract notions discussed in the preceding paragraphs more concrete by way of an example. The figure shows a series of thin lines of different orientations. For the majority of viewers, the lines of different orientation all appear to be equally visible. Yet, for some individuals, the lines of a particular orientation are blurred and appear to be of lower contrast. Panels B and C show how the lines of panel A might appear to such individuals. This visual defect is frequently the result of uncorrected astigmatism. Astigmatism is a clinical condition in which an individual's cornea is shaped like a lemon rather than like an orange (Mitchell, Freeman, Millodot, & Haegerstrom, 1973). Because the corneal curvature is unequal in the different directions, lines of different orientations cannot all be brought to focus at the same time. Such individuals cannot see lines of a particular orientation with clarity. If this condition occurs in adults, they eventually make their way to an ophthalmologist or optometrist, who prescribes a set of glasses in which the lenses are also lemon shaped but in the opposite direction to the natural astigmatism. The

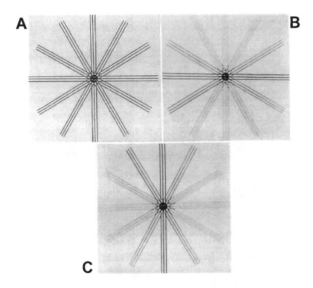

FIGURE 8.2. Photographs mimicking the appearance of the object (A) to an astigmatic eye that was emmetropic in either the vertical (B) or the horizontal (C) meridian. The lines parallel to the emmetropic meridian are blurred, whereas lines parallel to the focal line that is imaged on the retina are sharp apart from some blur at the extremities. From Mitchell, Freeman, Millodot, and Haegerstrom (1973). Copyright 1973 by Elsevier Science. Reprinted by permission.

glasses then optically correct the corneal defect, and clear vision is restored. However, if the astigmatism occurs in very young children, unless the optical imbalance is recognized early and appropriate steps are taken, then the process of Darwinian competition that was alluded to earlier takes place. We know from many studies of animal brains, that within our cortex we are born with a rudimentary set of cortical feature analyzers, each of which are involved with the analysis of lines of particular orientations. In the neonate this initial set of rudimentary connections are set up independently of visual experience, and in normal development each set of orientation-specific analyzers come to represent an equal area of cortex.

Figure 8.3 is a view of the surface of the visual cortex and illustrates with different shading the area of the cortical surface that is devoted to analyzing stimuli of different orientations. In the zone of cortex illustrated in Figure 8.3, there are roughly equal amounts of cortical territory devoted to analysis of each of the different ranges of stimulus orientation. However, with early astigmatism (like that described above) in which stimuli of one orientation are not seen as clearly as stimuli of other orientations, the number of neuronal analyzers for each orientation (which was initially equal) changes and the amount of cortical territory devoted to the analysis of the orientation that was not seen well during early visual exposure shrinks substantially.

Figure 8.4 (derived from Blakemore & Cooper, 1970) illustrates the

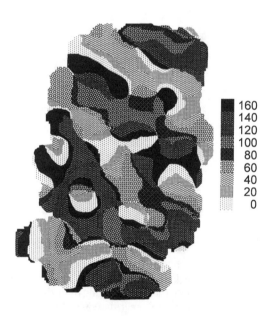

FIGURE 8.3. Reconstructed view of visual cortex showing how different areas respond to different orientations of lines.

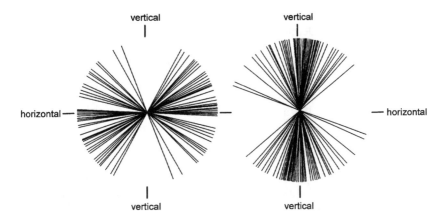

FIGURE 8.4. Polar histograms show the distribution of cortical orientation-specific analyzers from two kittens. The left is from a horizontally experienced cat, and the right from a vertically experienced cat. From Blakemore and Cooper (1970). Copyright 1970 by Macmillan Magazines Ltd. Reprinted by permission from *Nature*.

incidence of cortical orientation-specific analyzers in two kittens that were reared under environmental conditions which allowed a preponderance of either horizontal or vertical stimuli to be seen during postnatal development. In the left panel of Figure 8.4 is shown the cortical orientation distribution of the kitten reared in an environment containing preponderantly horizontal stimuli, whereas the animal whose cortical orientation distribution is illustrated on the right was reared in an environment in which vertical stimuli predominated. In Figure 8.4, each line represents the responses of a single neuron within the visual cortex, and the stimulus orientation to which that individual neuron was most sensitive is represented by the orientation of the line in the figure. As can be seen, for the left-hand panel most cortical neurons that are encountered prefer stimuli that are oriented near horizontal, with virtually no neurons responding best to stimuli that are near vertical in orientation. Thus, in the kitten reared in a predominantly horizontal environment, the distribution of analyzers within the visual cortex devoted to analyzing horizontal, as opposed to vertical, stimuli has increased dramatically. Just the opposite situation obtains in the kitten whose data are illustrated in the right-hand side of Figure 8.4. Here, there is a strong preponderance of neurons that respond best to vertically oriented stimuli, corresponding to the anisotropy in the postnatal visual exposure for this kitten. This example illustrates the principles alluded to above. If one does not get to use a set of analyzers within one's emerging brain early in life, then they will atrophy and other competing analyzers will grow at their expense.

A condition such as early childhood astigmatism is frequently not recognized until a child goes to school and displays various difficulties in reading or other visually demanding tasks. At this stage, the child may be tested and fitted with glasses that provide a perfect compensation for the peripheral optical defect. However, the ability to cure the peripheral defect may not be sufficient to cure the defect in the central nervous system. The use-dependent competitions described earlier depend on the exposure history of the organism, but only during a critical period early in postnatal development. During this critical period, the use to which a particular region of brain is put determines how it will function for the rest of the organism's life. If curative measures are applied only after the critical period has passed, then, even though the optical defect may be cured, the pattern of feature analyzers that has been set up by the unusual visual exposure to which this individual's brain was subjected early in life will result in a permanent imbalance.

The scenario described above is potentially of great generality. The competitions that are set up may occur between visual inputs representing different stimulus orientations or between visual pathways representing the two eyes within the cortex. Figure 8.5 shows a tangential (top) view of the surface of the visual cortex of the monkey (Hubel, Wiesel, & LeVay, 1977). Note the alternating stripes of light and dark. These stripes were visualized using a biochemical method to delineate the zones of cortex that respond to visual inputs represented by one eye or the other. In a normally raised animal, such as the one illustrated in Figure 8.5, equal areas of cortex are devoted to each eye. In addition, if the two eyes are used together, extensive

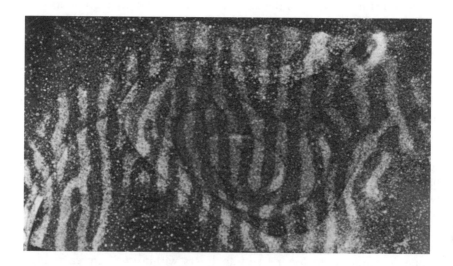

FIGURE 8.5. Tangential view of surface of the visual cortex of the monkey. From Hubel, Wiesel, and LeVay (1977). Copyright 1977 by the Royal Society. Reprinted by permission.

lateral connections that are initially present between each eye's territories are retained and the capabilities of stereoscopic vision result. Figure 8.6 illustrates the binocular responses of a single cell within the visual cortex of a normally reared animal. In this three-dimensional plot, one axis represents the spatial relationships between the two eyes, the second axis represents the timing relationships of stimulation to the two eyes, and the ordinate represents the response of the cortical cell. The spatial and temporal relationships between the two eyes are correlated with the depth of the visual stimulus and with its trajectory in three-dimensional space (Cynader, Gardner, & Douglas, 1978; Cynader & Regan, 1978). The main point that Figure 8.6 illustrates is that the responses of single cells within the cortex of normal animals are dramatically influenced by depth-related binocular inputs and that individual cells may respond well to stimuli only at a particular depth. The situation illustrated in Figure 8.6, in which inputs from the two eyes are processed in a synergistic manner, occurs in normal animals. However, if one eye for some reason does not provide a visual image which is as effective as that of the other eye, or if the two eyes for some reason provide different and incongruent visual images at the same time, then the binocular synergy illustrated in Figure 8.6 does not develop. It should be emphasized that conditions under which the two eyes provide different im-

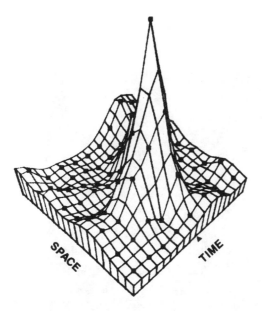

area:18
type:simple (binoc)
OD:4
space:12˚
time:−40 to +40

FIGURE 8.6. Space–time plot of an area-18 neuron in the visual cortex of a normally reared cat that responded poorly to monocular stimulation but showed strong binocular responses. From Cynader, Gardner, and Douglas (1978). Copyright 1978 by Springer-Verlag. Reprinted by permission.

ages are not uncommon. If, for instance, a child develops strabismus, either convergent (cross-eyedness) or divergent (wall-eyedness), then the two eyes are looking in different directions and provide incongruent inputs to the cortex. Under these circumstances, the binocular synergy illustrated in Figure 8.6 does not develop properly. In other situations, the inputs from the two eyes may be different and the image conveyed via one eye may be less salient for the organism. Figure 8.7 shows an autoradiogram comparable to that of Figure 8.5, illustrating the cortical surface in a monkey in which one eye was prevented from being used during development simply by patching the eyelid for the first few weeks of postnatal life (Hubel et al., 1977). In contrast to Figure 8.5 (in which inputs from each eye represent about 50% of the cortical territory), the vast majority of cortical territory in Figure 8.7 is occupied by the light-colored stripes, and the dark stripes are thin and broken up. The dark stripes represent the eye that could not be used for vision during early development, and Figure 8.7 shows that this eye's share of cortical territory was reduced from about 50% to only about 15–20%. The influence of the other eye's inputs within the cortex has expanded correspondingly. The situation illustrated in Figure 8.7 occurs quite frequently in the general population and appears to be part of the neural mechanism underlying amblyopia, or "lazy eye."

Like the problem of astigmatism, amblyopia has a strong "critical period." If one eye fails to send the brain a useful message during early development, then its inputs are simply disconnected from the cortex. Extensive studies have delineated the timing of this critical period in both human and

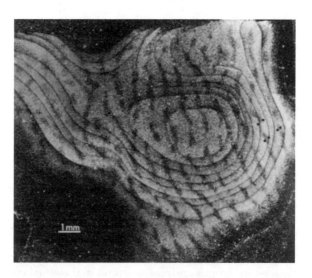

FIGURE 8.7. Autoradiogram of the cortical surface of a monkey in which one eye was prevented from being used. From Hubel, Wiesel, and LeVay (1977). Copyright 1977 by the Royal Society. Reprinted by permission.

nonhuman species. Figure 8.8 shows that the eventual visual acuity that is attained via a disused eye depends on the age of the organism and on the duration of the period of disuse (Mitchell & Timney, 1984). By disuse we do not necessarily mean blindness; reduced vision can result from cataract, or refractive errors such as myopia (nearsightedness) or hypermetropia (farsightedness). In Figure 8.8, the ordinate represents the eventual visual acuity (on a log scale) that is attained. An acuity of 1.0 represents normal vision, whereas an acuity of 0.1 would represent 20/200 vision, and an acuity of 0.005 would represent virtual blindness, or light perception only (denoted by LP at the bottom left of Figure 8.8). The horizontal black bars represent the duration of deprivation for individual subjects or groups of subjects. Thus, the subject illustrated at the top right of Figure 8.8 was prevented from using one eye for vision from 20 to 23 years of age. Despite this prolonged deprivation, visual performance through the deprived eye was essentially normal once the peripheral defect was corrected. By contrast, individuals who were prevented from using one eye between 1 and 2 years of age or just after 3 years of age showed devastating effects on visual capabilities (reduction to light perception levels only) even after the peripheral defect was repaired. Overall, Figure 8.8 makes clear that relatively

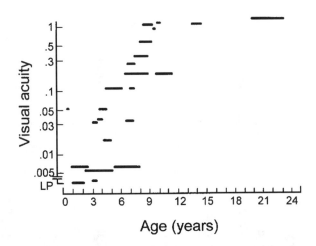

FIGURE 8.8. Visual acuity of 23 human subjects with unilateral cataract, measured immediately following restoration of normal visual input on removal of crystalline lens. Each subject is represented by a horizontal bar whose length spans period of monocular deprivation and whose position with respect to ordinate defines the first visual acuity score measured on careful optical corrections following surgical removal of lens. Ordinate shows the decimal score where a score of 1.0 represents an acuity of 6/6 and a score of 0.1 is equivalent to 6/60. Subjects able to perceive only absence or presence of light (light perception) are designated by LP. From Mitchell and Timney (1984). Copyright 1984 by the American Physiological Society. Reprinted by permission.

short periods of visual deprivation imposed on one eye early in life can have devastating effects on future visual capacities. Equivalent deprivations imposed later in life have much weaker effects. The effectiveness of therapy is also directly related to the critical period. Therapy begun after the critical period has ended is virtually ineffective.

What can we do about the problems illustrated above? First, we need better diagnostic approaches to pick up these disorders early in life, while therapy is still possible. In addition neuroscientists worldwide are working to increase the plasticity and flexibility of the adult brain, trying to extend the critical period so that therapeutic approaches can be undertaken later in life. We have evidence that the critical period is not entirely fixed. It is in fact not really a period; rather, it is a state of the brain. We know, for instance, that it is possible to extend the critical period in the visual cortex of animals well past its normal duration simply by rearing animals in the dark. When the visual cortex is not used throughout the naturally occurring critical period, it retains its capacity to be sculpted according to its eventual usage. Figure 8.9 illustrates the continuing plasticity of the visual

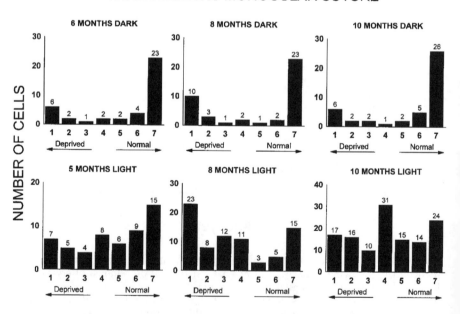

FIGURE 8.9. Effects of 3-month monocular deprivation (top, starting at 6, 8, or 10 months of age) of normally reared cats and light exposure (bottom, starting at 5, 8, or 10 months of age) of dark-reared cats on the distribution of ocular dominance in the striate cortex. From Cynader and Mitchell (1980). Copyright 1980 by the American Physiological Society. Reprinted by permission.

cortex in animals that had been placed in a dark room at birth and then kept in total darkness throughout the naturally occurring critical period (Cynader & Mitchell, 1980). These animals were thus prevented from using their visual cortex for vision during the normal critical period and then, after the normal chronological critical period was over, were allowed visual exposure through one eye only for a further 3-month period. The other eye was prevented from seeing by suturing one eyelid. In a normal animal of the same age, there would be no effect of disuse of one eye, but in these animals (which had been prevented from using the cortex throughout the critical period), the Darwinian competition that is described above occurs and the eye that fails to provide useful information is ruthlessly suppressed within the cortex. In Figure 8.9, the ordinate represents the number of cortical cells encountered (and therefore the amount of cortical territory allocated to each eye). The abscissa is a 1- to 7-point scale showing the relative strength of inputs from each of the two eyes. In the animals illustrated in the top histograms of Figure 8.9 (kept in the dark for 6 months, 8 months, or 10 months), the deprived eye (which was not allowed vision after the animal was taken out of the dark room) controls relatively few cells, while the normal eye influences a far greater number of cells. The lower histograms show that no substantial effects are observed in control animals that were reared in the light for comparable periods of time instead of in the dark. In these cases, even if one eyelid is sutured, the deprived eye still retains its share of cortical territory.

The data of Figure 8.9 make it clear that the critical period is not necessarily strictly linked to a particular chronological age. In this sense, it is not really a "period," but rather a state of the brain during which its long-term organization can be shaped by the input that it receives. Let us not imply that not using one's brain is good for you. Even though the visual cortex of a dark-reared animal retains plasticity after the end of the naturally occurring critical period, the functions of the cortex are compromised by this period of deprivation (Cynader, Berman, & Hein, 1976). Nonetheless, the finding that the critical period can be extended suggests that the critical period itself is not simply a biological clock that is ticking away as the animal ages. Rather, the use to which the brain has been put plays a role in determining its biochemical and physiological status, and hence its ability to learn and modify its circuitry according to usage.

NEURONAL SCULPTING
BY THE SOCIAL ENVIRONMENT

Not only are these neuronal sculpting mechanisms, with their sensitive periods gleaning information from the inanimate physical environment to optimize sensory and perceptual processing, but similar interactive genetic and environmental events unfold to specifically deal with the social world of young animals. Newborn vertebrates, across a wide range of species, need to form a bond or special attachment to their parents in order to obtain the sustenance, protection, comfort, and guided learning experiences necessary for their physical development, as well as their later competence as adults. Although it is common to attribute learning as the mechanism that forges these affiliative bonds through the association of reinforcing characteristics of feeding and comfort with the complex of stimuli that mothers and caregivers present, it is now abundantly clear that special dynamic neural mechanisms exist to facilitate the rapid, timely, and permanent construction of these bonds. Moreover, early filial and social bonding employ similar neuronal sculpting mechanisms to those described above for the assembly of a normally functioning visual system. As M. Leon (1992) has emphasized, young animals appear to learn only a limited number of things, but these things are absolutely necessary for their survival; typically this process involves attachment to their mother or parents. Research on precocial species—species that are mobile and self-feeding soon after birth—has been instrumental in identifying these special mechanisms that have evolved to ensure the mutual bonding of parent and offspring that forms the foundation in many instances for later learning of survival skills. Imprinting, which was first studied experimentally by Spalding (1873/1959), Heinroth (1911), and Lorenz (1935/1970, 1937), provides a classical example of this process. Young chicks shortly after hatching, quickly become attached to their hen and she to them. So powerful is this effect that chicks raised in an incubator will likewise quickly form a bond with, or become imprinted on, any stable (and preferably moving) object in their vicinity, especially 15–24 hours after hatching (Hess, 1964). Figure 8.10 from Hess (1973) illustrates the tight temporal occurrence of this effect in ducklings. While preference is normally shown to members of their own species, indicating a genetic predisposition to attach to the appropriate "mother figure," in the absence of this stimulus the chicks will become imprinted on any moving object.

Several important principles emerge from the imprinting example that we should emphasize here because they illustrate the operation of similar or common processes for building brains to competently handle particular environments:

First, imprinting in precocial species seems to have a well-defined "critical period" or sensitive period just as the visual cortex does. Recent evidence (Horn, 1995) indicates that c-fos activity, which reveals the expression of immediate early genes, occurs coincident with the onset of the imprinting period and terminates with its end. Thus the genome appears to control the readiness of the brain to recognize and become attached to a particular class of visual, auditory, and somatosensory inputs (and olfactory and gustatory inputs in other species), possibly arranged in a particular configuration (which under normal conditions would make their species image the most likely target for imprinting).

Second, the fact that chicks, ducklings, and many other precocial spe-

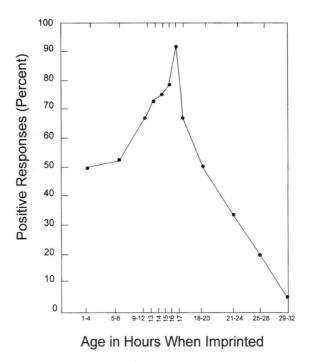

FIGURE 8.10. Critical age for laboratory imprinting in mallards. From Hess (1973). Copyright 1973 by Academic Press. Reprinted by permission.

cies will imprint on other objects indicates that a considerable portion of the information necessary to produce a typically normal adult hen or rooster, or duck or drake (etc.), resides in high-probability events that almost invariably occur in their environment. As discussed above, environmental events that are likely to occur with very high probability, which contain information critical for sculpting brain processes and therefore determining subsequent behavior, are absolutely necessary to produce normal adults. In a natural setting the first moving object that young newly hatched chicks encounter is their mother, and so a genetic tendency to follow a moving object will in all likelihood result in the brood following her. Given that auditory imprinting has been demonstrated to occur prior to hatching (Sedlacek, 1964), when presumably the hen's vocalizations set some of the filter characteristics in the chick's auditory brain structures, this could itself aid the initial species specific preference for hens. The hen's behavior itself obviously contributes substantial information to the process, as her attraction and attention to the nest and clutch serve as positive feedback, increasing the probability that she will be the object of her offspring's imprinting tendencies. Again, just as what newborn kittens, monkeys, and humans see during the critical period can influence the tuning of neurons in their visual cortex, so also are neurons in the intermediate medial hyper-striatum ventrale (IMHV), a telencephalic or forebrain structure in the chick, tuned to respond preferentially to the imprinted object.

The third principle that we wish to elucidate is that specific regions of the developing brain are involved in the imprinting process. Although there is now widespread acceptance that the brain controls all the complex be-havior and cognitive activity of animals and humans, the "folk" model that many people hold is more of the brain acting as a general processor, not unlike the central processing unit (CPU) of a computer, rather than as a large integrated collection of interacting specialized processors. With the incredible explosion of knowledge of the vertebrate brain over the past three decades, it has become clear that it consists of a large number of mod-ules that are relatively specialized in their function. Just as the structure of the body itself must proceed from the appropriate and tight timing and se-quencing of molecular and cellular events, the brain must also be morpho-logically differentiated and then programmed in the correct sequence to permit and optimize subsequent differentiation and programming of its various modules. In our imprinting example Horn (1991, 1995) has shown that individual neurons in the IMHV (shown in Figure 8.11) of the chick forebrain are intimately involved in imprinting. Neurons in this structure have been found to specifically respond to objects such as moving red boxes and blue cylinders that day-old chicks have been imprinted on. Obvi-ously, these specificities were not laid down by genetic information alone but by the interaction of the particular set of patterns presented to the chicks during the critical imprinting period, and the readiness and plasticity of this specialized area of the brain at that time. Figures 8.12 and 8.13 (Nicol, Brown, & Horn, 1995) illustrate data from some of Horn and his

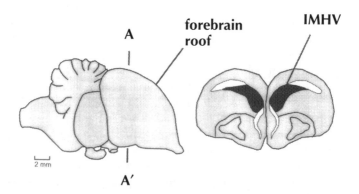

FIGURE 8.11. Drawing of the chick brain showing IMHV (the intermediate medial hyperstriatum ventrale). The vertical lines *AA'* above and below the drawing of the lateral aspect (left) indicate the plane of the coronal section outline (right) of the brain. From Johnson and Morton (1991). Copyright 1991 by Blackwell Publishers. Reprinted by permission.

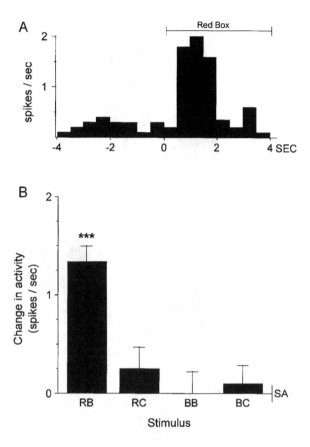

FIGURE 8.12. Excitatory response to the red box (RB) in a red box-trained chick. (A) Peristimulus time histogram of action potentials recorded at a site in the right IMHV. (B) The responsiveness of the same site to a blue cylinder (BC), a red cylinder (RC), and a blue box (BB). The response to the red box was significantly higher than this firing rate (***$p < .001$) and was significantly greater than that to any of the other stimuli ($p < .05$), indicating that neuronal activity at this site selectively signaled the presence of the training stimulus. From Nichol, Brown, and Horn (1995). Copyright 1995 by Blackwell Science Ltd. Reprinted by permission.

colleagues' experiments. Figure 8.12A shows how a neuron in IMHV increased its firing rate when presented with a red box, the moving object that the chick had been imprinted on in its "critical period." Figure 8.12B shows the selectivity of this response to the imprinted object in that increased firing of the neuron was only produced by a red box (RB) and not by a red cylinder (RC), a blue box (BB) or a blue cylinder (BC). Figure 8.13 shows that the specific type of stimulus chicks were presented with during their critical imprinting period resulted in more neurons that "preferred" that stimulus compared to dark-reared controls. Figure 8.13A shows that

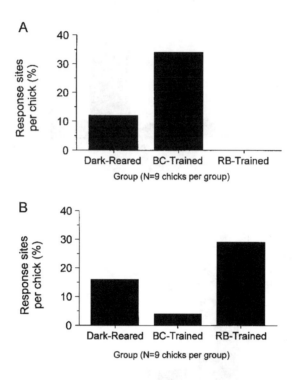

FIGURE 8.13. Selective training-induced change in responsiveness. Shown are the mean proportions of sites responsive to (A) the blue cylinder (BC) and (B) the red box (RB) in the three groups of chicks. From Nichol, Brown, and Horn (1995). Copyright 1995 by Blackwell Science Ltd. Reprinted by permission.

there were more sites in the IMHVs of chicks imprinted on a blue cylinder that preferentially responded to blue cylinders, while Figure 8.13B shows those chicks imprinted on a red box yielded more IMHV sites that specifically responded to red boxes. Interestingly, there was a clear reduction in responsiveness to the nonimprinted stimuli compared to dark-reared controls for both groups of chicks, suggesting that inhibitory processes play a vital role in producing populations of neurons specifically responsive to the imprinted object. Later we will show that other areas of the brain, or other specialized modules, likewise have their critical plastic periods, where presumably the genetic code and different high-probability environmental events interact in a dynamic pas de deux to sculpt and fashion structures to produce and control competent adult behavior.

The fourth principle to emerge from the imprinting example is that the "meaning" or functional significance of the phenomenon can only be understood by looking at the total ecological context. Thus, the critical period for imprinting evolved because the system conveyed advantage to these precocial birds in their particular ecological niche. Which sources of information are selected to reside in "the code" and which are selected to be lifted from the environmental store will obviously depend on the reliabilities and probabilities of these options and the advantages any particular solution confers to the species.

Finally, the fifth principle that emerges is that the appropriate unfolding of the developmental sequence of sensitive plastic periods and environmental tuning and programming is itself selected by the same principles of utility and evolutionary advantage that shape body structure and function. In precocial species like the domestic chickens used to illustrate mechanisms of bonding, early attachment ensures that the young follow and stay close to their mother. In this manner she can then be the agent for their subsequent development. Initially this may take the form of social imitation. Young chicks clearly engage in imitative learning, and the mother's behavior can direct their attention to features of the environment that ensure their survival. Thus, when a hen pecks at particular food objects, they are genetically programmed to do likewise, and presumably are reinforced (and programmed) by underlying neural mechanisms controlling operant behavior if they ingest nutritive items as a result. Likewise, when hens emit an alarm call for which there is a genetically determined behavioral response of freezing and/or running to the protection of the hen, the object of the mother's response become associated with fear and thus she teaches them what to be afraid of. Again it appears that this is not just standard avoidance learning, but *building on the affiliative bonding* established earlier in development, and indeed probably takes place in a different brain module, most likely the archistriatum, which may be homologous to the mammalian amygdala (which is crucial for fast emotional and motivational reactivity).

Although there is some debate about the relative potency and long-term effectiveness of these early filial bonding mechanisms that result from the aforementioned dynamic and interacting set of genetic instructions and high-probability environmental and social events, considerable evidence exists for nearly all vertebrate groups to show that they subsequently influence behavioral choices during adolescence and early adulthood. For example, Mainardi, Marsan, and Pasquali, (1965) have shown that female mice reared by perfumed parents preferentially chose perfumed to control males as mates. Likewise, lambs reared by humans tend to behave quite differently as adults and do not graze with the flock. Moreover, these effects are bidirectional and appear to influence the behavior of normally reared mature members of the group toward the early social isolate, as well as influencing the young isolates' behavior toward the flock (Klopfer & Gamble, 1966). Lorenz (1935/1970) considered imprinting a special form of learning because it appeared to have long-term effects that manifested themselves in adult sexual preferences as well as early filial attachment. While young testosterone-treated chickens and turkeys preferentially directed their courtship and sexual responses toward their imprinted objects (Bambridge, 1962; Schein & Hale, 1959), other studies have shown that under conditions of normal development adolescent experience can also be important and modify these early established preferences to some extent (Hinde, 1962, 1970). However, when there is no contact with other conspecifics between imprinting and adulthood, studies on turkeys (Schein, 1963) and pigeons (Warriner, Lemmon, & Ray, 1963) indicate that sexual preference is still powerfully directed at the imprinted object.

We have chosen to use primarily studies on precocial species where clear and early attachment to a mother or parental figure or object is easy to document and quantify by measuring following locomotor behavior. Also, we have not addressed the reciprocal question of critical or sensitive periods of attachment of mothers and parental figures of precocial birds to their offspring, a phenomenon equally striking in its robustness to the responses of the young. On the former point, there is abundant evidence available to show that early filial bonding and attachment also occurs in altricial species that have a prolonged posthatch or neonatal period of dependency before they are independently mobile (Hess, 1973; F. V. Smith, 1969).

MATERNAL BONDING

The attachment of mammalian mothers to their offspring appears to be controlled in a natural setting by a tightly orchestrated cascade of events that also results in a critical period for bonding and attachment. Klopfer's group (see Klopfer, 1971, 1988, 1996) and others, have shown that female goats are suddenly transformed from being disinterested and hostile toward kids to a nurturing caring mother immediately after parturition. Apparently the critical chain of events is cervical dilation during birth, which precipitates the release of the neuropeptide oxytocin from the hypothalamus. Then the olfactory bulb is "primed" (Kendrick, Keverne, Hinton, & Goode, 1992) and the olfactory features of her offspring are imprinted on the mother goat, so that subsequently she discriminates between her own and other kids, and dispenses care and nurturance selectively. Even artificial dilating the cervix with hydraulically inflated balloons dramatically switches virgin goats from attacking and showing hostility to kids at one moment to adopting and nurturing them minutes later. A considerable body of other research has confirmed that oxytocin release is intimately associated with filial bonding in a variety of vertebrate species and even highly correlated with different patterns of maternal behavior, including lactation, across species. Other reproductive scientists have been able to artificially transform indifferent female rodents into maternally responsive animals by injecting oxytocin into the brain near the hypothalamus.

Interestingly, oxytocin not only appears to mediate filial bonding and parental care, but it is also involved, presumably through interaction with other brain structures, with grooming sexual behavior and pair bonding. Carter (in a 1992 review) and her colleagues (J. R. Williams, Insel, Harbaugh, & Carter, 1994) have shown that in the monogamous prairie vole, oxytocin is released during physical contact and particularly after vaginal stimulation. When ovarectomized female prairie voles were injected with oxytocin and housed for 6 hours with a male partner, they preferentially chose this partner to a greater extent than did control females who had simply received artificial cerebrospinal fluid injections. The brain regions where oxytocin receptors are expressed include the prelimbic cortex, the stria terminalis, the nucleus accumbens, the midline nucleus of the thalamus, and the amygdala (Insel & Shapiro, 1992). Indeed, the amygdala appears to be essential for generating normal patterns of parental care in the prairie vole, because selective lesioning of the corticomedial area of this structure in males significantly reduced their levels of social contact and paternal behavior. Figure 8.14, taken from Kirkpatrick, Carter, Newman, and Insel (1994), shows this effect. It can be seen that lesions of the corticomedial zone of the amygdala clearly reduces the amount of time that males spend in side-by-side contact and in sniffing, grooming, and huddling in close contact with their pups, but it did not change their exploratory be-

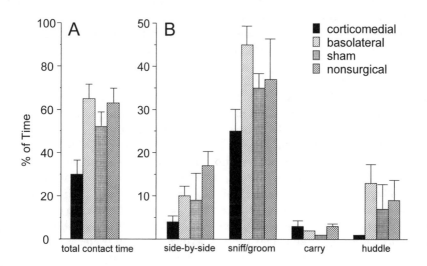

FIGURE 8.14. Parental care decreases after corticomedial but not basolateral amygdala lesions. (A) Total contact time of the four separate components from (B). From Kirkpatrick, Carter, Newman, and Insel (1994). Copyright 1994 by the American Psychological Association. Reprinted by permission.

havior, motor functions, fearfulness, performance on olfactory tasks, or general physical well-being or body temperature.

In slowly developing mammals there is also evidence that newborns and their mothers may share many of the same mechanisms of filial bonding. While in humans these effects may be masked by cultural practices and other associative learning effects that interactively reinforce and consolidate these behaviors, they nevertheless exist and indeed may drive infant and maternal behavior without the conscious awareness of the underlying causative events. In a paper on this topic M. Leon (1992) has reviewed experimental evidence that shows human neonates rapidly learn to recognize and preferentially respond to the smells, sights, and sounds of their own mother, which he suggests may indicate the operation of similar underlying neural mechanisms. Thus human newborns in the first week of life turn preferentially toward gauze pads containing the breast odor of their own mother compared to another mother's odor or to one containing cow milk odor (McFarlane, 1975; Russell, 1976). Subsequent research has shown that the appropriate pairing of tactile stimulation with a specific artificial odor is sufficient to produce a preferential turning response toward the odor source, suggesting that the nutritive reinforcement of milk is not the only reinforcer operating in this situation. Thus the findings on early human development of olfactory preferences associatively linked to parental care closely parallel findings in a variety of other species including rats, mice, deer, hamsters, gerbils, lambs, goats, and squirrel monkeys (M. Leon, 1992). The animal studies, however, permit neuroscientists to discover the underlying neural mechanisms that may be responsible for these early rapidly developed olfactory preferences that seem only to extend through the first week of life for young rats and are coincident with the period that noradrenergic neurons from the locus coeruleus project to the olfactory bulb (Shipley, Halloran, & de la Torre, 1985; Sullivan, Wilson, & Leon, 1989). Prolonged increases in dopamine may also play a role in this olfactory sensitive period since large increases have been found in the olfactory bulb after young rat pups have been stimulated with both odors and tactile stimulation (Coopersmith, 1967). These effects wane rapidly, probably marking the end of the olfactory imprinting critical or sensitive period.

Newborn human babies also appear to have a relatively mature auditory system at birth, and rapidly develop a preference for their mothers' voices. Interestingly, it appears that prenatal auditory experience can shape postnatal preferences, since DeCasper and Fifer (1980) have shown that newborns not only prefer their mother's voice but even prefer a particular narrative story their mothers have read repeatedly during pregnancy to a similar novel piece. Again, these findings are similar to those of animal studies where it has been shown that a particular area in chick forebrain is sensitive to species-specific auditory sounds during the period where auditory imprinting is optimal.

ATTACHMENT TO FACES

We have argued above that young animals' survival is dependent on recognizing their own species and in most cases their own parents or caregivers. A substantial body of evidence suggests that natural selection in higher vertebrates has resulted in the face or head having become the principal target area by which young animals recognize their mother and parents. There are probably many reasons for natural selection to have favored this part of the anatomy, including its spatial association with the voice or vocalizations, which often figure prominently as recognition markers in gregarious and social interactive species; its association with the directed attention of the head and eyes of the parent; and its association with directed nonverbal display of emotional responses. Interestingly, there is now also a substantial body of evidence to indicate that there are specific areas in the brain of a variety of species where "face stimuli" appear to be selectively processed. Although these findings were extremely controversial when they first appeared, there have been many replications in labs around the world and over a considerable range of species.

In human infants, presumably because of their quite poor visual acuity (Muir & Hains, 1993), face recognition in the first 2 months of life appears to be determined by large areas of high contrast, since the infant is incapable of resolving the finer (higher spatial frequencies) details. In fact, as we have described above, one of the necessary precursors for high-resolution vision that would enable fine details in faces to be fully resolved is the development of the initial stages of processing in the visual cortex, where we have shown that a critical period of plasticity sharpens up the feature detectors through interactive tuning by the early visual environment. However, as with findings of many other perceptual discrimination and preference capacities, newborns who are just a few hours old have been reported to exhibit more attentive tracking when following the movement of a high-contrast image of a face than when following the movement of control images where the features are scrambled (Goren, Sarty, & Wu, 1975; B. R. Johnson, Voigt, Merrill, & Atema, 1991), although this finding remains controversial (Muir, Humphrey, & Humphrey, 1994). Space limitations do not permit a full and exhaustive review of the human face recognition development here; however, the interested reader is referred to an excellent review by M. H. Johnson and Morton (1991).

Continuing our theme of specialized brain modules for processing ecologically important information, face- and head-specific neurons have been found in monkey temporal visual cortex along with other neurons that are sensitive to hands and other complex biological stimuli. Face-sensitive cells have been found clustered in columns in the inferior temporal lobe and in the banks and walls of the superior temporal sulcus (STS). Similar to the arrangement in lower parts of the visual system, where we find hierarchical connections between areas, it appears that neurons that are particularly sensitive to the identity of the face are located in the inferior temporal cortex whereas those responsive to emotional expressions, direction of gaze, and different perspective views are located in the higher STS (Hasselmo, Rolls, & Baylis, 1989; Perrett, Rolls, & Caan, 1982). For example, in Figure 8.15, taken from Perrett et al. (1982), we can see that this particular neuron recorded from the STS responded to faces but not to other arousing or interesting stimuli, or even other stimuli "with human meaning" such as a hand. The majority of "face neurons" in this study tended to give similar responses in spite of various transformations in the stimuli, as illustrated in Figure 8.16, where it can be seen that this particular cell gave very similar responses to a real face when it was both near and far, as well as the photo of the face, the same face viewed through colored filters, and when it was inverted. However, when the profile view of the face was presented, the response disappeared. In the more anterior pole of the inferior temporal cortex of monkeys, neurons have been identified that show stimulus invariant properties, including a subgroup that are view invariant; in other words, they respond to a face or specific group of faces independent of its orientation. Not only have face-sensitive cells been found in monkeys, but Kendrick and Baldwin (1987) have found similar populations of neurons in the temporal lobe of sheep that are sensitive to individual sheep faces, humans, and dogs. Figure 8.17 is taken from Kendrick and Baldwin's (1987) paper and illustrates the level of specificity for one particular neuron that responded maximally to sheep faces with large horns, less to faces of small

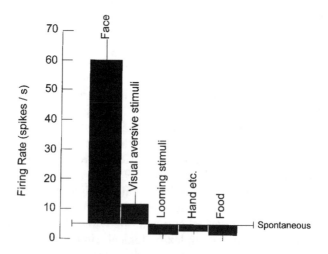

FIGURE 8.15. A comparison of the responses of one cell to the sight of faces and arousing or interesting stimuli. From Perrett, Rolls, and Caan (1982). Copyright 1982 by Springer-Verlag. Reprinted by permission.

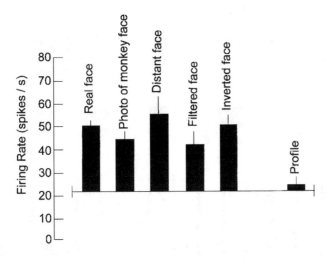

FIGURE 8.16. Responses of a face-selective neuron to transformed faces. From Perrett, Rolls, and Caan (1982). Copyright 1982 by Springer-Verlag. Reprinted by permission.

horned sheep, and not at all to humans or dogs. Taken together with the extensive work on the neural bases of imprinting and individual recognition in birds, it appears that these special processors, located in putatively homologous or similar brain regions, are either highly conserved in evolution or convergent pressures are so extreme that parallel solutions are formed.

In humans there is now very strong evidence for the existence of a very similar set of face-processing areas that has been obtained from brain damage studies where individuals with lesions in the occipitotemporal cortical region lose the ability to recognize faces (prosopagnosia). In patients undergoing brain surgery for relief of epilepsy, single-cell recording studies have also shown that the human temporal cortex contains neurons that selectively respond to human faces and facial expressions. Finally, these findings have been confirmed by positron emission tomography (PET) studies and evoked potential recording studies.

FACIAL EXPRESSIONS AND EMOTIONAL SIGNALS

Clearly the recognition of the identity and the nature of the emotional expression in a primate or human face is necessary before the appropriate social response can be produced. The amygdala receives a heavy input from these face-sensitive areas located in the inferior temporal cortex and also from many other visual auditory and somatosensory areas of the cortex, as

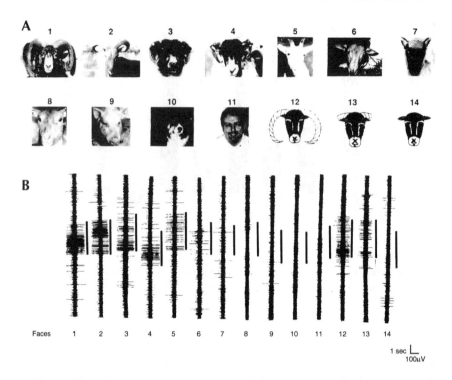

FIGURE 8.17. Responses of a sheep face-selective neuron in the temporal lobe of a sheep. (A) The facial stimuli that were used: 1, Mouflon; 2, Barbary; 3, familiar Dalesbreed; 4, unfamiliar Dalesbreed; 5, Saanen goat; 6, Welsh Mountain; 7, Clun Forrest; 8, Finn; 9, pig; 10, sheepdog; 11, human; 12, drawing of a sheep with big horns; 13, drawing of sheep with small horns; 14, drawing of sheep with no horns. (B) The responses of a single cell to the 14 facial stimuli in (A). A neuronal response was evoked by all the animals with horns, although small horns were less effective. From Kendrick and Baldwin (1987). Copyright 1987 by the American Association for the Advancement of Science. Reprinted by permission.

shown in Figure 8.18 (from Tovée, 1995). It subsequently projects its output widely to motor, autonomic, and endocrine output systems. From the pioneering work by Klüver and Bucy (1939) it is known that bilateral removal of the amygdala produces severe and permanent impairment to social and emotional behavior of monkeys, and recent evidence from a human patient with bilateral damage to her amygdala shows similar problems with reading emotional expressions from faces (Adolphs, Tranel, Damasio, & Damasio, 1994). This is illustrated in Figure 8.19 (taken from Adolphs et al., 1994), which shows that a woman (S.M.) with bilateral damage specifically to her amygdalae was seriously impaired in judging emotional expressions of faces, particularly those that portrayed surprise and fear.

While there is little evidence to date that shows the developmental his-

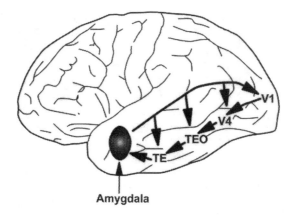

Amygdala

FIGURE 8.18. Illustration showing the relationship of the primate amygdala with the ventral stream of the visual system. Visual information is processed in hierarchical fashion from the primary visual area (V1) to the inferior temporal cortex. The amygdala receives a substantial input from the anterior inferior temporal cortex, and projections from the amygdala pass back to all visual areas: V4, visual area 4; TEO, posterior inferior temporal cortex; TE, anterior inferior temporal cortex. From Tovée (1995). Copyright 1995 by *Current Biology*. Reprinted by permission.

tory of these face-specific cells in either experimental animals or humans, it is interesting to speculate that the brain modules involved may also exhibit a sensitive period. These neurons in the inferior temporal cortex and amygdala may first require the prior development of lower feature detectors in the visual system. Then they too could be sharpened up and tuned through association with the mother's voice, odor, and tactile stimulation, so that they eventually would be involved in circuits to specifically recognize faces and the social signals semaphored through facial expressions.

MULTIPLE CRITICAL OR SENSITIVE PERIODS

How general are these critical period effects? The examples presented thus far have mainly been selected from the sense of vision, but there is no doubt that similar use-dependent selection of particular pathways and neural circuits goes on in other parts of the brain. Examples abound in other sensory pathways, including those of hearing and those of smell and touch (Brunjes, 1994). There is also strong evidence for critical periods in the development of higher cognitive functions such as language processing. For instance, the guttural sound "ch" is an important component of several languages, including Japanese, Spanish, and German, but it does not play an important role in English. During the "babbling phase" of language development in the first few years of life, all children make and use this gut-

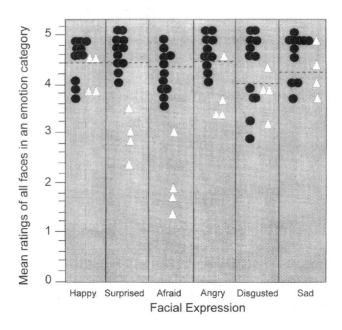

FIGURE 8.19. Emotional responses of subject S.M. with amygdala lesions, compared to those of normal subjects and subjects with brain lesions in other areas. Rating scores reflect the degree to which each subject judged the emotional adjectives to apply to photographs typical of each emotional category (0 = not very much; 5 = very much). Data are from 12 brain-damaged controls (black circles) and from 4 experiments with S.M. (white triangles). Mean ratings from 7 normal controls with no history of brain damage are denoted by the dashed lines. From Adolphs, Tranel, Damasio, and Damasio (1994). Copyright 1994 by Macmillan Magazines Ltd. Reprinted by permission from *Nature*.

tural sound, but in children who grow up in an "impoverished" environment (learning only English!) the ability to make this guttural sound is lost. At the crudest level, the expression "use it or lose it," while oversimplified, provides a strong metaphor to describe not only the use-dependent plasticity of vision but also the use-dependent plasticity of the articulatory apparatus of language.

There is abundant evidence that the best time to learn new languages is relatively early in life. Individuals who are exposed to a foreign language after they are 8–10 years old will eventually learn the foreign language, but they may never acquire the facility with this language that occurs naturally in young children. Abundant research shows that there is a time during early postnatal development when the brain is ready to accept language. The specifics of the language that is assimilated depends on the language (or languages) to which the developing brain is exposed. There is also evidence that other abilities which may be less obvious are regulated in development and show a clear critical or sensitive period during development. These can include complex motor skills such as riding a bike, or skiing, or swimming. In addition, there is strong evidence that abstract intellectual abilities such as musical and mathematical capabilities are strongly age related. By and large, if an individual mathematician has not shown flashes of great brilliance before the age of 25, then the probability is low that this individual will ever make important contributions to the discipline.

Importantly, it appears as though these critical periods that we have been studying do not occur in all parts of the developing cortex at the same time. Figure 8.20 illustrates a surface view of the cerebral cortex of the monkey. In this figure, the cerebral cortex, which is, after all, merely a crumpled sheet of tissue (about the size of a small coffee table in humans) surrounding the cerebral hemispheres, has been topologically unfolded and the many different individual cortical areas that have recently been discovered (Knierim & Van Essen, 1992) are depicted. As mentioned, there is growing evidence that not all of these areas go through their critical periods at the same time; in addition, there are suggestions that different layers of

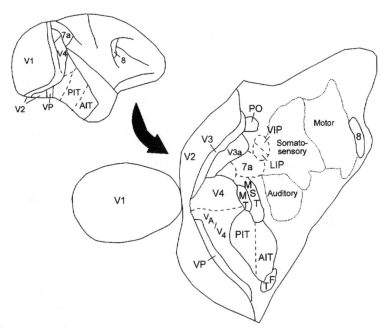

FIGURE 8.20. Surface view of flattened monkey cortex showing different processing areas. V1–V4, visual areas 1–4; MT, middle temporal area; MST, medial superior temporal area; VIP, ventral intraparietal; LIP, lateral intraparietal; PIT, posterior inferotemporal; AIT, anterior inferotemporal; PO, parietal occipital; VP, ventral posterior; TF, temporal field. Adapted from Knierim and Van Essen (1992). Original figure from Felleman and Van Essen (1991). Copyright 1991 by Oxford University Press. Adapted by permission.

the cortex may undergo critical periods at different times. Some of the cortical fields that are illustrated in Figure 8.20 show evidence of retaining plasticity even up to adulthood.

Some of the biochemical features that we have observed in the visual cortex (area V1) at one particular age are in fact present in other cortical structures only at other ages. Neuroscientists are now trying to visualize the parts of the brain that are most plastic at any given age and in particular circumstances. It is easy to imagine the implications of this visualization capacity, because it offers the opportunity to direct particular training strategies to those parts of the brain that are most ready to learn. In conjunction with emerging technologies such as functional magnetic resonance imaging (MRI), which enables us to visualize the activity of particular pieces of brain during specific tasks, it may become possible in the intermediate term to direct particular training and exercise to those parts of the brain that are most ready to accept it at any given age.

STRESS AND CRITICAL PERIODS

Stress can take many forms: it may be physical, resulting from prolonged exposure to cold or inescapable pain; or it may be mental, resulting from having a supervisor that doesn't value you as an employee, a spouse who nags you, or the general feeling of powerlessness that comes from being unable to control your own destiny. In the presence of short-term stressors, the body mounts an organized and normally effective response. A complex cascade of events controlled by the brain results in secretion of a series of releasing factors and hormones that increase the heart rate, alter the processing of glucose, dilate the pupils, and—stated most generally—prepare the body to meet that tiger lurking in the bushes or the slings and arrows of everyday corporate life. We need the short-term stress response in order to catch that bus that is moving away from us and to evade that tiger. However, while there is no question the short-term response of the body to stress is beneficial and necessary, there is growing evidence that long-term stress and the body's response to it is counterproductive and deleterious. The deleterious effects are seen both inside and outside the brain. First, a large body of literature has now shown that chronic stress can cause depression of the immune function, as well as other body systems that are controlled by the brain such as the cardiovascular system. Second, chronic stress has a deleterious effect on brain function. There is evidence that repeated and prolonged exposure to stress hormones causes neurons to die. Subjecting animals to chronic stress (e.g., by forcing them to endure inescapable shocks), results in cell death in various parts of the brain (Sapolsky, 1992). Interestingly, emerging evidence suggests that neurons in the brain that are most ready to learn (i.e., those that are within their critical periods) are the most vulnerable to the cell death and degeneration associated with chronic stress. As we know, the cortical plasticity of the critical period is due to a biochemical architecture within the cortex and to the expression of genes within individual neurons. This pattern of biochemistry and gene expression renders neurons ready to learn and alter their connectivity based on usage. Unfortunately it also appears to make them more vulnerable to the catabolic effects of stress hormones. This is an important point, because it suggests that the most plastic neurons will be those that will be most vulnerable to chronic stress.

In addition, stress and critical periods interact in another way. There is evidence (summarized in Chapters 2, 3, and 9, this volume) that the stresses to which we are exposed early in life, during a critical period, may modify our ability to modulate and control responses to stressors later on in life. There is evidence that rats that are subjected to mild stresses as neonates (e.g., by being handled repeatedly) show lesser, more controllable stress responses when tested as adults than do animals that have not been handled as infants. There thus appears to be a critical period for gaining effective neural control over the stress response.

GENERAL CONCLUSIONS

The skills, abilities, dreams, and prejudices that make up each individual result from the genetic history of the individual organism and also from the particular environmental stimuli, both physical and social, to which that organism was exposed. The feature analyzing and processing capabilities of the cortex are shaped by the input that it receives during particular critical periods early in development. Critical periods have been most extensively studied in imprinting and in sensory systems, but there is evidence for their role in higher brain functions as well. Even early sensory defects may cause devastating consequences for so-called higher functions. For instance, if a child cannot see well early in life because of uncorrected astigmatism, then later on there may well be reading difficulties in that same child. A child who cannot read is disadvantaged in learning relative to other children in his/her peer group. This can lead to low self-esteem and to a child who is turned off to school. Such a child is much more vulnerable to a large variety of poor outcomes including early pregnancy, low-wage employment, or unemployment—and therefore, as other chapters in this volume make clear, to poor health and enhanced mortality. Similarly, early auditory defects caused by transient episodes of otitis media may result in poor language acquisition. Poor verbal skills can lead to the same sort of deleterious cascade that is described above. We argue that inadequate and inappropriate social and emotional experiences in the early environment could likewise result in compromised higher level neural systems whose task is to provide information necessary to bond, imitate, and generally respond in socially appropriate ways. The best current strategies to prevent these deleterious cascades are to create sufficiently enriched environments so that critical period developments proceed optimally, or to diagnose problems early and attempt therapy promptly. A more ambitious long-term goal is to re-create the plasticity of the critical period in the older organism and then to try to cure long-standing deficits.

ACKNOWLEDGMENTS

Max Cynader is the Bank of Montreal Fellow, and Barrie Frost is the Max Bell Fellow of the Canadian Institute for Advanced Research. We wish to thank Ms. Sharon David for considerable help in preparing the manuscript.

9

Developmental Trajectories, Early Experiences, and Community Consequences

LESSONS FROM STUDIES WITH RHESUS MONKEYS

Stephen J. Suomi

PRIMATE COMMUNITY LIFE

A fundamental feature of virtually all advanced primates is their inherent sociality. Like humans, most monkeys and apes spend most (if not all) of their lives as members of distinctive communities of conspecifics, each typically characterized by complex kinship and status-defined social relationships (Novak & Suomi, 1991). These primate communities often encompass three or more generations within individual family units and usually retain their basic identity long beyond the lifespan of any one community member or generation of members. In most primate species the relationships between individual family members, between families within a given community, and even between different communities are far from static, and dramatic changes in each type of relationship can and do occur, often with long-term consequences for all involved. Yet even after events or episodes that result in major social disruption, most surviving individuals, families, and communities quickly return to species-normative patterns of social interactions, relationships, and overall group organization (Suomi, 1999).

An illustrative example of the complex and dynamic nature of primate social group life has been provided by extensive studies of rhesus monkeys (*Macaca mulatta*). Although rhesus monkeys are clearly not closest to us phylogenetically (that role falls to chimpanzees and bonobos—once called pygmy chimpanzees), in evolutionary terms they are probably our most successful primate relatives. Next to humans, rhesus monkeys live over a wider geographic range, encompassing a broader mix of climatic and habitat variation, than does any other species of primates with one or two possible exceptions. While the majority of nonhuman primate species are currently classified as endangered or threatened, some with rapidly dwindling natural populations for which almost certain extinction is forecast in the near future, rhesus monkeys are actually expanding their local populations in certain parts of their extensive range. They also thrive in a wide variety of captive environments and have long had a reputation for being unusually robust laboratory subjects (Novak & Suomi, 1991).

Although rhesus monkey communities in natural habitats vary widely in size, ranging from a few dozen to several hundred individuals, the basic social structure of each of these distinctive communities—termed "troops"—is remarkably similar from setting to setting. Rhesus monkey troops are always organized around multigenerational matrilines, that is, female-headed extended families. All troops, large and small alike, are composed of two or more separate matrilines, each encompassing three or more generations of close female kin. The long-term stability of these matrilines (and, indeed, of the troop as a distinctive whole) derives from the fact that all females remain in their natal troop throughout their entire lifetime, whereas virtually all males emigrate around the time of puberty (Lindburg, 1971). After leaving home, most adolescent males first briefly congregate in all-male gangs, then attempt to join other established troops. Some of the males who are successful in these efforts remain in their "new" troop for the rest of their lives, whereas others stay no more than a few years and then leave to seek membership in other established troops, sometimes repeating this pattern several times throughout their adult years (Berard, 1989).

It is thus the adult females and their female progeny who provide the long-term foundation for rhesus monkey communities. To be sure, every rhesus monkey troop contains numerous males of all ages—but troop membership for any one male is typically transitory, while it is always lifelong for all females. This is not to say that males play insignificant roles in rhesus monkey social group life; to the contrary, their presence is essential for the long-term survival of the troop as a whole. Nevertheless, it is the female matrilines around which most of the social activities of the troop are organized and the underlying social structure of the troop is defined and maintained.

A second feature characteristic of all rhesus monkey troops involves their multiple dominance hierarchies (Sade, 1967). To begin, there is a clear-cut linear hierarchy among the troop's different matrilines, such that all members of the highest-ranking matriline, including infants, are socially dominant over all members of the second-ranking matriline, including adults, who in turn outrank all members of the third-ranking matriline, etc. Such a hierarchy can be maintained only as long as all members of a matriline consistently support any member who is challenged by someone from a lower-ranking matriline, as when adult members of a high-ranking matriline come to the immediate defense of one of their infants whenever it is threatened or attacked by a nonfamily member. Another hierarchy can be found within each matriline; it follows the general rule that younger sisters outrank older sisters. Such status differences among female siblings most likely have their origin in the mother's consistent preferential defense of her female infant in the face of harassment by jealous older sisters; curiously, such status differences tend to remain remarkably stable throughout the rest of the sisters' respective lifetimes. A third hierarchy exists among the males that immigrate into the troop. Although male status superficially seems related to relative tenure (i.e., the longer a male has been in a troop, the more likely he is to be high in rank), in fact it appears to be more a function of the male's skills in joining and maintaining coalitions, not only with other males but with high-ranking females in the troop as well.

Rhesus monkeys are status seekers by nature, and a substantial proportion of their social activity is directed toward efforts to advance their own status in some troop hierarchies and/or to maintain their current status in others. However, it seems clear that social status in a rhesus monkey troop is less a function of an individual's relative size or strength than who its friends and relatives happen to be. Indeed, the complex familial and dominance relationships that characterize every rhesus monkey troop seemingly require any functioning troop member to have some knowledge of most if not all other members' specific kinship and dominance status—and to utilize such knowledge—in order to survive, let along thrive, in everyday troop life. How might such knowledge be acquired, maintained, and utilized in generation after generation of monkeys born into the troop? An impressive body of both laboratory and field data strongly suggests that it is an emergent consequence of the species-normative pattern of socialization that rhesus monkey infants experience as they grow up in their natal troops (Sameroff & Suomi, 1996). A description of this species-normative pattern follows.

DEVELOPMENTAL ASPECTS OF RHESUS MONKEY SOCIALIZATION

Rhesus monkey infants spend virtually all of their first weeks of life in physical contact with or within arm's reach of their biological mother, who provides them with nourishment, physical and psychological warmth, and protection from the elements, potential predators, and pesky older siblings. During this time a strong and enduring social bond inevitably develops between the mother and infant, recognized by Bowlby (1969) to be homologous with the mother–infant attachment relationship universally seen in all human cultures, the product of diverse evolutionary pressures over millions of years.

Rhesus monkey infants are also inherently curious, and like human infants, once they have become attached to their mother they quickly learn to use her as a secure base from which to organize the exploration of their physical and social environment (Harlow & Harlow, 1965). Unlike human infants, rhesus monkey infants are sufficiently precocious in their locomotor capabilities to be able to wander considerable distances away from their mother before the end of their first month of life (by comparison, weaning typically takes place during the fourth and fifth postnatal month). They are therefore physically capable of stumbling into potentially life-threatening situations from their second month on, and initially most monkey mothers spend considerable time and effort monitoring and often physically restricting their infant's early exploratory efforts (Hansen, 1966; Hinde & Spencer-Booth, 1967). However, in succeeding weeks the rhesus monkey equivalent of human stranger anxiety emerges in the infants' behavioral repertoire (G. P. Sackett, 1966), and thereafter it is the infant who is largely responsible for maintaining proximity to its mother (Hinde & White, 1974).

The usual result of this sequence—attachment formation, emerging exploratory tendencies (curiosity), and maturation of the capacity for developing social fears—is that rhesus monkey infants come to use their mother as a home base for virtually all of their environmental exploration. As they grow older these young monkeys are able and willing to spend increasing amounts of time at increasing distances from their mother, secure in the knowledge that whenever they become frightened or tired they will be able to return to her protective care without interruption or delay on her part. The presence of such a psychologically secure base clearly promotes exploration of both physical and social aspects of their immediate environment. On the other hand, when a rhesus monkey infant develops a less than optimal attachment relationship with its mother, its subsequent exploratory behavior is inevitably compromised, just as John Bowlby and other attachment theorists have described for human infants and young children (Suomi, 1995).

At any rate, during the course of their early exploratory forays away from their mother rhesus monkey youngsters inevitably come into contact with other troop members, including infants of similar age from other matrilines who have comparable physical, cognitive, and social capabilities as themselves. Interactions with these agemates begin to occur with increasing frequency in their third and fourth months of life, such that by the time of weaning most rhesus monkey youngsters are typically spending several hours each day playing with peers (Harlow & Harlow, 1965). These peer interactions continue to increase in both frequency and complexity throughout the rest of the monkeys' first year, and they tend to remain at high levels up to the onset of puberty (Ruppenthal, Harlow, Eisele,

Harlow, & Suomi, 1974). During this time the play patterns that dominate peer interactions become increasingly gender specific and sex segregated (i.e., males tend to play more with males, and females with females; Harlow & Lauersdorf, 1974). Moreover, these extended play bouts begin to encompass behavioral sequences that increasingly resemble prototypical adult social interaction patterns. As a result, by the end of their third year most rhesus monkey juveniles have had ample opportunity to develop, practice, and perfect activities that will be crucial for normal functioning when they become adults. Among the most important lessons learned through such play with peers is the appropriate expression—and control—of emerging aggressive capabilities, as well as knowledge about and respect for the various dominance hierarchies within the troop (Suomi, 1979).

The onset of puberty occurs for females near the end of their third year, when they have their initial menses (and regular 28-day menstrual cycles thereafter), and around the beginning of the fourth year for males, when their testes enlarge and begin to produce viable sperm. Adolescence in rhesus monkeys is associated not only with a pronounced growth spurt and altered hormonal activity but also with major social changes for both sexes. The biggest change occurs for adolescent males: during adolescence, they sever all ties with their matriline and emigrate out of their natal troop. Most of these males soon join "gangs" comprising of other adolescent and young adult males, and they typically remain in these all-male groups for at least several months before attempting to join another rhesus monkey troop. Field data have clearly shown that the process of natal troop emigration represents an exceedingly dangerous transition for adolescent males: the mortality rate for these males from the time they leave their natal troop until they have successfully joined another one approaches 50% (Dittus, 1979). Recent field studies have also revealed major individual differences in both the timing of male emigration and the basic strategy followed in attempting to enter an unfamiliar troop. Moreover, as already mentioned, once they have successfully joined a new troop, some males stay in that troop for the rest of their life, whereas others subsequently switch troops, often several times, although even these males never go back to their natal troop (Suomi, Rasmussen, & Higley, 1992).

Females, by contrast, never leave their natal troop. Puberty for rhesus monkey females is instead associated with increases in social activities directed toward their matrilinear kin, generally at the expense of interactions with peers. Kin-directed interactions are heightened even more when these young females begin to have offspring of their own. Indeed, the birth of a new infant (especially to a new mother) has the effect of invigorating the rest of the matriline, drawing its members closer both physically and socially and, conversely, providing a buffer from external threats and stressors for the new mother and infant. As they age, rhesus monkey females continue to be actively involved in family social affairs, even after they cease having infants of their own (Suomi, 1995).

INDIVIDUAL DIFFERENCES IN RHESUS MONKEY BIOBEHAVIORAL DEVELOPMENT

While the pattern of behavioral development described above is generally characteristic of rhesus monkeys growing up both in natural troops in the wild and in social groups maintained in captivity, there are nevertheless substantial differences among individual troop members in the precise timing and relative ease with which they make major developmental transitions, as well as how they manage the day-to-day challenges and stresses that are an inevitable consequence of complex social group life. In particular, recent research has identified two subgroups of individuals who tend to follow aberrant developmental trajectories that can potentially result in increased long-term risk for behavioral pathology and even mortality. Members of one subgroup, comprising approximately 15–20% of both wild and captive populations, consistently respond to novel and/or mildly challenging situations with extreme behavioral disruption and pronounced physiological arousal. Whereas most other monkeys typically find novel stimuli interesting and will readily explore them, usually with minimal physiological arousal, "high-reactive" individuals instead prefer to avoid such stimuli and, if that is not possible, they frequently react with obvious behavioral expressions of fear and anxiety and with significant (and often prolonged) activation of the hypothalamic–pituitary–adrenal (HPA) axis, sympathetic nervous system arousal, and increased noradrenergic turnover (Suomi, 1986).

High-reactive monkeys can be readily identified in their first few months of life. Most begin leaving their mothers later chronologically and explore their physical and social environment less than do other infants in their birth cohort. High-reactive youngsters also tend to be shy and withdrawn in their initial encounters with peers; laboratory studies have shown that they exhibit significantly higher and more stable heart rates and greater secretion of cortisol in such interactions than do their less reactive cohorts. However, when these individuals are in familiar and stable settings they are virtually indistinguishable, both behaviorally and physiologically, from others in their peer group. On the other hand, when high-reactive monkeys encounter extreme and/or prolonged stress, their behavioral and physiological differences from others in their social group usually become exaggerated (Suomi, 1991a).

For example, rhesus monkey juveniles inevitably experience functional maternal separations during the 2-month-long annual breeding season when their mothers repeatedly leave the troop for brief periods to consort with selected males (Berman, Rasmussen, & Suomi, 1994). The departure of its mother clearly represents a major social stressor for any young monkey and, not surprisingly, virtually all youngsters initially react to their mother's departure with short-term behavioral agitation and physiological arousal, much as Bowlby (1960, 1973) has described for human infants experiencing involuntary maternal separation. However, whereas most juveniles soon begin to adapt to the separation and readily seek out the company of others in their social group, high-reactive individuals typically lapse into a behavioral depression characterized by increasing lethargy, lack of apparent interest in social stimuli, eating and sleeping difficulties, and a characteristic hunched-over, fetal posture (Suomi, 1991b). Laboratory studies simulating these naturalistic maternal separations have shown that relative to their like-reared peers, high-reactive individuals not only are more likely to exhibit depressive-like behavioral reactions to short-term social separation but also tend to show greater and more prolonged HPA activation, more dramatic sympathetic arousal, more rapid central noradrenergic turnover, and greater immunosuppression (Suomi, 1991a). These differential patterns of biobehavioral response to separation tend to remain remarkably stable throughout prepubertal development and may even be maintained in adolescence and adulthood (Suomi, 1995). An increasing body of evidence has demonstrated significant heritability for these differences (e.g., Higley et al., 1993).

Recent field studies have shown that high-reactive rhesus monkey males usually emigrate from their natal troop at significantly older ages than those of the rest of their adolescent male cohort and, when they do finally leave their home troop, they typically employ much more conservative strategies for entering a new troop than do their less-reactive peers (Suomi et al., 1992). Laboratory research has shown that high-reactive young females are much more likely to exhibit inadequate care of their firstborn offspring than are other primiparous mothers (Suomi & Ripp, 1983). Thus, high reactivity appears to be associated with increased lifetime risk for a variety of biobehavioral problems.

A second subgroup of rhesus monkeys, comprising approximately 5–10% of the population, tend to be highly impulsive in their social interactions, especially those that involve aggression. Such impulsive individuals, male and female alike, also tend to have chronically low central serotonin metabolism, as reflected in unusually low cerebrospinal fluid (CSF) concentrations of the primary central serotonin metabolite 5-hydroxyindoleacetic acid (5-HIAA). These behavioral and neurochemical characteristics emerge early in life and are notably stable throughout development, as was the case for high-reactive monkeys. Impulsive individuals, especially males, seem to be unable to moderate their behavioral responses to rough-and-tumble play initiations from peers, and they often escalate initially benign play bouts into full-blown, tissue-damaging aggressive exchanges, disproportionately at their own expense (Higley, Linnoila, & Suomi, 1994). Impulsive juvenile males also show a propensity for making dangerous leaps from treetop to treetop, sometimes with painful outcomes (Mehlman et al., 1994).

Recent field studies have found that impulsive males are often permanently expelled from their natal troop prior to puberty, long before most of their male cohort begins the normal emigration process (Mehlman et al.,

1995). These males tend to be grossly incompetent socially and, lacking the requisite social skills necessary for successful entrance into another troop, most of them become solitary and typically perish within a year (Higley, Mehlman, et al., 1996). Hence, few if any of these males are likely to contribute to any troop's gene pool. Young females who have chronically low CSF levels of 5-HIAA also tend to be rather incompetent socially. However, unlike the males, they are not typically expelled from their natal troop (or even from their matriline) at any point during their lifetime, although studies of captive rhesus monkey groups suggest that these females usually remain at the bottom of their respective dominance hierarchies (Higley, King, et al., 1996). While most soon become mothers, recent research suggests that their maternal behavior often leaves much to be desired. In sum, rhesus monkeys who exhibit excessive impulsive and aggressive behavior (and who have low central serotonin turnover) early in life tend to follow developmental trajectories that often result in premature death for males and chronically low social dominance and poor parenting for females.

EFFECTS OF DIFFERENTIAL EARLY SOCIAL EXPERIENCE ON RHESUS MONKEY DEVELOPMENTAL TRAJECTORIES

Although considerable evidence from both field and laboratory studies has shown that individual differences among rhesus monkeys in stress reactivity and impulsivity tend to be quite stable from infancy to adulthood and are at least in part heritable, this does not mean that these behavioral and physiological features are necessarily fixed at birth or are immune to subsequent environmental influence. To the contrary, an increasing body of evidence from laboratory studies has clearly demonstrated that prototypical patterns of biobehavioral response to environmental novelty and stress can be modified substantially by certain early experiences, particularly those involving early social attachment relationships.

One set of studies has focused on rhesus monkey infants raised with peers instead of by mothers. These infants are permanently separated from their biological mothers at birth, hand-reared in a neonatal nursery for their first month of life, housed with same-aged, like-reared peers for the rest of their first 6 months, and then moved into larger social groups containing both peer-reared and mother-reared agemates. During their initial months these infants readily develop strong social attachment bonds to each other, much as mother-reared infants develop attachment relationships with their own mothers (Harlow, 1969). However, because peers are not nearly as effective as is a typical monkey mother in reducing fear in the face of novelty or stress, or in providing a "secure base" for exploration, the attachment relationships that these peer-reared infants develop are almost always "anxious" in nature. As a consequence, while peer-reared monkeys show completely normal physical and motor development, their early exploratory behavior is somewhat limited. They seem reluctant to approach novel objects, and they tend to be shy in initial encounters with unfamiliar peers. Moreover, even when they interact with their same-aged cagemates in familiar settings, their emerging social play repertoires are usually retarded both in frequency and complexity. One explanation for their relatively poor play performance is that their cagemates must serve as both attachment objects and playmates, a dual role that neither mothers nor mother-reared peers have to serve. It is also difficult, if not impossible, to develop sophisticated play repertoires with basically incompetent play partners. Perhaps as a result, peer-reared youngsters typically drop to the bottom of their respective dominance hierarchies when they are grouped with mother-reared monkeys their own age, and they usually stay at the bottom of the hierarchy as long as these mixed groups remain intact (Suomi, 1995).

In addition, throughout development peer-reared monkeys consistently exhibit more extreme behavioral, adrenocortical, and noradrenergic reactions to social separations than do their mother-reared cohorts, even after they have been living in the same social groups for extended periods (Higley & Suomi, 1989). Such differences in prototypical biobehavioral reactions to separation persist from infancy to adolescence, if not beyond. Interestingly, the general nature of the separation reactions of peer-reared monkeys seems to mirror that of "naturally occurring" high-reactive mother-reared subjects. In this sense, early peer rearing appears to have the effect of making rhesus monkey infants generally more highly reactive than they might have been if reared by their biological mother (Suomi, 1997).

Early peer-rearing has another long-term developmental consequence for rhesus monkeys—it tends to make them more impulsive, especially if they are males. Like the previously described impulsive monkeys growing up in the wild, peer-reared males initially exhibit aggressive tendencies in the context of juvenile play, and as they approach puberty the frequency and severity of their aggressive episodes typically exceed that of mother-reared group members of similar age. As adults, peer-reared females tend to groom (and be groomed by) others in their social group less frequently and for shorter durations than do (and are) their mother-reared counterparts and, as before, they usually stay at the bottom of their respective dominance hierarchies. These differences between peer-reared and mother-reared agemates in aggression, grooming, and dominance remain relatively robust when the monkeys are subsequently moved into newly formed social groups, and they generally are quite stable throughout the preadolescent and adolescent years (Higley, Suomi, & Linnoila, 1996). Peer-reared monkeys also consistently show lower CSF concentrations of 5-HIAA than do their mother-reared counterparts. These group differences in 5-HIAA concentrations appear well before 6 months of age, they persist during the transition to mixed-group housing, and they remain stable at least throughout adolescence and into early adulthood. Thus, peer-reared monkeys as a group resemble the impulsive subgroup of wild-living (and mother-reared) monkeys not only behaviorally but also in terms of decreased serotonergic functioning (Suomi, 1997).

An additional risk that peer-reared females carry into adulthood concerns their maternal behavior. Peer-reared mothers are significantly more likely to exhibit neglectful and/or abusive treatment of their firstborn offspring than are their mother-reared counterparts, although their risk for inadequate maternal care is not nearly as great as is the case for females reared in social isolation; moreover, their care of subsequent offspring tends to improve dramatically (Ruppenthal, Arling, Harlow, Sackett, & Suomi, 1976). Nevertheless, most multiparous mothers who experienced early peer rearing continue to exhibit nonnormative developmental changes in ventral contact with their offspring throughout the whole of their reproductive years (Champoux, Byrne, Delizio, & Suomi, 1992).

In summary, early peer rearing seems to make rhesus monkey infants both more highly reactive and more impulsive, and their resulting developmental trajectories not only resemble those of naturally occurring subgroups of rhesus monkeys growing up in the wild but also persist in that vein long after their period of exclusive exposure to peers has been completed and they have been living in more species-typical social groups. Indeed, some effects of early peer rearing may well be passed on to the next generation via aberrant patterns of maternal care, as appears to be the case for both high-reactive and impulsive mothers rearing infants in their natural habitat (Suomi & Levine, 1998). As noted by John Bowlby and other attachment theorists for the human case, the effects of inadequate early social attachments may be both lifelong and cross-generational in nature.

What about the opposite situation: are there any consequences, either short or long term, of *enhanced* early social attachment relationships for rhesus monkeys? A recent series of studies attempted to address this question by rearing rhesus monkey neonates selectively bred for differences in temperamental reactivity with foster mothers who differed in their characteristic maternal "style," as determined by their patterns of care of previous offspring. In this work specific members of a captive breeding colony were selectively bred to produce offspring who, on the basis of their genetic pedigree, were either unusually highly reactive or within the normal range of reactivity. These selectively bred infants were then cross-fostered to unrelated multiparous females preselected to be either unusually nurturant with respect to attachment-related behavior or within the normal range of maternal care of previous offspring. The selectively bred infants were then reared by their respective foster mothers for their first 6 months of life, after which they were moved to larger social groups containing other cross-fostered agemates, as well as those reared by their biological mother (Suomi, 1987).

During the period of cross-fostering, control infants (i.e., those whose pedigrees suggested normative patterns of reactivity) exhibited essentially normal patterns of biobehavioral development, independent of the relative nurturance of their foster mother. In contrast, dramatic differences emerged among genetically high-reactive infants as a function of their type of foster mother: whereas high-reactive infants cross-fostered by control females exhibited expected deficits in early exploration and exaggerated responses to minor environmental perturbations, high-reactive infants cross-fostered to nurturant females actually appeared to be behaviorally precocious. They left their mothers earlier, explored their environment more, and displayed less behavioral disturbance during weaning than not only the high-reactive infants cross-fostered to control mothers but even the control infants reared by either type of foster mother. Their attachment relationships with their nurturant foster mothers thus appeared to be unusually secure.

When these monkeys were permanently separated from their foster mothers and moved into larger social groups at 6 months of age, additional temperament–rearing interaction effects appeared, marked by optimal outcomes for those high-reactive youngsters who had been reared by nurturant foster mothers. These individuals became especially adept at recruiting and retaining other group members as allies during agonistic encounters and, perhaps as a consequence, most rose to and maintained top positions in their group's dominance hierarchy. In contrast, high-reactive youngsters who had been foster-reared by control females tended to drop to and remain at the bottom of the same hierarchies (Suomi, 1991a).

Finally, some of the cross-fostered females from this study have since become mothers themselves, and their maternal behavior toward their firstborn offspring has been assessed. It appears that these young mothers have adapted the general maternal style of their foster mothers, independent of both their own original reactivity profile and the type of maternal style shown by their biological mother. Thus, the apparent benefits accrued by high-reactive females raised by nurturant foster mothers can seemingly be transmitted to the next generation of offspring, even though the mode of transmission is clearly nongenetic in nature (Suomi & Levine, 1998). Clearly, high reactivity need not always be associated with adverse outcomes. Instead, following certain early experiences high-reactive infants appear to have relatively normal, if not actually optimal, long-term developmental trajectories, which, in turn, can be amenable to cross-generational transmission. Whether the same possibilities exist for genetically impulsive rhesus monkey infants is currently the focus of ongoing research.

These and other findings from studies with monkeys demonstrate that differential early social experiences can have major long-term influences on an individual's behavioral and physiological propensities over and above any heritable predispositions. The nature of early attachment experiences appears to be especially relevant: whereas insecure early attachments tend to make monkeys more reactive and impulsive, unusually secure early attachments seem to have essentially the opposite effect, at least for some individuals. In either case, how a rhesus monkey mother rears her infant can markedly affect its biobehavioral developmental trajectory, even long after its interactions with her have ceased (as is always the case for males living in the wild).

MATERNAL BEHAVIOR AND TROOP DEMOGRAPHICS

Numerous studies carried out over the past 30 years have demonstrated that most rhesus monkeys mothers, no matter what their characteristic maternal style might be, are usually highly sensitive to those aspects of their immediate physical and social environment that pose a potential threat to their infant's well-being, and they appear to adjust their maternal behavior accordingly (see Higley & Suomi, 1986). For example, both laboratory and field studies have consistently shown that low-ranking mothers typically are much more restrictive of their infant's exploratory efforts than are high-ranking mothers, whose maternal style tends to be more "laissez-faire." The standard interpretation of these findings has been that low-ranking mothers risk reprisal from others if they try to intervene whenever their infant is threatened, so they minimize such risk by restricting their infant's exploration. High-ranking mothers usually have no such problem; hence, they can afford to let their infant explore as it pleases.

Other studies have found that mothers generally become more restrictive and increase their levels of infant monitoring when their immediate social environment becomes less stable, such as when major changes in dominance hierarchies take place or when a new male tries to join the social group. Changes in various aspects of the physical environment, such as the food supply becoming less predictable, have also been associated with increases in maternal restriction of early infant exploration. For those infants whose opportunities to explore are chronically limited during their first few months of life, their ability to develop species-normative relationships with others in their social group, especially peers, can be compromised, often with long-term consequences for both the infants and the troop.

The extent to which mothers' rearing styles can affect not only their offspring but also their troop as a whole can be seen in a long-term study by Berman, Rasmussen, and Suomi (1997) of free-ranging monkey troops living on Cayo Santiago, an island off the eastern coast of Puerto Rico, where rhesus monkeys were first introduced more than 50 years ago and have been thriving ever since. This particular population, like many on the Indian subcontinent, has been steadily growing in number over the past few decades, as reflected in the tendency of individual troops to increase in number of residents over time—but only up to a point, after which each troop typically fissions into several smaller "splinter" troops (Kessler, 1989).

Berman et al. (1997) found that in small troops mothers generally tended to be laissez-faire in their maternal style relative to mothers living in troops with larger populations. Mothers in small troops rarely restricted their infants' early exploratory efforts, seldom intervened in their subsequent social activities, and indeed spent relatively little time monitoring their behavior after weaning. In turn, their infants actively sought out peers from neighboring matrilines and spent increasing amounts of time in mutual play bouts as they were growing up. These youngsters typically established strong, positive social relationships with their nonkin peers prior to puberty, and those positive relationships tended to be maintained, at least among the females, throughout adolescence and into adulthood. Perhaps not surprisingly, Berman et al. (1997) found these small troops to be quite cohesive and relatively peaceful, at least with respect to relations between matrilines within each troop.

However, in succeeding years most of these small troops increased in population, one result of which was an increase in the relative density of nonkin (i.e., members of other matrilines) within each mother's effective social "space" (which Berman and colleagues operationally defined as activity within a 5-meter radius of the mother, a well-established metric in the rhesus monkey field literature). As this "crowding" ratio of nonkin to kin within this space increased, so did these mothers' propensity to restrict their infants' exploration, intervene in their social activities, and indeed monitor their every move. As a result, their infants had fewer opportunities to seek out agemates from other matrilines, and when they did manage to interact with these nonkin peers their play bouts were often truncated by the mothers' interventions. The play that did occur tended to be less frequent, briefer in duration, and less positive in affective tone than was the case when the troop had been smaller. These youngsters thus did not have the same opportunities to develop extensive social relationships with peers from other families during their juvenile years as did their counterparts from earlier cohorts. Moreover, their relations with nonkin did not markedly improve as they grew older, remaining relatively infrequent and often hostile by the time they became adults. Not surprisingly, Berman et al. (1997) found that the general atmosphere within these now-larger troops was more tense and involved less cooperation between matrilines than in previous years when the population per troop was substantially lower.

As these troops continued to grow in population, the ratio of nonkin to kin within each mother's effective social space likewise increased and mothers tended to become even more vigilant in their efforts to restrict their infant's exploration and social interaction opportunities, to the point where almost all of their offspring's play and affiliative activities were limited to partners within their matriline. The few interactions a youngster might have with peers from other families were mostly negative in nature, with aggression the rule rather than the exception, as when the troop had been smaller in population. These negative interactions with nonfamily members generally were continued into adulthood, adding to the overall tension and lack of cohesion characteristic of these larger troops.

Berman et al. (1997) found that in time each of these large troops broke up, usually after an episode of intense interfamily aggression. The breakup always occurred along matrilines, inevitably resulting in several small "splinter" troops that quickly developed their own distinctive individual identity. Of great interest was the finding that within each new splinter group the ratio of nonkin to kin within each mother's effective social space dropped to levels comparable to those of the original troop back in the days when it was still relatively small. As before, mothers in these new, small splinter troops tended to be laissez-faire in their respective maternal styles, and once again their offspring developed extensive, basically positive play partnerships with peers from other families within each splinter troop. However, as these small splinter troops started expanding in population themselves, the mothers once more began restricting their infants' social world, starting the cycle anew.

The findings of Berman et al. (1997) provide powerful evidence that rhesus monkey mothers are indeed capable of adjusting their maternal behavior to deal with changes in their troop's social demographic characteristics. But the larger lesson from this study is that these mother's adaptations had important long-term consequences not only for their offspring but also for the basic identity of the troop as a whole. This case demonstrates that while changes at the community level can affect interactions between specific dyads, changes in those individual social relationships can ultimately influence the nature of the community itself. Thus, at least for rhesus monkeys living in groups that grow in size over time, individual relationships and community characteristics appear to be inextricably linked in a system involving long-term reciprocal feedback.

IMPLICATIONS FOR THE STUDY
OF HUMAN DEVELOPMENT

This chapter has summarized findings from many years of studies investigating biobehavioral development in rhesus monkeys. These studies have described species-normative patterns of development that unfold across a wide range of field and captive environments, characterized variations in developmental trajectories that appear to persist across multiple generations, demonstrated the influence of early social experiences on both short- and long-term outcomes of these different developmental trajectories, and uncovered a complex and dynamic relationship between demographic aspects of a community and interactions at the level of individual mother–infant dyads within the community. What implications might these findings have for advancing our understanding of human development?

One must begin with the caveat that rhesus monkeys are clearly not furry little humans with tails but instead are only close phylogenetic relatives who share much of our genetic heritage but lack certain capabilities, for example, spoken and written language, that make us uniquely human. It is therefore unlikely that specific findings from studies with rhesus monkeys or any other nonhuman primates will generalize across all levels of analysis to specific aspects of human development. On the other hand, a number of general principles can be gleaned from studies involving this highly successful primate species that arguably can provide meaningful insights to our general understanding of basic human developmental phenomena.

First and foremost is the general principle that early social experiences, especially those with primary attachment figures, can have profound consequences for both behavioral and physiological functioning throughout the lifespan. Sigmund Freud and John Bowlby, among others, always emphasized the long-term importance of the initial relationship with one's mother, but the primate data clearly demonstrate that the impact of that first important social relationship encompasses not only social, emotional, and cognitive domains but also affects specific aspects of a remarkably wide range of physiological functioning throughout much (if not all) of the lifespan. These effects of early experience occur in the absence of any apparent linguistic capabilities or specific cultural traditions among the individuals involved. It is hard to believe that most humans would not be at least as sensitive to differences in that initial attachment relationship as are most rhesus monkeys, and one could easily argue that the unique linguistic and memory capabilities of humans might even enhance the long-term impacts of specific early social experiences over those found for rhesus monkeys.

Secondly, both short- and long-term consequences of specific events that occur in a social context are seldom (if ever) uniform across all individuals experiencing those particular events. Rather, some individuals, owing to heritable predispositions, previous experiences, or (most likely) both, may be more sensitive behaviorally and/or physiologically to the fallout from such events than are others. Not all young monkeys respond in a depressive manner to their mother's brief departures that are specifically devoted to the conception of their next sibling, and not all infants blessed with unusually nurturant (foster) mothers subsequently exhibit obvious enhancement of their respective biobehavioral developmental trajectories. These differential effects of early experiences are readily expressed without the benefit of self-reflecting capabilities that are universal among humans but apparently lacking in rhesus monkeys. One might surmise that self-reflection could well enhance differential perceptions of the same or similar events, such that the range of different long-term consequences for particular events experienced early in life might actually be greater (and perhaps even more stable) for developing humans than for developing monkeys.

Finally, the discovery of an apparent feedback system involving mother–infant dyadic relationships, on the one hand, and basic demographic features of the larger social community, on the other, raises a series of conceptual, methodological, and analytical challenges for subsequent basic research in the realm of human development. Scientists studying rhesus monkeys have not been the first to link characteristics of the community to specific relationships between particular individuals within that community—the idea of such a linkage has been promoted by philosophers and politicians alike throughout recorded history. However, these new findings from long-term study of expanding monkey populations suggest that neither unidimensional nor unidirectional models of social influence are likely to be adequate for predicting and understanding the dynamic features of social life within complex communities. Such simplistic models do not do justice to the complexity of developmental processes routinely exhibited by rhesus monkeys, and it is hard to see how they would be any more appropriate for advancing our understanding of the even larger complexities that underlie human developmental phenomena.

ACKNOWLEDGMENT

Most of the research described in this chapter was supported by funds from the Division of Intramural Research, National Institute of Child Health and Human Development, National Institutes of Health.

10

Psychosocial Factors and Psychoneuroimmunology within a Lifespan Perspective

Christopher L. Coe

W hen discussing the relationship between psychosocial processes and health, it is important to consider the biological factors underlying this association, because an understanding of the basic physiology is usually helpful in focusing our attention on the issues of more global significance. Success with this type of multidisciplinary approach has been most evident with respect to cardiovascular disease, where we have gained considerable insight into the genetic and physiological factors within the individual that mediate disease risk, as well as lifestyle and societal variables accounting for disease prevalence at the population level. Over the last two decades, there has been growing interest in the interaction between psychosocial factors and a different dimension of health that involves immunological well-being and disease. This chapter reviews some of the salient physiological and psychological issues that have emerged in studies investigating this relatively newer field of psychoneuroimmunology (PNI).

Although empirical support for the idea that psychological factors influence immunity can be traced back to many studies for over 70 years (e.g., Ishigami, 1919; Mora, Amtmann, & Hoffman, 1926; Marsh & Rasmussen, 1960; Weinman & Rothman, 1967), most researchers attribute the coalescing of the scientific discipline to the publication of a book with the name *Psychoneuroimmunology* (Ader, 1981). This anthology brought together a sufficient body of research to demonstrate convincingly that environmental and psychological factors affect many immune responses in animals and humans. In addition, it served to stimulate the integration of previously disparate research, an effort that has continued up to the present (Jemmott & Locke, 1984; S. Cohen & Williamson, 1990). Since 1981 there has been significant progress in delineating the neural and hormonal processes that mediate environmental and psychic influences on the cellular events of the immune system (A. J. Dunn, 1989; Maier & Watkins, 1998). Some of these neuroendocrine processes accounting for psychological influences on immunity are briefly reviewed in this chapter.

The field of PNI has also been forced to tackle the question of how alterations in immunity actually result in disease, because not every small shift in immune responses necessarily has this negative outcome. We still need to learn more about which events are capable of compromising our immune competence to such a degree that it initiates an immune-related disease. Examples of stress-responsive immune measures are discussed later, but at this point it is important to emphasize that advances in PNI will also require refining our knowledge about which immune responses are most critical to study for each immunological disease of interest. Just as we must distinguish between cardiovascular disease and immunological disorders in a general discussion of health, within PNI one must make distinctions between the three major categories of immune-related disease: infectious illnesses, autoimmune disorders, and cancer. Each type of disease involves different immune processes, and it is likely that the nature and strength of the relationship between psychosocial variables and the specific cellular mechanisms will vary. The importance of these seemingly subtle distinctions becomes more apparent when discussing PNI within a lifespan perspective, because most immune responses and the prevalence of different diseases vary with age.

While it has been possible to show that extrinsic and intrinsic factors influencing the integrity of the body can affect immune competence at any point in the lifespan, it has been a guiding hypothesis of my own research program that there are two major periods of vulnerability. We know that the susceptibility to infectious disease is highest in children, reflecting the immaturity of the immune system, and thus it is likely that psychoneuroimmunological relationships will prove to have a special health relevance in childhood. In contrast, immune responses are relatively more robust and resilient in young and middle-aged adults; as a consequence, the second period of vulnerability does not emerge again until old age, when we see a return of the morbidity and mortality associated with infectious disease. The two other major categories of immune-related disease, autoimmune disorders and cancer, also become more common in older individuals. This profile of disease across the lifespan reflects the two periods of significant developmental change in immunity: the maturation of immune competence during infancy, and subsequently the decline in immunological vigor in old age, a process termed immune senescence (Pawelec & Solana, 1997).

In a book such as this one, discussing how economic and social policies influence the health of whole populations, it is important to keep the developmental perspective in mind. The health relevance of PNI should be considered with respect both to the potentially vulnerable populations and to the resilient individuals, people in the prime of healthy adulthood. On a positive note, we might expect that this large, latter segment of the population would show only transient and relatively moderate changes in immunity in response to psychosocial events, with few disease sequelae. We reached this conclusion in part through our experiences with evaluating immunity in healthy and asthmatic students before and after academic examinations: students showed significant changes in immunity with little increase in disease symptomatology (Kang, Coe, McCarthy, & Ershler, 1996). In the following pages we provide support for these hypotheses about the potential importance of *developmental PNI* after considering some basic tenets of PNI applicable to individuals at any age.

CONCEPTUALIZING THE LINK BETWEEN PSYCHOSOCIAL FACTORS AND IMMUNOLOGICAL HEALTH

There are a number of different models one can envision to characterize the relationship between psychosocial factors and health (Figure 10.1). A simple model would describe the direct and immediate effect of a psychosocial factor, such as stress, on basic physiological functioning, which would in turn translate into disease pathology. For example, in research on rats it was found that physical restraint or electric shocks increased stomach acid secretion and ulceration of gastrointestinal tract evident within a day (Weiss, 1984). A comparable illustration from PNI studies would be the way stressors impair the ability of white blood cells to travel normally through the blood stream and to make their way to the site of infection or inflammation (Dhabhar, Miller, McEwen, & Spencer, 1995). However, even in animals, it is not easy to demonstrate that these changes will lead to a direct elicitation of disease processes, unless the events are sustained over a long duration or are recurrent. With respect to the relationship between psychosocial factors and immune-related disease, therefore, it is probably more appropriate to consider several indirect models.

One type of indirect model is based on the idea that small alterations in immunity do not usually result in illness by themselves unless the host is simultaneously exposed to a disease-causing agent (Figure 10.1). That is, in keeping with "germ theory," a bacterial or viral pathogen is the actual vector of infectious disease; the psychosocial event is influential because it creates a window of opportunity by compromising the host's ability to mount an effective immune response. A similar impairment of other aspects of immune competence might allow a metastatic process or incipient tumor to escape containment by the immune system. For example, Riley, Fitzmau-

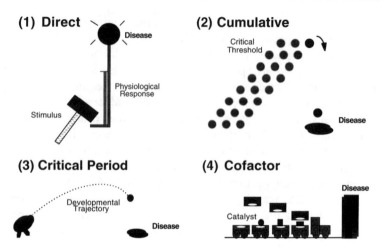

FIGURE 10.1. Direct and indirect models commonly used to explain the relationship between psychosocial factors, immunity, and health. (1) A direct and immediate effect on physiology may result in pathology, but in most instances the influence is more indirect. (2) Negative effects may accumulate in an incremental manner until a critical threshold is reached. (3) Perturbations during a sensitive period may alter development or the set points at which immune responses are established. (4) Alternatively, psychosocial factors may serve as a catalyst or permissive cofactor aggravating a pathogenic process.

rice, and Spackman (1981) showed that mice were unable to contain the growth of an experimentally introduced tumor if they were subjected to 2 hours of daily stress for 6 days after it had been implanted. While this type of vulnerability model is relatively easy to demonstrate in animal models, it is likely that alternative explanations emphasizing even more indirect relationships may actually occur more frequently in humans. One can hypothesize that the long-term negative consequences would result from an accrual of many small alterations over time, in which case the actual effect on health might appear to be delayed from the antecedent events and emerge only if the events were recurrent. Although detectable physiological changes might occur after each episode, only the aggregate toll would eventually have health implications. This type of *cumulative* (or wear-and-tear) model has become more popular recently, in conjunction with the idea that psychosocial processes help to balance or imbalance the regulatory set points of the body (sometimes described as an allostatic load model: McEwen & Stellar, 1993; Seeman, Singer, Rowe, Horwitz, & McEwen, 1997; see also Hertzman, Chapter 2, this volume).

The cumulative and allostatic models are particularly applicable to the developing individual. Our studies in young monkeys, for example, have indicated that psychosocial processes influence the developmental trajectory of the immature organism, altering the rate of maturation and/or the set points at which certain physiological responses eventually become established in the adult. Both prenatal and postnatal rearing conditions affect the number and type of cells in circulation, as well as the immune responses to challenge with a virus or foreign protein (Coe, 1993). Because this type of effect appears to be more common in the young animal, when even single events appear to have more lasting physiological effects, it may be important to add the notion of *critical periods* of vulnerability to the cumulative model.

Finally, under the heading of indirect models we must consider the situation in which psychosocial events are not the initiating cause of disease, nor even exert a major or predominant effect, but just serve as a *cofactor,* catalyzing or augmenting the actions of another variable. Here one might list those studies showing an influence of psychological factors on an illness with a strong genetic basis, possibly accelerating or worsening the expression of symptoms in a sick individual. For example, it has been reported that family functioning may influence the age of asthma onset in children genetically prone to this respiratory condition (D. A. Mrazek, Klinnert, Mrazek, & Macey, 1991). Similarly, retrospective surveys of certain patient populations suggest that stressful life events can be associated with the first clinical expression of autoimmune disease in children and adults (Grant et al., 1989; Heisel, 1972) or that psychosocial factors can influence the course of breast and skin cancer (Levy, Herberman, Maluish, Schlien, & Lippman, 1985; Temoshok & Fox, 1984). As these longer-duration effects become better understood, it will be possible to determine whether they are mediated indirectly through the immune system, by psychological factors tilting the balance of immunity toward health or illness.

ACCOUNTING FOR THE ASSOCIATION BETWEEN PSYCHOSOCIAL FACTORS AND IMMUNITY

Considerable effort has been expended to determine the physiological pathways involved in mediating psychosocial influences on immunity. The flow diagram presented in Figure 10.2 illustrates the major systems through which an external event or psychic experience might act and thereby alter cellular processes within the immune system. Presumably these PNI effects emanate largely from the brain and are passed via the endocrine and autonomic nervous systems to the immune system. We have become increasingly knowledgeable about the actual steps, which include the nerves that innervate the major immune sites, such as the thymus and the spleen, and many stress-responsive hormones including cortisol and epinephrine (adrenaline) that can influence immune responses. By injecting various hormones or by administering drugs that block the activity of certain physiological systems, it has been demonstrated unequivocally that these pathways have the potential to mediate meaningful changes in immune

PNI

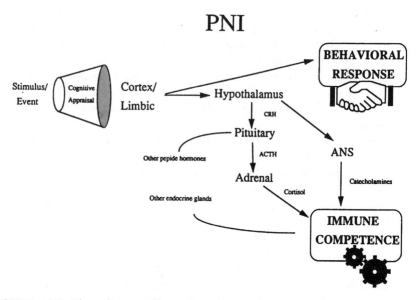

FIGURE 10.2. Flow diagram illustrating the brain, autonomic nervous system (ANS), and endocrine pathways through which environmental and psychological events might act to impinge upon the immune system (CRH, corticotropin-releasing hormone; ACTH, adrenocorticotropic hormone). Behavioral responses can augment this effect or obviate the need for physiological activation.

responses (Benschop, Rodriguez-Feuerhahn, & Schedlowski, 1996; Crary et al., 1983; Landmann et al., 1984; Munck, Guyre, & Holbrook, 1984). Of course, beyond the controlled experiments in the laboratory, it is still sometimes difficult to know which physiological pathways are the primary cause of immune or health changes in the outside world.

While ongoing studies are continuing to provide more details on neural or hormone processes involved in mediating immune alterations, it is already a significant development that the majority of scientists are now convinced there is a logical and plausible basis for the effects of stressful, and even some positive, events on immunity. Changes in the number, type, and ability of white blood cells to function have been found to occur routinely in a variety of experimental paradigms (for review, see Herbert & Cohen, 1993). The ability of cells to grow and divide or to perform normal functions, from releasing soluble substances to killing virally infected or mutagenic cells, all appear to be compromised during times of adversity. Similar types of immune changes have been found following a variety of stressful life events—after environmental disasters, bereavement, divorce, loss of a job, and school examinations—suggesting that the day-to-day functioning of immune cells is responsive to our psychological well-being on a regular basis (Bartrop, Luckhurst, Lazarus, Kiloh, & Penny, 1977;

Ironson et al., 1997; Solomon, Segerstrom, Grohr, Kemeny, & Fahey, 1997; Irwin, Daniels, Smith, Bloom, & Weiner, 1987; Kiecolt-Glaser et al., 1984; Kiecolt-Glaser, Glaser, et al., 1987). Table 10.1 lists some of the life events, lifestyle, and psychological variables that have been associated with changes in immunity. This listing is not intended to suggest that each type of experience elicits independent immune alterations through unique pathways; rather, there is likely some commonality in the emotional reactions (dysphoria or anxiety) and changes in lifestyle (health-promoting or disease-causing habits) that cause changes in immune responses.

Elucidating the psychobiological processes involved in PNI has been made both more interesting and more complex by another important realization that emerged early in research on the brain–immune system relationship. There also appears to be a strong reciprocal influence of the immune system on the brain, at least during times of immune activation and illness. We now know that many substances made by white blood cells, such as the interleukins that are released primarily to facilitate cell growth and cell-to-cell interactions, also have secondary effects on the digestive, endocrine, and nervous systems, influencing appetite, body temperature, sleepiness, and even mood. These soluble blood-borne products provide feedback about the immune system to the brain via the vagus nerve and through chemical signaling at the blood vessels and tissues surrounding the brain (Maier & Watkins, 1998; Reyes & Coe, 1996). Recent studies indicate further that these cytokines affect neurotransmitter activity in important brain regions (e.g., the hippocampus, locus ceruleus) and alter the hypothalamic control of the endocrine system, and thereby can influence behavioral and emotional processes (A. J. Dunn, 1989). This immune feedback could also play a role in mediating fatigue, a feeling of malaise, or loss of motivation, and thus has even been hypothesized to contribute to symptoms in the mentally ill. Knowledge about this two-way communication between the brain and the immune system has served to validate the importance of PNI; in time, it may help to guide us to incorporate new measures in research on psychosocial factors and health.

TABLE 10.1. Life Events, Lifestyle Variables, and Psychological Processes That Have Been Associated with Alterations in Immunity

Events	Lifestyle	Psychological processes
Bereavement	Diet	Perceived stress
Divorce	Drug use	Optimism/pessimism
Unemployment	Alcohol consumption	Expression of emotion
School exams	Smoking	Stoicism/fatalism
Caregiving	Sleep	Social support
Hurricanes/earthquakes	Exercise	Mental illness

ASSESSMENT OF IMMUNE MEASURES
IN PSYCHONEUROIMMUNOLOGICAL RESEARCH

Even a brief introduction to PNI normally requires some complex immunological terms, but before presenting difficult jargon, it is possible to distill the function of the immune system down to a few primary goals, such as the need to distinguish between the "self" and "other," and to protect the "healthy self" from harm caused by the "other." From this perspective, one can point out the commonality between the three major types of immune-related disease and the many cellular responses that are coordinated to accomplish these goals. Bacterial and viral pathogens are "other"; they must be recognized as distinct from oneself and eliminated from the body in order to prevent and limit infectious disease. Autoimmune disease, in contrast, reflects a failure in this recognition process; in this case, the immune system treats healthy tissue as "other" and begins to attack it inappropriately (e.g., multiple sclerosis, rheumatoid arthritis). Finally, in the interest of maintaining a healthy body, immune processes must remain vigilant and detect abnormal changes in mutagenic cells. These cancerous tissues should be attacked as if they were "other." A failure in this immune surveillance or a weakened ability to stop metastatic growth may allow an incipient cancer to reach an advanced stage when it can no longer be contained by the immune system.

To accomplish these diverse tasks, the activities of several types of white blood cells, including phagocytic cells and lymphocytes, each of which numbers in the millions, must be coordinated. Initially, immunity in primitive organisms was based primarily on phagocytes engulfing the foreign substance and either destroying it directly or externalizing it from the body. Phagocytic cells, such as the neutrophil and eosinophil, still play an important role in infectious and parasitic disease. With the evolution of vertebrate animals, more advanced responses developed, including the release of antibody to help label and neutralize the target. Antibody production by one type of lymphocyte (B cells) is still a critical aspect of humoral immunity; when we are administered vaccines, the primary goal is to boost antibody responses by those lymphocytes that can recognize the particular antigen in that vaccine. But when the task involves the containment and killing of cancerous cells, the immune system must rely on other types of lymphocytes (natural killer cells and cytotoxic T cells) for a direct cellular response to lyse the cancer cells. The activities of the B lymphocytes and killer cells are coordinated, in turn, by regulatory cells from the thymus, which can up- and down-regulate their responses. Two types of regulatory lymphocytes—T helper and suppressor cells—are often measured in studies of PNI because of this pivotal role.

There are many ways to assess immunity, but unfortunately no general consensus exists with regard to the how best to measure the different types of cells (Table 10.2). Studies with human subjects have most commonly opted for assays on cells found in the bloodstream, although other body

TABLE 10.2. Examples of Immune and Immune-Related End Points Utilized in Studies of Psychoneuroimmunology

In vitro	*In vivo*	Immune-related measures
Number and type of leukocytes	Cell trafficking	Inflammation
Helper/suppressor	Distribution	Swelling
Natural killer cells	Homing	Tissue repair
Cell functioning	Cell responses	Sickness behavior
Proliferation	Cell activation	Fever
Chemotaxis	Cytokine release	Anorexia
Cell products	Antibody production	Sleep
Disease modeling	Disease induction	Symptomatology
Cell killing	Infectious agents	Morbidity
Apoptosis	Tumor growth	Mortality

fluids such as saliva offer alternative possibilities, providing a less invasive means to assess antibody and interleukin (cytokine) levels. Research with experimental animals allows for other, sometimes better opportunities, such as the collection of cells from the major immune sites (e.g., the thymus, spleen, or lymph nodes), which can not be easily or ethically done in humans. Early papers in PNI were usually satisfied with any demonstration of a change in immunity, regardless of the cell type or source. A better guiding principle today would be to tailor measures to the specific disease or psychosocial question of interest. For example, in a cancer study one should evaluate different cells than those evaluated in an investigation of an inflammatory condition such as asthma or rheumatoid arthritis.

Because of the incredible advances in immunology, many different approaches and assays are available. Among the arsenal of possible measures are increasingly sophisticated analyses of the different types of cells found in body fluids and tissues. A first step might be a tallying of the total number of white blood cells and an enumeration of the various lymphocyte subsets. Cells can be labeled and grouped together by their surface markers or functional properties. Thus, it is common today to see reports on the ratio of CD4 to CD8 cells, markers of the two regulatory lymphocytes derived from the thymus, usually described as the ratio of helper cells to suppressor cells. Stressors typically lower this ratio of T cells, which would presumably have a negative effect on the overall regulation of immunity. Even more elegant would be a refined analysis of just the T helper cell population, subdividing them into Th1 or Th2 cells, frequently done on the basis of which cytokines (interleukins and interferon) they produce in cultures *in vitro*. This delineation could be important because Th1 cells are biased to promote cellular immune responses, whereas Th2 cells shift the body toward a reliance on an antibody response. Such an analysis is very valuable in a disease like AIDS, where the cellular immune responses may be more critical than is antibody production for containing the spread of the virus.

Once the blood sample has been obtained and the cells are available, a number of routine assays can also be conducted *in vitro* to assess the ability of the cells to function. Traditionally, two assays were commonly employed in PNI research: (1) the proliferation assay, which assesses cell growth after stimulation with plant proteins (mitogens); and (2) the cytolytic assay, which measures the ability of natural killer and cytotoxic T cells to kill cancerous or virally infected target cells after coincubation of the cells for 4–6 hours. Both assays continue to be utilized, but increasingly they are being supplemented with others, including assays that measure the release of substances from the stimulated or activated cells (e.g., levels of cytokines in the supernatant fluid around the cells). For example, it is possible to show that when cells are collected from stressed humans or experimentally manipulated animals, they are less able to release important cytokines and are less responsive to stimulation by these cytokines (Glaser et al., 1990; Pavlidis & Chirigos, 1980).

In PNI studies with research animals, a large number of *in vivo* measures have also been utilized, ranging from infection with pathogens to implanting tumors. The value of this approach is that it is easier to designate a good or bad response, and what entails a significant health-impacting change after the experimental manipulation. If the induced disease has a lethal end point, then the mortality rate and duration of survival provide a clear metric of immune competence, beyond just the quantitative measure of the functioning of a single cell type. Obviously, the options for employing *in vivo* measures are more limited with human subjects, although some investigators have creatively used vaccine paradigms. In several studies, the efficacy of vaccines to elicit an antibody response has been shown to be influenced by our psychological state (Glaser, Kiecolt-Glaser, Malarkey, & Sheridan, 1998). In a few cases, PNI studies with humans have utilized actual infection with viruses—for example, permitting the unique demonstration that psychological factors influence the likelihood of infection and the occurrence of cold symptoms after a controlled exposure to rhinoviruses (S. Cohen, Tyrell, & Smith, 1991). Other creative *in vivo* approaches in human research have included (1) the study of the stress-induced reactivation of latent herpes viruses (Glaser, Kiecolt-Glaser, Speicher, & Holliday, 1985; Kasl, Evans, & Niederman, 1979), and (2) prospectively tracking patient populations with a particular immune-related disorder, correlating measures of immunity with either disease progression or mortality (Levy et al., 1985).

IMMUNITY AND STRESSFUL LIFE EVENTS

As illustrated in Table 10.1, many different types of stressful life events have been shown to alter immune responses, at least for a period of time. One early PNI study focused on bereavement and reported a decreased ability of lymphocytes to proliferate *in vitro* for at least 1–2 months after loss of a spouse (Bartrop et al., 1977). The lytic activity of natural killer cells was also shown to be reduced in grieving individuals (Irwin et al., 1987). These immune changes appear to concur with the marked increase in overall morbidity and mortality during the first year after losing a spouse (Klerman & Izen, 1977; Kraus & Lilienfield, 1959; Maddison & Viola, 1968), although the proliferative activity of lymphocytes in bereaved individuals was observed to recover by 1 year (Schleifer, Keller, Camerino, Thornton, & Stein, 1983). Similar types of immune alterations have been found following other stressful life events, including environmental disasters, unemployment, and divorce (Ironson et al., 1997; Kiecolt-Glaser, Fisher, et al., 1987; Solomon et al., 1997).

However, the most comprehensive immune evaluations have been conducted on a more modest and common life stressor, the effect of school examinations. During exam week, there are pervasive shifts in many lymphocyte responses, including proliferative and killing ability (Kiecolt-Glaser et al., 1984). In our studies on high school students, we were interested in whether some other responses might also be inappropriately increased, especially cellular processes that are pro-inflammatory, because inflammatory disorders are often thought to get worse during stressful times. Specifically, we found that the production of superoxides by neutrophils, the most common phagocytic cell, was much higher during final exam week and for 2 weeks afterward in both healthy and asthmatic adolescents (Kang et al., 1996). Although superoxides can serve a useful function in fighting off bacterial infections, when overproduced they can be irritating to healthy tissue; we hypothesized this could be one physiological mechanism linking stress with increased symptomatology, at least if the asthma is not well managed with medication. In a subsequent study we found that the pattern of cytokine secretion by lymphocytes also changed during exam week, in a direction that could aggravate lung tissue in asthmatics (Kang et al., 1997).

In a number of PNI studies, investigators have attempted to understand the basis for individual variation in the amount of immunological change seen after various life events. Several factors have emerged as important in determining how an individual will respond, including the way we perceive a stressor, our coping strategies, and the adequacy of our social resources (S. Cohen, 1988; S. Cohen & Williamson, 1991; Herbert & Cohen, 1993; Strauman, Lemieux, & Coe, 1993). To emphasize the positive aspects of this relationship, we can state that certain types of appraisal processes, optimistic attribution styles, the ability to express emotion, and the capacity to take advantage of social support all appear to buffer the individual against adversity—first at the psychological level, but then also at the physiological level. These observations are not unique to PNI research; although comparable findings in studies with immune measures reinforce the view that a consideration of personality variables is critical for characterizing the overall relationship between psychosocial factors and health.

While these studies have uncovered many important biological consequences of psychosocial events, I was struck in my own research with both
humans and animals that most immune alterations appeared to return to
normal within a few days or weeks without precipitating disease. Even in
the case of the latent herpes viruses, which become partially reactivated
during stressful times, the immune system is often capable of containing the
virus before the expression of a clinical symptom (e.g., a cold sore or genital sore).[1] These observations led us to consider the possibility that more
health-significant immune changes might occur during certain phases of the
lifespan and that some disease sequelae might emerge temporally distant
from the antecedent events.

CRITICAL PERIODS
FOR PSYCHONEUROIMMUNOLOGY

Development

Having provided some general background information on the field of PNI,
we turn now to evidence indicating that psychosocial factors may prove to
be particularly relevant to the development of immunity in the very young
(Figure 10.3). Interestingly, many seminal studies in PNI were conducted
with this perspective in mind and demonstrated that early rearing conditions in rats could influence immunity or affect later responses to disease in
the adult (Ader, 1983; Solomon, Levine, & Kraft, 1968). One study on tu-

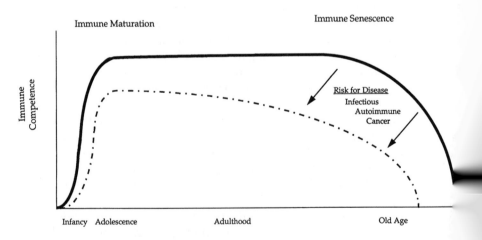

FIGURE 10.3. Environmental and psychosocial events may alter the developmental trajectory of the immune system, reducing immune competence and increasing
the risk for immune-related diseases. At the end of the lifespan, psychosocial factors
may influence the occurrence and progression of immune senescence.

mor containment dramatically illustrated the health consequences of weaning rat pups prematurely from their mother at 2 weeks rather than at the more typical 3 weeks of age: when a tumor was implanted later in adulthood, mortality was markedly accelerated in the rats separated at the younger age (Ader & Friedman, 1965). One of the better studies evaluating a PNI-type relationship in children was also conducted more than three decades ago. Meyer and Haggerty (1962) showed that poor family functioning influenced the incidence of streptoccocal infection over a period of 1 year, increasing the likelihood of a positive throat culture and symptom expression. Similarly, environmental and familial stability were found to influence the severity and duration of upper respiratory illness in children (Boyce et al., 1977). While much more controversial, psychological and familial factors have also been implicated in the occurrence and onset of many other diseases, including asthma, juvenile rheumatoid arthritis, and cancer (Greene & Miller, 1958; Heisel, 1972; Jacobs & Charles, 1980; D. A. Mrazek et al., 1991).

Notwithstanding these important pediatric studies, the preponderance of the evidence in support of a developmental emphasis must be derived largely from animal research. Here we find extensive studies in laboratory rodents, farm animals, and monkeys indicating that early rearing conditions can affect immune responses (Coe, 1993; Kelley, 1985; Laudenslager, Reite, & Harbeck, 1982). The findings can be clustered in two general categories: (1) acute immune alterations that occur as a consequence of disturbances in the parent–offspring relationship, and (2) enduring immune alterations that persist following disruption of normal rearing conditions. For example, we and others have documented that many immune changes occur in infant monkeys after they are removed from their mothers at 6 months of age, at a point when they are no longer nursing but still emotionally dependent upon her. Lymphocyte proliferative and cytolytic responses, and antibody responses to antigens, were compromised for a few days to several weeks. While it is not ethical to conduct comparable controlled studies on the effects of separation in children, similar types of immune changes were found in young children who evinced the most distress at starting kindergarten (Boyce et al., 1993). Interestingly, even in monkeys, the magnitude of the immune suppression that occurs after separation from the mother can be modulated and largely ameliorated by providing a more benevolent separation environment (e.g., by having the separation occur in familiar surroundings or by allowing the separated infant to remain with other social companions).

But it is the second more permanent category of early rearing effects—those involving changes in the trajectory of immune development—that are likely to be of greater consequence. Typically, these more profound and prolonged immune alterations are evident when the precipitating events are experienced at a younger age. To investigate this phenomena, we characterized the immunological impact of rearing infant monkeys by humans instead of by their biological mothers. The human caregivers were benevolent, providing all essential health and hygiene needs, but it became very clear that a failure to completely fulfill the natural psychological needs of the young monkey resulted in a number of physiological alterations. A chronic change in several immune responses was apparent, indicative of a maturational derailment beyond that of an acute stress effect. One unexpected result was that their lymphocytes proliferated more than normal when stimulated with plant proteins (mitogens) in the *in vitro* assays (Coe, Lubach, Ershler, & Klopp, 1989). This proved to be associated with a permanent lowering of the CD8+ lymphocytes in the bloodstream of the human-reared monkeys, which raised the CD4/CD8 cell ratio across the first 2 years of life (Lubach, Coe, & Ershler, 1995).

Although this finding could be considered simply as the pathological response to an abnormal environment—the consequences of being reared in a clean but psychologically inappropriate world—we believe it highlights the positive and not always visible influence that parenting can have on many aspects of development. In addition to promoting cognitive and emotional growth, good parenting may be critical for facilitating the maturation of normal immunity. We have not yet had the opportunity to assess this relationship in humans with respect to the benefits of typical types of parenting, but unfortunate sociopolitical circumstances did create an opportunity to test the veracity of our conclusions about the immune effects of socially deficient rearing conditions. At the end of the Ceaușescu regime in 1991, the world was shocked to discover that nearly 2% of the children in Romania were being reared in institutional settings (Holden, 1996). While adequate food and health care were provided, these institutions were woefully understaffed and the children were deprived of normal psychosocial stimulation. To document the effects of this neglect and in the hopes of calling international attention to their plight, several researchers visited these orphanages to assess the children's cognitive and behavioral development. In addition, Dr. Mary Carlson (Harvard University Medical School) and Dr. Megan Gunnar (University of Minnesota) collected saliva samples from a group of 3-year-old children as a means to measure their adrenal hormone levels. A subset of 59 samples were subsequently provided to our laboratory to determine if the children showed signs of immunological dysregulation. Sadly, as the lessons from animal research had suggested, these children showed evidence of both disease exposure and an inability to contain one type of herpes virus. We measured antibody levels in the saliva against two pathogens: *Hemophilus influenzae* (Hib), the bacteria that causes meningitis, and herpes simplex (Hs), the virus that causes cold sores. Over 55% of orphanage children had antibody against Hib in their saliva, indicating they had been exposed to a bacteria not found in any of the home-reared children. But even more revealing of their immune status, 39% of the children expressed high levels of antibody and other proteins against Hs in their saliva, a prevalence level above that seen in the saliva of family-raised Romanian and American children, who typically contained this virus in a latent state.

These findings on institutionalized children go beyond basic science issues and compel us to advocate political solutions when we find children being raised in such adverse conditions. However, the results also indicate the need to learn more about the potentially positive and negative ways in which normal parenting can affect the development of physiological systems. In our own research program, this interest in the influence of early experience led us to consider whether there might be an even greater vulnerability during fetal development. Again, we began by modeling this scientific question in monkeys and initiated a series of studies to assess the possibility of lingering postnatal effects after disturbance of the fetus (Coe, Lubach, Karaszewski, & Ershler, 1996; Schneider, Coe, & Lubach, 1992; Schneider & Coe, 1993). At this juncture, we have evaluated the impact of several different types of pregnancy conditions on the infant: changing the social environment of the pregnant female monkey; eliciting daily periods of arousal during early or late pregnancy; and activating the maternal endocrine system via injection of hormones. Following these different types of prenatal disturbance, we have found that immune responses are altered in the infant monkey after birth and some effects continue to be evident through the second year of life (Coe et al., 1996; Reyes & Coe, 1997).

One can only speculate as to whether the human fetus is equally susceptible to prenatal perturbations, but the suggestion from rodent and primate research would be that the psychosocial environment can impact the development of immune responses from the fetal stage through the weaning age. In the absence of equivalent information on prenatally induced immune effects in humans, we can hope that our species will prove to be more resilient. Humans have a particularly extended period of postnatal development compared to animals, which may provide us with more opportunity for recovery during childhood. Prenatal events initiate a developmental course, but the postnatal rearing environment is probably more critical for fine-tuning immune competence. When both stages are severely impacted, as in the case of extreme poverty and malnutrition, we already know that immune responses can become significantly compromised (Chandra & Newberne, 1977).

Immune Senescence

As discussed briefly at the start of this chapter, we and others have been investigating whether a similar perspective is appropriate for understanding changes in immunity at the other end of the lifespan. While an eventual decline in immunity with age is inevitable, studies of the elderly reveal a wide range of individual variation, and the course of immune senescence does not always coincide with chronological years (Naliboff et al., 1991; Solomon et al., 1988). Genetics, nutritional status, concurrent disease of a nonimmune nature, as well as earlier life events account for some of the individual differences in the immunological vigor of older people. In addition, psychological well-being or distress can be influential. For example, prolonged stressful experiences, such as caregiving for a spouse with a chronic illness, have been shown to exert a debilitating effect on immune processes and other physiological systems, including the tissue repair required for the healing of wounds (Kiecolt-Glaser, Glaser, et al., 1987; Kiecolt-Glaser, Marucha, Malarkey, Mercado, & Glaser, 1995; Kiecolt-Glaser, Glaser, Gravenstein, Malarkey, & Sheridan, 1996). On the positive side, certain psychological and lifestyle variables may facilitate the maintenance of more youthful immune responses in the elderly. One of the most dramatic demonstrations of the labile nature of immunity in the elderly involved an assessment of the benefits of relaxation therapy (Kiecolt-Glaser et al., 1985). After just 1 month of such an intervention program, there were marked increases in natural killer cell activity and a reduction in Herpes antibody titers, suggesting that the virus was now under better immune containment.

In our research with nonhuman primates, we were interested in determining if psychosocial factors had equivalent effects on immune responses in old monkeys (more than 20 years of age). In collaboration with Dr. William Ershler, a gerontologist, we began by demonstrating that lymphocyte proliferative and cytolytic responses were typically lower in old monkeys than in young and middle-aged monkeys (Ershler et al., 1988). By comparing immunity in old monkeys of identical age, however, we subsequently found that, as in humans, there was wide variation in the extent to which old animals exhibited signs of this immunological decline. Further, when we investigated the effects of minor surgical procedures (e.g., laparoscopic examinations) or changes in their social housing conditions, these events exerted large effects on immunity in the older animals (Lemieux, Coe, & Ershler, 1996). One social manipulation that yielded particularly interesting results involved the addition of one or more juvenile monkeys to the cage of the aged monkey (Figure 10.4) (Coe, Ershler, Champoux, & Olson, 1992). Initially, we expected that the presence of a social companion would be immune enhancing, but to our surprise it resulted in a lowering of proliferative and cytolytic responses in the old monkey. After several iterations of this experimental paradigm, we discovered that to prevent the immune-suppressing effects of this social stimulation, it was necessary to provide the old female monkey with "psychological control" over her exposure to the juvenile, which we facilitated by designing a two-compartment cage with a small tunnel. Still, when compared with other social housing options, the best immune responses in old monkeys were found when they were housed with just one other old animal.

While these specific findings are obviously unique to primate research, when considered in the context of comparable studies on humans, we can draw some general conclusions about psychosocial processes, immunity,

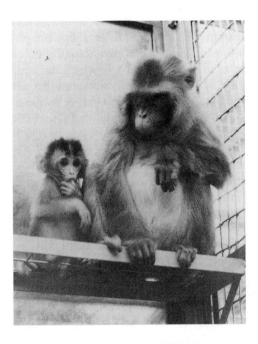

FIGURE 10.4. Studies in many types of animals have indicated that psychosocial factors significantly influence immunity. In our research on monkeys, social housing conditions had particularly pronounced effects on lymphocyte proliferation and cytolytic responses in the very young and old, suggesting that these stages may be especially vulnerable points in the lifespan.

and aging. Clearly, there appears to be a biological imperative, an "aging clock," that will tend to reduce immune competence toward the end of the natural lifespan. However, the onset of this senescence process may be influenced both by prior experiences that occurred earlier in the lifespan and by contemporaneous events. Some elderly individuals still have vigorous immune responses, similar to those seen in middle age, and do not evince overt signs of the immune decline typically associated with age. Even in these individuals, however, there may be a greater vulnerability to the adverse effects of negative life events, because of an inherent tendency for the age-related immunological decline.

IMPLICATIONS OF PSYCHONEUROIMMUNOLOGY FOR HEALTH PROMOTION AND SOCIAL POLICY

The field of PNI has made significant progress over the last two decades, from a new and controversial scientific discipline to an endeavor increasingly well regarded by biological and medical researchers. During the early phase of the research it was critical to establish the physiological mechanisms accounting for the influence of psychological processes on immunity. Much has been learned about the ways in which the brain can influence immune responses, and it is now generally accepted that neural and endocrine processes can modulate immunity. Similarly, it was essential to document the wide range of environmental and life events that could alter immunity to establish the generality of this relationship. While the focus has been largely on the adverse effects of negative events, it has opened the door to the possibility that positive interventions and health-promoting lifestyles can facilitate immune responses. We need to learn much more about the potential health implications that improvements in diet, sleep, and exercise habits have for immune function. Following disease onset, there is also compelling evidence that psychological processes, including the expression of emotions and the capacity to utilize social support, may be instrumental in facilitating immune changes of value for retarding disease progression. Here there is also a need to learn more about the purported immune-enhancing effects of less conventional treatments, including relaxation, visual imagery, and biofeedback therapies, which while the subject of considerable speculation, have relatively less empirical support. Considering the popularity of these "alternative" complementary medicine approaches, it will be critical to establish their efficacy for immune-related disorders, especially as an adjunct therapy to conventional medical treatments.

But there are also additional lessons from PNI research that echo messages from studies of cardiovascular disease. The findings demonstrate that psychosocial and lifestyle factors are important in accounting for variation in immune responses, and probably immune-related disease, across individuals and populations. This brief chapter has provided just a partial summary of the available information indicating that decisions we make about the rearing of children may be critical for promoting their health and well-being. Thoughtful and compassionate social policy decisions may be able to facilitate health at many phases in the lifespan, especially the particularly vulnerable periods of pregnancy, childhood, and old age highlighted in this chapter. It must be acknowledged, however, that with regard to immunity and immune-related diseases, we still have much to learn about the antecedent events that increase risk or promote health. Only a few community and large population studies have incorporated a PNI perspective, and primarily these have evaluated the impact of environmental disasters (Ironson et al., 1997; McKinnon, Weisse, Reynolds, & Baum, 1989; Solomon et al., 1997). Therefore, we are currently unable to compile a list of the major risk factors that result in poor immune competence and immunological disease, as has been done for the known effects of obesity, smoking, high cholesterol levels, or Type A personality traits on cardiovascular disease (but see Thomas, Duszynski, & Shaffer, 1979, and Solomon, 1981, for attempts to do so for cancer and autoimmune diseases).

We can speculate that age and socioeconomic status (SES), the two major risk factors evident in almost all types of disease, will also emerge as salient ones in PNI research. Morbidity and mortality in both historical and contemporary disease epidemics continually remind us of the importance of the age variable. In this chapter we have argued further that the age-related risk for immune disorders concurs with our understanding of the basic biology of the immune system and the developmental changes in immunity across the lifespan. To keep the scope of this review manageable, we did not tackle the possible contribution of SES. SES has also not been systematically addressed as a variable in PNI research, but it is reasonable to speculate from the prevalence of immune-related diseases, such as asthma in low-income groups that SES should be considered in any future study of population health with a PNI orientation. Because the negative events associated with impaired immunity are more common (Gennaro, Fehder, Nuamah, Campbell, & Douglas, 1997) and the opportunities for positive, health-promoting lifestyles and resources are more limited in low-SES groups, we should anticipate finding gradients between economic factors and immune well-being similar to those described for other outcome measures considered in this book. The challenge will be to distinguish whether these disease gradients across social and economic classes reflect primarily increased exposure to environmental risk factors or a synergistic influence with the lifestyle and psychosocial factors found to be particularly important in PNI research.

ACKNOWLEDGMENTS

Partial salary support comes from National Institute of Mental Health (NIMH) Grant No. MH41659, which also provided the funds for the developmental research on immunity in infant monkeys. Acknowledgments are also due to the many authors who collaborated with me on the primate studies cited in this review.

NOTE

1. Here there may be some important exceptions, including individuals who do show recurrent expression of herpes symptoms such as cold sores and genital sores during times of stress (Kemeny, Cohen, Zegans, & Conant, 1989). In addition, there are instances when stressful events appear to facilitate the ability of Epstein–Barr virus to induce mononucleosis (Kasl et al., 1979) or in the elderly may lead to reactivation of varicella zoster (herpes zoster), latent for years since chickenpox in childhood and subsequently reemergent as the disease shingles.

11

Individual Pathways in Competence and Coping

FROM REGULATORY SYSTEMS TO HABITS OF MIND

Daniel P. Keating
Fiona K. Miller

T he research reported in the preceding chapters of this volume provide substantial support for several major findings about human development. These findings, in turn, point to a number of crucial challenges, both to our understanding of human development and to effective action in support of human development. The major findings can be readily summarized. The first is that an individual's experiences during development have a profound impact on the brain and on general physiology. In other words, one's experiences become embedded in one's biology. Second, early development is of particular importance for this biological embedding by setting in place key conditions for subsequent growth and development. Some of the effects of early development may occur as *critical periods*, when the presence or absence of particular experiences makes a biological system functional or nonfunctional. Others are better described as *sensitive periods*, during which the quality of particular experiences shapes developmental outcomes, but in less absolute ways than in critical periods. Third, the effects of these early developmental processes can be observed in the health and competence of populations, as noted in the discussions of gradient effects in Part I.

This summary suggests strong evidence for the *existence* of a linkage between early development and the subsequent well-being of populations, but it does not explain *how* that linkage is created. For this, we need to examine more closely the underlying developmental processes, including how they become organized within an individual. This effort, however, introduces tremendous complexity in two related ways. On the one hand, we have only begun to identify and understand the numerous pathways and circuits of neural, neuroendocrine, and neuroimmune development. On the other hand, it is increasingly clear that these circuits are highly interactive and mutually influential. But it also seems clear that individual behavior and development is more coherent and organized than might be expected if one considered only the isolated development of multiple systems and their interactions. Understanding the coherence and continuity of individual behavior poses an important challenge for developmental scientists.

The study of regulatory systems and their development may provide one lens through which the coherence of individual behavior can be resolved out of the complexity of underlying neurophysiological processes. In other words, regulatory systems offer one route for studying the expression of underlying biological processes in observable behavior. They are grounded in biological functioning and likely serve to structure the everyday behavior of the individual. Regulatory systems have recently received considerable attention from a number of researchers interested in how these systems develop and how they are related to the development of individual competence.

In this chapter, we outline a framework for understanding the role of regulatory systems in the development of competence. First, we review some recent work on regulatory systems in early development and highlight research that has explored the connection between regulatory systems and competence. Next, we explore the developmental pathways that link them together. We then describe an ongoing longitudinal study designed to explore these pathways, which offers initial support for our proposed framework. Finally, we suggest that the integration of the developmental pathways of regulatory systems and competence can be viewed productively as emerging habits of mind.

REGULATORY SYSTEMS AND COMPETENCE

Recent theory and research have identified a potentially critical role of regulatory systems in both normal and atypical development (Cicchetti, Ackerman, & Izard, 1995; Cicchetti & Tucker, 1994; Cummings & Davies, 1996; Derryberry & Reed, 1996; Eisenberg et al., 1996, 1997; Fox, 1994; J. Garber & Dodge, 1991; Rothbart, Posner, & Rosicky, 1994; Rubin, Coplan, Fox, & Calkins, 1995; Thompson, 1994; Thompson & Calkins, 1996). In general, regulatory systems organize a set of processes "through which one system modulates or governs the reactivity of another system" (Derryberry & Reed, 1996, p. 215). It seems likely that these systems become integrated over the course of development, moving from more basic perceptual or sensory tendencies toward eventual executive control systems involving the goal-directed regulatory functions of the frontal lobe (Cicchetti & Tucker, 1994; Derryberry & Reed, 1996).

Contemporary findings suggest that the emotion, attention, and social regulatory systems are rooted in neurophysiological processes and that they are manifested in observable behaviors such as babies' visual focusing and disengagement (Derryberry & Rothbart, 1997), preschoolers' internalizing and externalizing behaviors (Fox, Schmidt, Calkins, Rubin, & Coplan, 1996), affective bonds between caregivers and receivers (Derryberry & Rothbart, 1997; MacDonald, 1992), and indices of social competence in school-age children (Eisenberg et al., 1997).

Emotion Regulation

Emotion regulation has been the focus of much recent work on regulatory systems. At least three systems appear to be involved: the neuroendocrine, the autonomic, and the central nervous systems (Fox, 1994). At the same time, emotion regulation is a broad construct that includes not only physiological arousal and neurological activation but also cognitive appraisal, attention processes, and behavioral response tendencies. Thompson (1994) identified the processes involved in his definition of emotion regulation as the "extrinsic and intrinsic processes responsible for monitoring, evaluating, and modifying emotional reactions, especially their intensive and temporal features, to accomplish one's goals" (pp. 27–28). This and other definitions have several features in common: emotion regulation involves the modulation of arousal, a process that is rooted in neurophysiological systems and is observed in behavior; it involves processes in the cognitive, affective, social, and behavioral domains; it occurs in the service of individual goals; and perhaps most importantly, it leads to individual coping and adaptation.

In particular, the role of emotion regulation in competent social functioning has been explored by a number of investigators. Significant associations between emotion regulation and social competence in preschool have been reported such that well-regulated children are good problem solvers, more able to compromise and meet mutual needs when playing with peers, able to make new friends (Frankel & Bates, 1990), likely to develop peer interaction skills through higher levels of play (Gottman & Katz, 1989), more popular, and more likely to engage in positive peer relationships (Eisenberg et al., 1993). In contrast, dysregulated preschoolers express anger as aggression, are less sociable, and are less likely to receive positive responses from their peers after displaying helping behavior (Eisenberg & Fabes, 1992). They are also more likely to make hostile attributional biases when presented with ambiguous information about a peer (Dodge, 1991). They could be at risk for delinquency, may feel anxious and lonely (Rubin, Hymel, Mills, & Rose-Krasnor, 1991), and may be denied opportunities for social–cognitive development (J. Garber & Dodge, 1991).

Of course, different investigators have used a variety of definitions and operationalizations of emotion regulation in exploring the links between emotion regulation and competence. As we have used it, the construct of emotion regulation is also informed by a functionalist perspective that emphasizes, in addition to the internal modulation of affect, the fact that the "manifestation of an emotion creates the setting for new person–environment transactions" (Campos, Mumme, Kermoian, & Campos, 1994, p. 296). As such, the way in which emotion regulation functions in the service of goals is theoretically observable in specific behaviors and expressions, as long as those behaviors are interpreted with respect to their contextual appropriateness (Campos et al., 1994; Thompson & Calkins, 1996).

Attention Regulation

Akin to emotion regulation, attention regulation involves a complex pattern of processes arising from neural development and neuromodulator activities (Derryberry & Rothbart, 1997) that "regulate the arousal and reactivity of the cortex in ways that are integral to both attentional and emotional processes" (Cicchetti & Tucker, 1994, p. 542). Several different attentional circuits have been identified, and their processes are hypothesized to be evident in observable behaviors (Derryberry & Rothbart, 1997). First, general alertness and focused attention are hypothesized to be functions of the vigilance and tonic activation systems (Cicchetti & Tucker, 1994; Derryberry & Rothbart, 1997). Second, attentional orienting, involving the engagement or disengagement at or between different locations, as well as the breadth or depth of attention at those locations, is thought to be a function of a posterior attention system involving several brain regions (Derryberry & Rothbart, 1997; Rothbart et al., 1994). Third, attentional processes involved in the effortful control of behavior and in attentional flexibility and efficiency are hypothesized to be a function of an anterior attention system (Derryberry & Rothbart, 1997; Posner & Rothbart, 1992).

In general, the hypothesized function of attention regulation is to recruit various elements of the attentional system in a flexible way that enables the individual to pursue goals and respond to challenges to those goals. Orienting, focused attention, and effortful processing are likely to be operating simultaneously in complex situations. Thus, the observable behaviors reflective of the attentional system likely represent a mixture of these attentional components.

Again, research supports the view that attention regulation and competence are connected. Four-month-old infants who were better able to disengage their attention from an attractive stimulus were rated by their mothers as more easily soothable and less sensitive to negative affect (Rothbart, Ziaie, & O'Boyle, 1992). In school-age males, attentional focusing and shifting has been related to popularity, constructive responses to anger, and to social competence, including ratings of prosocial behavior (Eisenberg et al., 1996; Eisenberg, Fabes, Nyman, Bernzweig, & Pinuelas, 1994). In a series of studies on children's responses to error, Shafrir and his colleagues (Shafrir & Eagle, 1995; Shafrir, Ogilvie, & Bryson, 1990) compared the speed with which children displaying more or less defensive styles initiated a subsequent test trial following an error. Children with more defensive styles initiated a subsequent trial more quickly than their less defensive peers. This difference in time to request a new trial was also associated with cognitive performance, in that the children who more systematically attended to their errors—and thus took more time to investigate them—showed overall higher levels of task performance.

The close interplay between emotional and attentional processes is illustrated in the research described above. Some theories seem to subsume emotion to attention, or vice versa. Whether these systems are reducible to each other, however, remains an open question. An initial working presumption might be to view them as distinct, given the evidence noted above that they are based in different neuroanatomical systems. Whether these distinctions are functionally significant and can be observed behaviorally is one of the questions for ongoing research.

Social Regulation

Many of the regulatory processes discussed above are typically regarded as occurring principally within the individual, although they are frequently relied upon in social contexts. It is likely, however, that elements of both emotion and attention regulation play a significant role in the regulation of social interaction as well. A third domain of regulatory processes, one specifically social in nature, has been proposed by several investigators (Derryberry & Rothbart, 1997; Kochanska, 1995; MacDonald, 1992). This regulatory system involves several aspects of social interaction, including affiliativeness, mutual affection, and warmth, particularly in nurturing relationships. Panskepp (1992) has proposed two key neural circuits that support this regulatory system: (1) a set of inhibitory connections that suppress defensive aggression and are enhanced through social play, leading in turn to increased social bonding; (2) a system that is activated during reunion with the caregiver following separation distress, at which time opiate neurons provide warming comfort and is perhaps also activated during caregiver interactions through oxytocin release (Derryberry & Rothbart, 1997; Panskepp, 1992). MacDonald (1992) proposed that this parent–child bond plays a significant role in the transmission and adoption of parental values. Kochanska and her colleagues (Kochanska, 1995, 1997; Kochanska, Aksan, & Koenig, 1995) have hypothesized that positive affect between parent and child is associated with compliance and internalization of conscience in the child.

DEVELOPMENTAL PATHWAYS LINKING
REGULATORY PROCESSES AND COMPETENCE

As we have seen, recent theory and research have begun to delineate the relationships among regulatory processes and social, cognitive, and behavioral competence. There are several developmental pathways through which early patterns of regulation (attentional, emotion, and social) might influence later competence. One pathway may be through early regulation to subsequent regulation, with indirect effects via the influence of regulatory capabilities on the ease or fluency of performance at a later time. Another pathway may involve direct effects of early regulation on later competence, attributable to a more effective "learning system" in operation during the intervening period. In this pathway, optimal patterns of regulation may enable the more rapid acquisition of developmental skills, through more effective habits of learning, including more readily self-directed attention, more balanced regulation of one's emotions, or greater opportunities for learning through easier social engagement. It is possible, perhaps even likely, that both direct and indirect effects operate across this sensitive period of development during which many critical cognitive and other competencies are being acquired. This combined pathway would tend to amplify the effects of regulatory systems on competence over the course of development by increasing the amount of learning across developmental time and by enhancing the ability to access that competence under challenge in a real-time task.

Infant attentional and emotional regulatory capacities have been identified by a number of researchers as key systems that are predictive of later social and cognitive competence (Fogel & Thelen, 1987; L. Katz & Gottman, 1991; Kopp, 1989; M. D. Lewis, 1993a, 1993b; Tamis-LeMonda & Bornstein, 1989). During the first 6 months of life, infants display a shift from sole reliance on internally directed regulatory mechanisms to the inclusion of externally directed regulatory behaviors (Brazelton & Yogman, 1986; Mayes & Carter, 1990). Internal mechanisms include self-soothing behaviors such as sucking, rocking, and ear rubbing, as well as those behaviors that limit an infant's perception of external stimuli, such as gaze aversion. However, an infant's repertoire of internal behaviors is limited in the comfort they provide. Hence, externally directed behaviors are also required for regulation (Gianino & Tronick, 1988; Mayes & Carter, 1990). To regulate externally, the infant signals the caregiver for help through behaviors such as smiling, cooing, babbling, crying, and fussing. Here, the success of the infant's regulation is dependent on sensitive caretaking (Thompson, 1990).

As Gianino and Tronick (1988) posit in their mutual regulation model, the responsivity of the caregiver has a strong impact on the development of the infant's external regulatory abilities. The infant's attempts to modulate emotion pass through a feedback loop that includes the caregiver. Hence, the infant's regulatory success is dependent on his/her ability to emit cues and the caregiver's ability to read them. In order to regulate, an infant must recruit and organize components from a repertoire of internally and externally oriented behaviors.

Current research suggests that well-regulated infants tend to do the following: attend to their surroundings; experience the positive affect required to explore their environment; and produce clear emotions and appropriate levels of emotionality. Similarly, well-regulated infant–caregiver dyads enable infants to develop the following: a regulated and reparable representation of the dyad that can be used during interactions with others; a positive affective core; a clearly defined notion of self and others; and mutually coordinated infant–parent schemes (Gianino & Tronick, 1988; L. Katz & Gottman, 1991; Kopp, 1989; M. D. Lewis, 1993a, 1993b; Parke, Cassidy, Burkes, Carson, & Boyum, 1992). In contrast, dysregulated infants have difficulty attending to their surroundings (Kopp, 1989; Sroufe, 1979). If an infant cannot regulate disorganizing negative affect, he/she may focus too heavily on the source of the felt emotion (the caregiver) and thus experience fewer opportunities for exploring the environment (M. D. Lewis, 1993a).

In a challenging situation, then, well-regulated infants may be more likely to recruit a creative balance of internally and externally oriented behaviors in the service of regulation and, consequently, task completion. This pattern of approach to the task is also generally characterized by positive affect. In contrast, dysregulated infants may not effectively recruit behaviors to serve emotion and attention regulation goals, which are in turn central to task performance. Dysregulated infants may show a pattern of approach to a task that is characterized by an abundance of either internal or external behaviors (rather than a modulated balance), negative affect, and inadequate task completion. As noted above, regulated and dysregulated infants may follow different developmental pathways, such as early differences associated with gender in the ability to modulate arousal (Weinberg, Tronick, Cohn, & Olson, 1999).

These and other differences during infancy may lead to diversity in subsequent regulatory capabilities and in social, behavioral, and cognitive competence in early childhood. In preschoolers, observed levels of social interaction moderate the relationship between emotion regulation and behavioral competence, as assessed by the Child Behavior Checklist (Rubin et al., 1995). Specifically, those children who engaged in low levels of social interaction and who were also poor emotion regulators were more likely to display increased internalizing behaviors. Conversely, those children who engaged in high levels of social interaction and were poor emotion regulators were more likely to show increased externalizing behaviors (Rubin et al., 1995). The overlap between these findings and those arising from the study of nonhuman primates (see Suomi, Chapter 9, this volume) reinforce the view that early experiences play a key role in subsequent regulation and competence.

There is evidence that regulation influences attentional processes and that differences in attentional style have implications for children's capacity to control and redirect their emotions (Bornstein & Sigman, 1986; Cicchetti, Ganiban, & Barnett, 1991; Kopp, 1989; Rothbart et al., 1992). Because early social environments mediate emotional experience and supply and support particular strategies for regulating emotions, they should have considerable impact on the development of attention, learning, novelty seeking, and so forth.

There is also good evidence that parental characteristics and the quality of the relationship between parent and child are good predictors of developing competence. Maternal responsiveness has been found to influence cognitive competence directly (Estrada, Arsenio, Hess, & Holloway, 1987; Olson, Bates, & Bayles, 1984; Wachs & Gruen, 1982), whereas attachment style, a function of both parent and child contributions, predicts concurrent or subsequent cognitive differences (Hazen & Durrett, 1982; Main, 1983; Matas, Arend, & Sroufe, 1978; Schneider-Rosen & Cicchetti, 1984). While much of this influence may be mediated by emotional processes, there is increasing emphasis on parents' and families' roles in organizing the child's learning environment, and some of the effects of maternal responsiveness on competence may reflect the mother's role as teacher rather than caretaker (Barocas et al., 1991; R. Bradley, 1989; R. H. Bradley et al., 1988; Dunham & Dunham, 1990; Tamis-LeMonda & Bornstein, 1989).

Recent research suggests that emotion-regulation and parent-mediated pathways to competence are initially independent (M. D. Lewis, 1993a), but their convergence over development is undoubtedly a critical factor (e.g., Barocas et al., 1991). A fine-grained analysis of development in the preschool years is capable of tracking these independent influences and recording how and when they intersect for children with different histories. Most important, when researchers look at early social influences on competence, they find that each potential influence is mediated by the individual characteristics of the child (e.g., Belsky & Rovine, 1987; Gunnar et al., 1989). Also each path of influence is reciprocal: changes in social and cognitive competencies feed back to the social environment, both enhancing and constraining subsequent influences (Sroufe & Jacobvitz, 1989). These two types of interaction make developmental causation sufficiently complex to defy simple, linear research strategies.

A seminal longitudinal study by M. D. Lewis (1993b) assessed the relations between distress regulation and cognitive competence, and found that infant distress, particularly with mother present, was a good predictor of cognitive competence both in infancy and in the year before school entry—much better than infant measures of cognitive capabilities. The pattern of results suggested two socioemotional roots of competence: the age-specific style of emotion regulation and parental response and facilitation. The results also suggested that social and emotional influences on cognitive competence are far more important than early cognitive differences themselves. As in other studies, infant temperament in isolation was not a useful predictor of competence, but interactions between infant characteristics at particular ages and maternal behaviors showed strong predictive power.

Several implications arising from this work can be highlighted. First, relationships between early predictors and later cognitive performance are generally stronger for *interactions* than for main effects, even when the main effect predictions are within the same domain. This fits well with a second point: studies of the *integration over time* of various developmental subsystems are likely to be more informative than those restricted to a single domain. Similar critiques of "direct correspondence" theories have emerged from work in other domains of development such as cognition (Keating, 1996), emotion (Campos, 1994; Camras, 1992), and attachment (Rosen & Rothbaum, 1993). Drawing on the conceptual framework and research described above, we have pursued a study of regulation and competence in early development to explore some of these connections.

A LONGITUDINAL STUDY OF REGULATION AND COMPETENCE IN EARLY DEVELOPMENT

The research described above makes it clear how crucial it is, if one is interested in the developmental pathways of regulatory systems and competence, to observe the same individuals across time and their interplay. In this respect, the existence of critical or highly sensitive periods in early development is an advantage to the investigation. It affords the opportunity to target attention on specific domains of development at specific points in time when key aspects of organization are in progress (Cicchetti, 1989). In our laboratory, we have focused on specific aspects from the concepts introduced above: emotion regulation, attention regulation, and social regulation as predictors of competence, which is assessed in multiple domains.

We selected entry into formal schooling as the initial target of our longitudinal investigation because schools are society's formal institutions for educating and socializing the next generation. Readiness to learn in school is a major factor in subsequent success. Substantial evidence demonstrates that early school performance is highly predictive of long-term achievement (Entwisle & Alexander, 1990; Kellam, Brown, Rubin, & Ensminger, 1983) and that early behavioral problems in school are associated with increased risk of subsequent dysfunction (Offord et al., 1992; Tremblay, Mâsse, Peron, & LeBlanc, 1992). In the last two decades, it has also become clear that environmental, emotional, and motivational factors have been assigned a greater role in cognitive outcomes (Ceci, 1990; Keating, 1996), and researchers of social and personality development have increasingly emphasized the impact of children's close relationships on their cognitive functioning (Belsky, 1981; Wachs & Gruen, 1982).

Several considerations guided our investigation. The first is that it required a longitudinal approach because the hypothesis is about development within individuals. The second is that the identification of behaviors associated with regulatory processes should be neurophysiologically plausible, even if we are not yet in a position to routinely include direct, on-line assessments of neural or neuroendocrine function. The third is that the crucial aspects of progress on these developmental pathways can be observed in behavior, if we use a functionally relevant and sufficiently fine-grained approach.

Children in our longitudinal investigation had participated as infants in a series of studies on the object concept, using a traditional "*A not B*" task paradigm. After several trials in which the experimenter "hides" a toy at one location (*A*) and the infant finds it there, the toy is then hidden in a new location (*B*). (The "hiding" is done in plain view of the infant.) We have observed individual differences in infant regulatory styles during this task. This task affords a potentially valuable opportunity to examine the key organizers of emotion, attention, and social regulation for several reasons: it presents a challenging set of demands to the cognitive system; it requires the infant to engage in a moderately intense but positive and game-like social exchange with a stranger; and embedded within this standard task are several episodes likely to induce some distress in most infants (such as removing the toy from the infant after he/she has retrieved it from the hiding location; or the mother's restraint of the infant to inhibit premature reaching to the hiding location).

We developed measures of infant attentional, emotional, and social regulation among infants who were seen at 9 and 12 months of age. Measures of regulation were coded for each infant for every 10-second interval in each hiding episode: positive affect (smiling, cooing, laughing); negative affect (crying, fussing, frowning); social referencing (the infant's use of another person to seek information); social enjoyment (amount of social pleasure that the infant experiences from engagement in the game); social attention (the infant's degree of interest in objects vs. interest in people); and intensity of task engagement (degree of the infant's interest and participation in the game). We also developed assessments of regulation among these children as preschoolers while they were performing a cognitively demanding task, Block Design. This task presents similar challenges to the preschooler as the object permanence task does for infants: the child must follow the social script of the task, that is, the child must attend to the experimenter's instructions and wait until permitted to examine the design, touch the blocks, and begin working on the design. Further, the child cannot work on the design until he/she is finished because each design must be completed within an allotted time. In a similar fashion, we developed detailed coding schemes for key aspects of regulation in this developmental period, coded in 30-second segments of four episodes that have different levels of challenge. The behaviors coded were positive affect (happiness toward self or other), anxious affect (self-directed anxiety), angry affect (irritation, resistance, defiance), focused attention (attention to the task), orientation to error (perceives error, monitors performance), attentional efficiency (appropriate attention shifting), social play (social involvement in the game), and sociability (enjoyment of social interaction with experimenter). Using the detailed coding schemes, it was possible to obtain reasonable agreements between independent coders of these behaviors during infancy and early childhood. In this study, early childhood competence was defined to include cognitive competence using standardized assessments, social–cognitive competence using tasks designed to tap inferential skills in social and psychological domains, and behavioral competence as assessed by parental report.

Our findings support the notion that regulatory systems have both indirect and direct effects on competence (F. K. Miller, 1995; F. K. Miller, Keating, & Marshment, 1996, 1997; F. K. Miller & Marshment, 1998). Infant regulation is related to preschool cognitive and behavioral competence, accounting for significant variance in several measures across this 5-year period; it is also significantly related to theoretically similar aspects of preschool regulation; and preschool regulation is clearly associated with preschool competence. By statistically controlling the effects of regulation on competence at each developmental period, we found that regulation at each period made independent contributions to the prediction of competence. This pattern of longitudinal and concurrent relationships establishes a connection between patterns of regulation and competence during the developmentally sensitive early years of life. These results build on and extend previous research that has illuminated important connections among patterns of social, emotional, and cognitive development.

In addition to establishing these broad connections, this investigation also provided evidence of consistent and interpretable relationships among specific processes and outcomes. The significant role of positive affect in infancy and early childhood, assessed during socially and cognitively challenging situations, suggests an important role for overall emotional tone in regulation and competence. This developmental pathway may be related to constructs such as defensiveness, in that openness to experience may be a key factor in both regulation and the acquisition of cognitive and behavioral competence. Among preschoolers, to take another example, children whose parents reported them as having more behavior problems showed a pattern of higher sociability or extroversion upon first encountering a novel situation but were generally more distractible and less likely to maintain positive social interactions when challenged. As a final example, we found a strong connection between preschoolers' anger and their ability to take another's perspective in a social cognition task. A developmental history of angry interactions with others may make it difficult to attend to the social and personal cues from which perspective taking ability is constructed.

These examples illustrate the value of including detailed process analyses in longitudinal investigations. Another benefit arises from the ability to contrast longitudinal and concurrent relationships. Infant regulation makes a significant contribution to preschool competence, independent of preschool regulation. Similarly, preschool regulation makes a significant contribution to preschool competence, independent of infant regulation. Together, they account for a significant amount of variance in competence. This is not to say that regulatory processes at the two developmental periods are unrelated; rather they are modestly related to each other.

The developmental pathway that captures these patterns may be described as follows. Infants who have developed good emotion, attention, and social regulatory capabilities are more likely to have habits of learning that contribute to their subsequent cognitive and behavioral development. They are also more likely to continue to acquire other developmentally appropriate regulatory capabilities. Preschoolers with good emotion, attention, and social regulation are likely to perform better in challenging situations, have better perspective taking skills, and be reported by their parents as having fewer behavior problems.

If patterns of competence and coping present at school onset have their roots in earlier development, as our preliminary findings suggest, there are two key implications. One is that improving the prospects for success across the whole population of children requires attention to the quality of the social environment before children even get to the school door. The other is that for schools to deal effectively with the increasing diversity with which they have been challenged in recent years, we require a more complete understanding of the developmental pathways leading to that diversity, the developmental processes that give rise to those various pathways, and hence the multiple pathways to further expertise that need to be designed for children with a range of developmental histories (Keating, 1990).

It is important to recognize that the empirical basis for the developmental linkages among neurophysiology, regulatory systems, and competence is preliminary, but it is plausible and consistent with the available evidence. But the real story is in the details, and future research will need to take these questions much further to establish the developmental pathways. Methodological advances in neuroimaging and neuroendocrine assays, which proceed ever more rapidly, will be especially crucial in moving the study of these linkages from plausibility to firm empirical grounds. A conceptual framework that encompasses the developmental integration of biology, behavior, and context is also crucial because the complexity arising from multiple systems, developing in mutual interaction with each other, may otherwise prove hard to resolve.

HABITS OF MIND

The rapidly emerging work on regulatory systems and their association with competence and the particular longitudinal investigation of infancy to early childhood summarized here provide support for the view that one key pathway to competence and coping is through the development of regulatory systems. We also have reason to believe, as noted above, that the development of these regulatory systems is substantially influenced by the quality of the social environment, especially the quality of the interpersonal relationships experienced early in life. Although we have only begun to identify some of the key pathways, it is already clear that these findings are consistent with the notion that early experience becomes biologically embedded, especially during sensitive periods, and has pervasive and enduring effects on later development.

We have sought a way to capture in simple terms this developmental integration of neurophysiological patterns, the regulatory systems through which those patterns are expressed in behavior, and competence in multiple domains, which depends in turn both on the patterns of regulation and the activity of the individual in specific learning contexts or habitats. We describe this developmental integration as *habits of mind.*

We see habits of mind as the dynamic system that links together biology and behavior over the course of development, as expressed in and supported by various contexts throughout development. It thus includes both the styles of behaving, learning, interacting, perceiving, and thinking that are rooted in underlying neurophysiology and are the result of the integration of different regulatory systems with each other, as well as the patterns of competence and expertise these developmental processes yield as the individual navigates various habitats (such as family, school, community, and the many expectations arising in these contexts). This complex feedback loop generates biobehavioral "attractor states," which likely have great stability within the individual, but also undergo reorganizations at critical or sensitive periods and sometimes as a result of nonnormative but highly salient individual life events.

These attractor states can be seen in habits of learning, for example, when some children react defensively against the perception of error. This habit of mind likely serves the goal of reducing anxious arousal from negative self-judgment but has the unfortunate consequence of blocking out information from error feedback, which may be critical for learning. They can also be seen in habits of perception, such as the psychological mindedness of clinicians who "automatically" see patterns of relationships or of individual functioning. Indeed, most habits of mind have an automatic, noneffortful character that serves the individual well when there is a match between the habit of mind and the context in which the individual functions (as in a scientist's critical habit of mind or a novelist's literate habit of mind) but serves the individual poorly when there is a mismatch (as in an

anxious child's fearful habit of mind that does not distinguish between secure versus threatening contexts).

Prevention or intervention efforts that do not take this dynamic system of development into account may yield less than optimal outcomes.
For example, behavior change may occur in one context but not generalize
to other contexts due either to its superficiality (that is, not affecting the
underlying regulatory system) or to the expectations of others in different
contexts, which promotes regression to the original habit of mind. Exploring the complexity of these developmental integrations of neurophysiology, regulatory systems, and competence is challenging but potentially worthwhile both for our understanding and for our efforts to create
more optimal conditions for human development. It also becomes a more
accessible goal with the marked advances in the various disciplines and
methods needed for such an exploration. A conceptual framework that
seeks the integration of these developmental dynamics, such as the one outlined here, may also serve to move such an exploration forward more effectively.

ACKNOWLEDGMENTS

This work has been supported by the Canadian Institute for Advanced Research
(where Daniel P. Keating is a Royal Bank Fellow), the Natural Sciences and Engineering Research Council of Canada, and the Social Sciences and Humanities Research Council of Canada (from whom Fiona K. Miller has received a doctoral fellowship). We also thank Robin Marshment, who has collaborated on various
aspects of the research reported in this chapter.

Part III

*Human Development
and the Learning Society*

After considering the evidence for pervasive socioeconomic gradient effects in developmental health in Part I, which raised the strong possibility of biological embedding to account for those effects, we reviewed in Part II the scientific basis for that claim which could be found in the impact of early experiences on brain and behavioral development. In Part III, we take up the social implications of the linkages identified in Parts I and II. If the developmental health of populations is substantially a function of the quality of the environments that we create for children and youth, we need to address the social and cultural aspects of human development that determine whether those supports of development will be present. The outcomes in developmental health are viewed as crucial not only for societal adaptability but also for future economic prosperity in the Information Age.

In Chapter 12, Daniel P. Keating explores the notion of "experiments in civilization" as a method for understanding the dramatic social and technological changes we are now experiencing. In particular, an innovation dynamic is identified that operates as a feedback loop between technological and social innovation. The thrust of this analysis is that for societies to support developmental health during this period of dramatic transformations, they will need to become "learning societies," that is, societies placing a premium on human development.

In Chapter 13, Thomas P. Rohlen argues that, in both the workplace and the school, the way in which learning occurs is central. It is also closely related to much that has been discussed in preceding chapters, notably how social processes, feelings, and attachments mediate intellectual growth. Many new insights are emerging about how to restructure learning contexts to improve learning in several senses, including wider participation and greater integration with normal problem solving. Innovations in manufacturing, the rise of knowledge industries, new technologies, the experiences of Japanese organizations, and new research into schools and classrooms all cast important light on these aspects of "learning software." The vision of a learning society rests on such changes and will require new approaches to child development and human resources.

By focusing on an innovative approach to learning, in Chapter 14 Marlene Scardamalia and Carl Bereiter raise questions about how we can transform North American schools into learning organizations, taking account of the social embeddedness of learning. When their chapter is read alongside Chapters 11–13, we are left with the question of how changes in the cultural and technological environment of learning may change the apparent developmental capabilities of children. These expanded capabilities, which capitalize on the potent process of collaborative knowledge building, may be the precise tools needed in the knowledge-based economies of the Information Age.

12

The Learning Society

A HUMAN DEVELOPMENT AGENDA

Daniel P. Keating

In Parts I and II, we learned that socioeconomic gradients in developmental health appear to constitute a valuable social diagnostic: the flatter the gradient, the better the overall developmental health of the population. We identified a strong contender for the origin of this phenomenon: the biological embedding of developmental experiences, especially in early life, in neural systems. The lifelong effects of this process can be observed—in increasing detail in both human and nonhuman populations—in a wide range of health and behavioral outcomes, including competence and coping. The quality of the developmental experiences available to children and youth thus has a profound effect on individuals and populations.

If this conceptual framework is sound, based on the logic and evidence presented in Parts I and II, then it seems prudent, even essential, to look more closely at the ways in which societies provide supports for developmental health throughout the population. In this critical examination, we can use the gradient effect and the biological embedding of early experience as touchstones for the analysis. As noted in Chapter 1 and elaborated in this and subsequent chapters, the impact of the quality of the social environment on human development likely goes beyond its effect on individuals and populations. The ability to function as a civic society with self-renewing "social capital" (Putnam, 1992), to generate the human capital necessary for economic prosperity in the Information Age, and to adapt to the rapid social and technological changes we now confront depends heavily on how a society organizes itself to support human development.

This seems, and no doubt is, a tall order. It is particularly daunting in the context of rapidly shifting environments. One productive approach may be to understand the nature of the changes we are experiencing from an even broader perspective on human development. This expanded conceptual framework would encompass both the evolutionary—hence biologically encoded—origins of human social interaction and organization (see Chapters 8 and 9, this volume), on the one hand, and the social and cultural histories that shape contemporary patterns of social functioning, on the other. These are of course on quite different time scales. The biological predispositions and constraints of the social functioning of our human primate species, *Homo sapiens,* have much in common with those of our close cousins, nonhuman primates. But our ongoing "experiments with civilization" (Keating & Mustard, 1993) have yielded a wide variety of ways in which these inherent predispositions can be channeled and reorganized. On an evolutionary timescale, these experiments have proceeded with lightning speed and at an accelerating pace.

It is useful to think about not only what we have learned from these experiments but also how we have learned it. In doing so, we should be aware of a common cognitive bias: the propensity to view change as progress. This may be a fundamental cognitive bias for humans, given our preference for narratives as a way of organizing experience and the emotional satisfaction they provide, both of which may have an evolutionary basis. This tendency, however, may lead us to experience the cultural and social "software" (see Rohlen, Chapter 13, this volume) of our own developmental histories as "second nature" and thus beyond question. What any society has learned is embedded in its interlocking social institutions and practices and its cultural patterns of making meaning. Currently successful societies are by definition those that have prospered, or at least survived. How they learned to do so is largely through trial and error, along with occasional efforts at systematic planning. The culmination in "modernism" of central social planning has not been notably successful, however, diminishing the general enthusiasm for systematic or scientific approaches (Harvey, 1989). Thus, the forms of social and cultural organization that are currently successful likely embody essential and accidental features, as well as evolved and planned elements. Moreover, social and cultural forms that are currently successful may be adapted to current circumstances but not necessarily adaptable to a shifting terrain.

On a smaller scale, many organizations and enterprises have confronted a similar challenge in recent years: how to benefit from what one has learned in order to adapt to a changing environment. The "learning organization" has emerged as a concept that brings together many of the key features of groups trying to meet this challenge (see Chapters 13 and 14, this volume; J. S. Brown & Duguid, 1991; Senge, 1990). We have explored the possibility of generalizing this notion of a learning organization to the broader scale—a learning society (Keating, 1995, 1996b, 1998). Many of the key features are similar across this scale transformation: clear goals; the active participation of all in achieving them; understanding the core dynamics of the system within which the group is operating; continuous improvement based on reliable feedback regarding progress; and effective means for nonjudgmental internal communication and collaboration.

Even if we grant that the building of a learning society is a desirable goal, we may well ask whether it can be achieved. Predicting the future is of less value in this regard than attempting to create it. A better question is, "What principles might help in its construction?" In this and the next two chapters, we take up that challenge and try to identify some social and cultural factors that may be crucial in this effort. We begin with a broad historical perspective within which we may better understand the current dynamics of change.

CONTEMPORARY SOCIAL CHANGE IN HISTORICAL CONTEXT

It has become commonplace to note that we are experiencing rapid, perhaps unprecedented, social, technological and economic change as we approach the 21st century. The perceived rapidity of these changes not only generates a sense of disorientation among many individuals but also presents major challenges to societal adaptability. Societies must cope simultaneously with global economic competition, the demand for new competencies in the population, the provision of opportunities for health and wellbeing throughout the population, and the maintenance of the social fabric for nurturing, socializing, and educating the next generation. We have argued that successfully meeting these challenges sets the foundations for future population health and competence, economic prosperity, and social cohesion. But many of the traditional societal forms and practices may experience difficulty in adapting to change, and new forms that may be able to meet these challenges have yet to emerge clearly.

The pace, magnitude, and complexity of social change are often perceived as overwhelming and uncontrollable. This perceived lack of control can then distort our perceptions of the challenges and opportunities, further diminishing our ability to respond and adapt to change. This dynamic—accelerating change and decreasing sense of control—makes thoughtful social responses difficult to achieve.

We may start to break this cycle by appealing to a combined evolutionary and historical perspective that takes note of the fundamentally social nature of humans, particularly focusing on the many different patterns of organizing social life with which we humans have experimented. Like almost all of our close relatives—nonhuman primates—*Homo sapiens* is a social species. We play, work, interact, learn, and reproduce in social groups throughout our lives. We develop in social relationships from the earliest period of life, as do most other primates, but we remain dependent on the caretaking of others for a longer time than does any other primate. At the core, then, we need social groups to survive.

Moreover, as we have seen, our early experiences—most of which occur through social interactions—play a critical role throughout life in how we cope, how we learn, and how competent we become. The nature of the social environment in which we develop is thus a key determinant of our quality of life. Diverse life outcomes, positive and negative, are closely associated with identifiable differences in early social experiences (see Keating & Miller, Chapter 11, this volume). In turn, the quality of the human social environment is partly a function of the competence that is available within the society. The nurture, education, and socialization of new members of the group depend on the skills and commitment of more mature members and on social arrangements that facilitate high-quality interactions among generations.

Many of these demands are neither historically new nor species specific. But we face additional challenges unknown to our human and prehominid ancestors. Although we share much in common with our primate cousins, we humans appear to be unique in having developed the capabilities of conscious self-reflection, cultural transmission of skills and knowledge through language and other symbolic means, cumulative technological development, and civilization. In evolutionary terms, these are quite recent changes in our lives (Keating, 1995; Keating & Mustard, 1993).

We can get a better sense of how recent they are by using a calendar year analogy. Let us take 100,000 years as an estimate of the time elapsed since the emergence of fully modern humans and place it on the scale of a single year. Using this baseline, we can note that our species first moved into small urban centers, supported by agriculture, about the end of November, and started the industrial revolution on the afternoon of New Year's Eve. Only a few minutes ago, we launched experiments in instantaneous global communication, information technology, and multicultural metropolism. This recency is further exaggerated if we use the earlier starting point of the emergence of consistent toolmaking and tool use by hominids, which may go back as much as 2.5 million years.

The origins and mechanisms of this evolutionary process remain controversial (Dennett, 1995), but several important features have gained fairly broad consensus. Consider first the social sophistication of nonhuman primates. From this perspective, we can see that complex social arrangements and behaviors among humans are not merely a function of cultural experiences; other primates are also skilled social strategists (see Suomi, Chapter 9, this volume; Tomasello, Kruger, & Ratner, 1993). Much of our "intuitive" understanding of how to function in groups thus has a lengthy evolutionary history, which has embedded in us many elegant "designs" for social interaction, although some of them may present obstacles to further adaptation—excessive wariness of "others" may be one such obstructive design feature.

At some critical juncture, we humans added language capabilities to this already rich social mix, yielding virtually infinite potential for complex communication. Language enables much more complex social communication and may even have arisen initially out of a need to maintain cohesion in larger groups (Donald, 1991; Dunbar, 1992), although there is much controversy at the moment regarding the evolutionary history of human language (Dennett, 1995). The larger group size may have contributed economic benefits of organization and specialization of work, permitting more effective exploitation of harsh habitats as well as a primitive form of shared risk.

The teaching and learning of special skills were also enhanced by language, and an accelerating cycle of technological innovation and development ensued. Apparently unique to *Homo sapiens,* this unification of language and tool use was put forward by Vygotsky (1978) as the starting point of fully human intelligence, both phylogenetically and ontogenetically.

At a later critical juncture, the evidence suggests that we humans drew on our increasing symbolic and instrumental sophistication (i.e., better language and tool use) to establish connections *between* troops and tribes. This is a signal accomplishment, which we might justifiably designate as the initiation of human "experiments with civilization" (Keating & Mustard, 1993), on two grounds: (1) the organization of social life was no longer exclusively within the troop, and (2) culture emerged as an explicit means of intergroup cohesion and identification. We can date the origins of this new design pattern in human activity to about 40,000–50,000 years ago (Stringer & Gamble, 1993), when the remarkable onset and spread both of symbolic forms (particularly cave painting and sculpture) and of more complex stone technologies, which had been previously unchanged for perhaps 2 million years, coincided. The rapidity and coincidence of these emerging forms suggests the innovation of language-based cultural diffusion, which implies in turn the capacity to work with others outside one's own group and to innovate on a collaborative basis.

It is important, however, not to romanticize this prehistoric past. Ample evidence supports the pervasive nature of human conflict, among individuals and between groups, then and now. Cooperation did not displace conflict, but new designs for intergroup collaboration and diffusion are likely to have afforded substantial material advantages to groups who took it up, even against the backdrop of persistent intergroup conflict. A contemporary manifestation of the romantic misconception is the belief that cooperation is a natural and desirable state of humanity for which only the educational opportunities to exercise it are needed in order to induce it. The evidence suggests rather the contrary. Both competition and cooperation represent potential human activities, but persistent and effective cooperation has to be highly supported by well-designed structures and practices that acknowledge and account for the equally human propensities toward competition and conflict. As in most complex systems, it is the tension between cooperation and competition that is a source of creative self-organization.

Without going into great detail, we can refer to another shift that occurred some 30,000 years later, about 10,000 years ago: the agricultural revolution, when we humans began to learn how to make and cultivate our own resources rather than foraging for them. That set of innovations enabled us to store up resources, which permitted humans to congregate in ever larger groups in relatively more stable settings. That congregation in turn gave rise to the organization of state structures, as well as to the organization of knowledge and the origins of science. Our attempts to understand the world systematically and to generate new knowledge can be traced in many ways to the confluence of these technological and social innovations.

The agricultural revolution first enabled the congregation and settlement of large groups of humans in specific places over a durable period of time—in other words, cities. The organization of production in agricultural societies demanded that a relatively large proportion of the population was needed to provide direct physical energy—plowing, sowing, reaping, and so on. Thus, only a small portion of the population was directly involved in the acquisition and expansion of knowledge, a shift in social organization that was potentiated by the agricultural revolution. Literacy and numeracy, for example, remained rare skills over long historical periods—and into the present in less affluent societies. Yet the potential for rapid and systematic accumulation of knowledge owing to the opportunities for collaborative learning was historically realized, as was the onset of new social designs, including formal education and cumulative science.

The next major revolution in social forms occurred very recently, as the industrial revolution carried this process even further. It represents another major qualitative shift in how we dealt with the world in material ways. The technology story is one that is well known. The industrial revolution removed human labor from the direct energy loop required for material production but created a demand for ever more complex arrangements for the organization of labor. Rosenberg and Birdzell (1986) have identified the social innovations that were equally important to the technological innovations: new ways of organizing labor, new ways of sharing financial risk, new ways of establishing trade relationships, and so on. The culmination of this matching of technological and social innovation in the industrial era may well be the advanced stages of "Fordism" in production. More complex forms of automated production and the design of work organization have begun to take advantage of the next likely shift, the one toward a knowledge economy (see Rohlen, Chapter 13, this volume). Note again that these technological innovations were mutually dependent upon concomitant changes in social structures and practices.

These examples thus illustrate an ongoing, mutually causal interplay between technological and social innovation. This may be difficult to visualize initially, as we are more accustomed to linear or main-effect models, in which an isolated cause yields a specific outcome. But as we trace these major transformations in our species' history, we can see that changes in technology generated demands and opportunities for changes in societal functioning, and changes in society generated demands and opportunities for technological innovation:

- Language and complex communication within the group (100–50K years before the present [BP]; Donald, 1991)
- Intertribal communication and cultural diffusion (about 40K years BP)
- The agricultural revolution and settled urban civilizations (about 10K years BP)
- The industrial revolutions (about 0.5–0.1K years BP), from steam to electrical power
- The information and knowledge revolutions (now)

Another such transformational moment thus seems to be upon us, in the form of currently expanding information technologies and knowledge media: instantaneous and thoroughly diffused global communication; unlimited knowledge storage and retrieval; sophisticated techniques for data analysis, simulation, and visual representation; and artificially intelligent design with robotic manufacture. Unique among species, then, we humans have created what systems theorists call an iterative feedback loop between our ways of using material resources and the ways in which we organize our social lives. This new pattern of cultural and social change continually reshapes the ecological habitats in which we live and work, and in which subsequent generations will develop (Keating & Mustard, 1993). The essence of this "innovation dynamic" is shown in Figure 12.1.

The accelerating pace of technological and social change appears to be based, then, on our species-specific penchant for collaborative learning across (formerly rigid) group boundaries. Enhancing this new design for learning through progressively more efficient cultural means—oral histories, formal instruction, writing, and now information technologies—contributes directly to this acceleration (Dudley, 1991). Changes in the means of communication also have nontrivial consequences for cognitive activity: how we think, what we know, and how we learn. A well-understood example is the connection between the practice of literacy and the development of logic, argument, reflection, and metacognitive understanding (Cole & Scribner, 1974; Olson, 1994). As literacy spreads, so do literate habits of mind. This analysis suggests that the combination of a new technology for communication with new capabilities in the population creates a potent new medium for discourse among previously isolated groups and individuals—and thus new opportunities for innovation.

The mutual feedback system of technology innovation and social innovation is thus an extremely important dynamic. It is that dynamic which now apparently leads us to the cusp of yet another major qualitative shift,

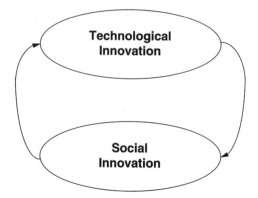

1. **Precision Stone Tools**
   Intergroup Learning

2. **Agricultural Resource**
   Urban Congregation

3. **Industrial Manufacture**
   Taylorism / Urban Linkages /
   Market Mechanisms

FIGURE 12.1. The innovation dynamic.

which has been variously referred to as the Information Age or the knowledge revolution. Note how rapidly the pace of change appears to be accelerating: the Neolithic revolution occurs about 40,000 years ago; the agricultural revolution, about 10,000 years ago; and the earliest phases of the industrial revolution (e.g., Johannes Gutenberg's invention of printing with movable type), roughly 550 years ago.

POTENTIAL PATHWAYS
OF THE INNOVATION DYNAMIC

One of the things that may be different about this change, even compared to previous major historical shifts, is its capacity for almost infinite acceleration, because the technology innovation is precisely about knowledge. It builds on the notion that information in an ideal sense becomes totally accessible and very inexpensive or free. Communication becomes a universal phenomenon. Artificially intelligent systems begin to replace a whole host of human activities in the economic space. What we may be entering is a quite unprecedented kind of change, but the phenomenon of change is one whose key dynamics we may nevertheless be able to grasp.

Can we use this understanding of the innovation dynamic to get a better grasp of the challenges facing modern societies? Many observers have suggested that we appear to be at the cusp of change, but we may envision different possible paths for the future. One path (path B in Figure 12.2) has captured the attention of science fiction writers and social science prognosticators alike. This path is put forward by many as the most likely outcome on the path of least resistance. Simple inertia from our current directions seems to lead toward the separation of a technology or cognitive elite from increasingly marginalized mass populations. And, of course, that division is not just within societies in the advanced world but also certainly between the developed and the developing world. To the extent that this change goes along in the direction that we see it going now, in terms of deskilling and unemployment, that path seems to have a high probability.

Conceptually, at least, there are alternative pathways. One alternative would suggest that we need to think about a way of introducing technology that would in fact encourage mass or universal participation in collaborative knowledge building, not only about our material and economic existence but also in terms of our social functioning and societal structure. The generic concept, then, that holds these ideas together is the notion of a learning society, represented as path A in Figure 12.2.

As already noted, many would predict that path B is the almost inevitable route from where we now stand. But we can take note of the fact that when systems are at major change points, as we know from looking at many different dynamic systems in many different domains, the variance increases dramatically. In such circumstances, small pushes to that system can move it down different paths—the well-known "butterfly effect." Thus, another way

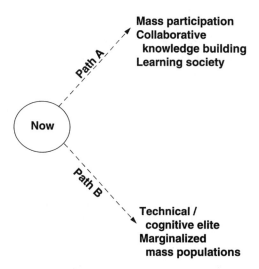

FIGURE 12.2. Schematic view of possible future pathways.

of phrasing the task that we have attempted is that we are trying to understand the key dynamics of human development in such a way that it might be
possible to push humankind on a more virtuous cycle, onto a path that has
more of the positive features of path A and therefore enables us to avoid some
of the very worrisome features of path B. Among the most worrisome features
of path B, of course, is that it calls into question the stability of society itself, if
it were to remain sharply divided, and it would likely worsen the negative gradient effects discussed in Part I of this volume.

Many of the central aspects differentiating these two possible pathways invoke important features of human development. A knowledge
economy relies heavily on the human resources of its population, including
health, coping, and competence. These, in turn, may well arise from the
quality of the social environment in which those developments occur across
the life course, with a particular impact attaching to the quality of the social environment in early childhood. Making effective use of these well-
developed human resources requires attention to the social organization of
those resources, whether in support of the economy (i.e., workplace organization for production) or the society (i.e., community coherence). It may
now be possible to employ a conceptual framework on human development to move toward a learning society—a framework that would focus
both on promoting developmental health and making use of those human
resources to achieve these goals.

THE LEARNING SOCIETY

We have used the term "learning society" to capture this idea. Although
this term is fraught with the potential for misinterpretation, it does connect
a number of key themes essential for constructive change. Among these are
that change is a continuous process, that it can be brought to conscious
awareness in which goals are made explicit, that it involves the broader society and not just communities of experts, and that collaborative learning is
crucial to effective societal adaptation.

It is important to clarify potentially major misconceptions that may
arise from the use of each of the constituent terms. Learning is not to be restricted to the individual acquisition of knowledge or skill already attained
by others (as in, say, "learning to read"); rather, it also will include activities better described as collaborative knowledge building and innovation
(see Chapters 13 and 14, this volume). Traditional psychological notions
that viewed learning as a purely internal set of processes describing the adaptation of the individual to a relatively fixed external environment (the
"to be learned" material) represent one type of obstacle to this broader understanding.

Society is to be seen as not only a collection of institutions and practices but also as a culturally integrated organization of those institutions and practices; that organization is in itself capable of adapting and learning from experience. As noted above, it has become commonplace to speak of learning organizations capable of effective institutional memory, collaborative goal seeking, and continuous improvement, all of which occur in a real sense at the group rather than the individual level. A learning society can be usefully regarded as a generalized form of the learning organization.

This introduces one further potential misconception, which is that collaborative efforts depend on uniformity of goals among the individual members of a group. From this misconception, it is easy to dismiss the notion of an effective learning organization (or learning society) merely by taking note of the ubiquity of conflict and competition in human activity. The heart of this misconception is the view that competition and cooperation are exclusive states. It can be observed in many well-functioning complex systems that cooperation and competition are linked in a dynamic tension that is essential to the system's functioning. Neural competition at the level of cells and cooperation at the level of systems is but one well-documented example.

This is, of course, the now familiar competition–cooperation dynamic in yet another guise. When rewards are distributed (partially) on the basis of individual accomplishment, the risks of cooperation are magnified. But knowledge building, as opposed to knowledge transmission, occurs far more effectively in collaborative networks than as individuals. It grows increasingly clear that knowledge of all types is always a social and cultural product. As advanced information technologies spread, this social nature of knowledge will become ever more apparent. The emerging picture of science as a collaborative and cumulative discourse captures the essence of one key self-organizing social system. Differences among societies in how well they are able to make use of the social nature of knowledge may determine, in part, how effective they will be in building successful, innovation-based economies. In other words, socially distributed intelligence may become increasingly central to societal success. It depends, in turn, on the diversity of talent available in the population *and* on the ways in which human groups interact to become units of learning.

Recent work on human groups supports the notion that organizations which grow and adapt best tend to learn collaboratively (J. S. Brown & Duguid, 1991). As noted above, key ingredients include the following: shared and clearly understood goals; open, lateral networks for the flow of information and expertise; and reasonable distribution of gains from group efforts. A legitimate social expectation of institutions from schools, to workplaces, to the delivery of human services, to community development is that they should examine the ways in which they might increase their adaptability and effectiveness through reorganization along these lines (see Chapters 13 and 14, this volume).

LEARNING ORGANIZATIONS: KEY PRINCIPLES

The systematic study of learning organizations is relatively recent. Thus we have many descriptions and case studies but little comparative or systematic research. Nonetheless, key elements noted by thoughtful observers can be summarized. They all start with the recognition that learning occurs not just within individuals but also by groups and organizations of all sorts. As the world to which we need to adapt becomes more complex, it is only when knowledge and expertise are distributed across individuals that effective learning can occur.

A first characteristic of collaborative learning organizations is that they tend to emphasize coordinated group effort toward commonly shared goals rather than purely individual accomplishment. One might say there is a coherent conceptual framework among the members of the organization. This presumes, of course, that enough people in the organization have chosen to participate actively in the organization's success. This is enhanced when individuals believe that they will get a reasonable return for their investment of effort. Steep gradients, in an organization or a society, may well mitigate against this desirable characteristic of full, mindful participation.

Second, there is active commitment to continuous improvement and to the diffusion of best practices throughout the organization. Part of each individual's contribution is to discover ways of doing the task better or more efficiently. Collaborative learning organizations are characterized by horizontal networks of information flow rather than vertical/hierarchical structures for top–down decision making. In vertical systems, there are "checks" on the flow of information at many points, both on the way up and the way back down. Decentralized decision making makes an organization more nimble, as the information can find a most effective route. This does, of course, place a burden on the first element, a widely shared understanding of the organization's goals. The horizontal networks, when effective, bring together all the expertise of an organization. This, in turn, raises the value of diversity of expertise within the organization, as there will thus be more contact points with the external world to which the group need adapt. In North America, one often overlooked resource is multicultural diversity. Although often viewed as a difficulty to be overcome rather than as a strength, and although some advantage may accrue at present to more monocultural societies, the potential strength of a diverse storehouse of useful cultural solutions is not to be overlooked.

Third, a hallmark of many learning organizations is that they understand and can analyze the dynamic system within which they are functioning (Senge, 1990). This permits an organization to act at the points of greatest leverage and, equally important, to avoid reactions to specific events that have negative impact in the long run.

Improvements and refinements in information technology, such as the emerging platforms for telelearning, will likely create new opportunities for the building of learning organizations (see Scardamalia & Bereiter, Chapter 14, this volume). Supporting effective learning by organizations in all sectors of society will be a critical factor in the building of a learning society. Societies with cultural traditions that emphasize a balance between the individual and the collective are likely to be better prepared to organize in this fashion, compared with societies that have a stronger emphasis on the individual apart from society.

It is useful to think of the learning society we hope to achieve not as a static structure toward which we are headed but as a continuing process that we will improve on as we proceed. The two key steps for building a learning society are to (1) start functioning like one as soon as possible, recruiting available resources and networks, and (2) learn from this experience as we go, to enhance the effectiveness of the learning networks that emerge.

Understanding is only one step toward effective change. Understanding in the absence of action has no practical consequence. Can we design a coherent strategy for becoming the kind of learning society we have described? We hardly need reminding of how catastrophic the failures of grand central plans for society have been in this century (Harvey, 1989). We are wise to be wary of such grand social designs. We also note that as the complexity of available information expands, the adaptability of institutions that rely on centralized decision making decreases, in part because it cannot be maximally sensitive to local conditions. For all these reasons, there can be no central blueprint to specify the steps for building a learning society.

In addition to a conceptual framework, then, we need a plan to create the infrastructure for collaborative learning in a learning society. This infrastructure needs to incorporate several elements: (1) that the human resources of the population are an integral part of a successful learning society; (2) that the range of competencies to be developed must also shift to include the abilities to learn and produce collaboratively; and (3) that the maintenance and expansion of effective learning organizations and networks (in the public, private, and intermediate sectors) is the essence of the learning society.

One of the essential features of a learning society is the continuous monitoring of the developmental health of its members, a system incorporating this knowledge into policy and planning, both public and private. It is distressing to realize how much more attention currently is paid to monitoring economic performance and environmental impacts than is paid to monitoring human development (Keating & Mustard, 1996). In order to make effective use of such information, however, we need to provide both the technological and conceptual infrastructure for informed community discourse on how best to adapt to the changing needs of contemporary societies (see Offord et al., Chapter 15, this volume). It is only through such ongoing societal investment that there is any real hope of lasting (i.e., self-renewing) change. In other words, achieving the goal of a learning society requires acting as if it were so and learning how to do it as we proceed.

We should beware of hubris as we attempt to meet these challenges. We have been shaped by thousands of millennia of hominid evolution, which gives us much potential but also many constraints, only some of which we understand very well at this time. We have even less experience of knowing how to adapt to the experiments in civilization that the innovation dynamic keeps churning up. The hubris would be that, despite these inherited constraints and limited experience, we should expect to be able to solve these complex problems forthwith. As they remain unresolved, we sometimes lapse into looking for someone or some group to bear the blame, rather than recognizing the inherent difficulty and complexity of the problems. Solution-focused discourse seems, under these circumstances, to be a better use of human resources than identifying the blameworthy. Although resistance to productive change may arise from self-centered goals, such as retaining power, or from personal apprehensions, such as fear of change, we should recognize that some of the most formidable obstacles to change lie in the inertia of complex systems themselves. It is, however, at points of fundamental change that new ways of surmounting old obstacles are most possible. Being prepared to take advantage of these opportunities for societal adaptability is the essence of the learning society.

13

Social Software for a Learning Society

RELATING SCHOOL AND WORK

Thomas P. Rohlen

Learning and unlearning occur throughout the human realm, but not at the same rate and not automatically. Learning better ways to do things is the very essence of innovation. If we view learning and unlearning as central to problem solving and therefore to adaptive processes of all kinds, then it follows that differentials in systems of learning are of enormous consequence for individuals, organizations, and whole societies. This implies that a key challenge before every society is the improvement of the basic processes of learning upon which it depends. Despite our focus on individuals as learners, learning processes are primarily social in nature; that is, it is the patterns by which we interact in organized environments such as schools, workplaces, and communities that determine how much and what kind of learning occurs. To what degree these patterns encourage or inhibit regular feedback, fresh thinking, open communication, and so forth is a fundamental question before every society. As the world adjusts to increasing rates of change, adapts to new technologies, and adjusts to the globalization of economic competition, the topic of learning and particularly its encouragement becomes of central importance.

This chapter is largely about the linkages between learning processes in schools and those at work. It argues that the ways we work are changing, that as a result a gap exists today between our schools and our work organizations, and that this gap is growing as the problem-solving component of work is emphasized and as information technologies are defining new possibilities for cooperative learning in the workplace. In essence, the message is that our schools need to teach learning processes that better fit the way work is evolving. Above all this means teaching the skills and habits of mind that are essential to problem solving, especially where many minds need to interact.

Let me clearly state at the outset that I am not going to focus on new instructional technologies. While computers and information networks are obviously important elements of the changing workplace, they are neither the essence of the matter nor even a necessary prior condition. What is most fundamental to the evolving nature of learning as a central ingredient of work are the understandings and the social arrangements that define the learning process itself. New information technologies greatly enhance the possibilities of cooperative problem solving, but only if the more fundamental understandings and social arrangements are in place.

By equating learning to problem solving, we highlight its relevance to activities that add value in the course of adult working and living. Problem solving means learning to make improvements large or small in how things are done. The opportunities to problem solve are ubiquitous in the workplace and in everyday life. What is remarkable is how infrequently we perceive these opportunities and/or are encouraged to act on them. The culprit is not human ignorance or laziness nearly so much as it is the institutional expectations that frame our world.

A simple example will help illustrate this point. Two cars collide at an intersection. Let's assume the light had just changed. What do both drivers immediately begin thinking about? That is, what is the problem for them? If no one is seriously hurt, they are almost certain to begin worrying about who will be judged at fault. And, related to this, they will each immediately start worrying about insurance claims, legal penalties, and so forth. Typically, these worries lead each driver to a defense of his/her own actions with all the associated matters of favorably adjusting the evidence, accusations of the other's carelessness, and protestations of his/her own innocence. Perhaps the parties will be civil, perhaps not. Perhaps they will clear the road quickly, and perhaps they will be more concerned with their own circumstances. The point is that anomalous events such as this are almost certain to be quickly classified into a framework that defines "the problem." In this instance a legal/moral framework sets everyone to thinking about matters defined by terms like "blame," "fault," "guilt," and "error." If we stop to think about it, a very large proportion of our work and school activities are similarly shaped by a similar framework. Patently, it is not the drivers' job to attend to the more basic "problem," one typical of traffic intersections, that the way lights change is readily anticipated and this tempts drivers to make small but dangerous miscalculations.

The police officer arriving on the scene also sees a set of "problems." His/her job is to clear up matters—first, by restoring traffic to normal; then, by recording the facts, and perhaps by assigning blame. The problem of disputing drivers must be dealt with. Experience has shown that separating the two drivers and taking down their stories separately is the best means of reducing the tensions and obtaining a degree of accuracy in the reporting. The police officer's job is thus part traffic manager, part referee, and part judge—all practical and legal roles. He/she clears things up and restores matters to the status quo ante.

Interestingly, the issue of why such accidents occur as frequently as they do and what might reduce their occurrence is a job assigned to someone somewhere else, perhaps a traffic engineer or an analyst for an auto insurance think tank. This division of labor, between a world of routine behavior measured in terms of right and wrong (where an anomaly is rarely experienced as an opportunity to improve a situation) and a distant world of experts charged with finding solutions, is a ubiquitous part of our social existence. It is profoundly commonplace to separate routines from the expectation of improvements. One is tempted to say we have inherited a world that institutionalizes a fundamental barrier between doing and thinking, between routines and their improvement. An anomaly in a routine is a "mistake," "someone's fault," or a situation to be "cleaned up," rather than an opportunity to stop and examine what it can tell us about the possibility for improvement.

In the foregoing example a number of other considerations separate the world of routines from that of innovation. First, job definitions separate those on the scene from those whose task is analysis. Second, the authority to solve the deeper problem is not delegated to anyone on location. Third, the information that would likely become the basis of a solution (such as how often has a similar accident occurred at this intersection at what times and under what conditions) is collected and analyzed somewhere else. For such reasons the people directly involved are neither responsible for nor empowered to act upon the problem. This state of affairs is commonplace throughout organizations: the more complex the society or the organization is, the further removed problem solving (i.e., learning) becomes from the great majority of workers.

The critical point here is that our basic institutional understandings frame our perceptions and expectations and in so many cases transform an "opportunity" to learn into something else. That something else very often becomes a matter of blame and fear, keeping score, punishments for wrongdoing (and its associated denial), and, often enough, cover-up.

In the more advanced realms of work today, however, this situation is gradually changing as a new approach is being tried, one that is encouraging average workers to view themselves as responsible for improvements in the very routines they are performing. This shift is quite revolutionary if we understand that it is shifting the definition of work—delegating responsibility more widely and putting thinking back into doing. From this shift arises the prospect that average work will become part of inclusive, interactive efforts at problem solving and innovation.

It is paradoxical that while we are very concerned with improving education today, we rarely examine the fundamental assumptions about learning taught in our schools. Are we, for example, helping students see mistakes as opportunities to learn, or are they made to feel afraid of making mistakes? Are we giving them a sense of their own problem-solving responsibilities, or are we encouraging them to think their job is to support routines for the sake of those very routines? Are we encouraging children to work effectively together to solve problems, or are we rewarding them exclusively for individual achievements? Most importantly, are we teaching them to master problem solving as a process, or are we teaching them to master information as a routine?

THE INFORMATION AGE
AND THE LEARNING SOCIETY

There is a critical historical shift to consider in this regard. In a little more than 100 years the advanced nations have gone from largely an agricultural existence to a fundamentally industrial and organizational one, from a rural population to an urban one, from an elite to a mass culture, from nation-states and colonialism to economic globalism, and from a time of information scarcity to one of information overload (see Drucker, 1994, for a succinct overview of these changes). The meaning of space and time has been transformed by technology. If in 1990 it was the modern factory, the public school, and the nation-state that symbolized the future, as we approach the year 2000 the reigning signposts are such things as the global corporation, the Internet, and a deepening skepticism about the basic assumptions and values we have inherited as the "modern" agenda. Visionaries preparing us for the future point to the rise of a single global economy, to the microchip revolution, to new systems of telecommunications, to the increasing pace of change in technology and new product development, to the explosion of knowledge, and to the superabundance and availability of information as defining characteristics of this new era. Value, once added via advances in energy use and economies of scale, is now enhanced primarily by the application of intelligence. Whether it is a smarter machine or a smarter medicine or a smarter business policy, the general trend is toward rapid change due to the intensified application of intelligence to problem solving. This coincides with a growing perception that the most economically dynamic elements of our society are its "knowledge workers" and its "learning organizations" (Davis & Davidson, 1991; Drucker, 1988, 1993; Reich, 1991; H. Smith, 1995; Zuboff, 1988). How we create knowledge, who has information, and the way we organize ourselves to learn and innovate are very much at the heart of these changes.

As innovation becomes more and more critical to organizational success, companies are reevaluating their priorities and organizational makeup in order to enhance their internal rates of learning. They are talking about and coming to view knowledge and knowledge creation capabilities as crucial assets.[1] This may sound as though they are preoccupied with research and development (R&D), but the reality is that increasingly managers are viewing knowledge creation as everyone's job. The idea is that problem solving can and should occur routinely at all levels and in regard to every kind of issue. The ideal is that learning ought to be ubiquitous throughout the organization.[2] The ways this will happen are only beginning to be perceived, and much R&D and experimentation lie ahead; nevertheless, the direction of change is clear. It is also clear that schools must adapt to this new direction. So far the rate of innovation has been much greater in the business world, where external pressures for change are more severe and persistent than they are in the world of education.

Already there is a growing wage gap between those with skills of growing relevance in this environment and those lacking such skills. Significant parts of our populations are in jeopardy of being left out or left behind for want of the relevant education and skills, intensifying the crisis of human development much of this book is about. We rightly are concerned about the prospect that many in the next generation will not be ready to participate effectively. In this regard it is critical that we develop as clear a picture as possible of work as it is evolving under these new conditions (Reich, 1991; Zuboff, 1988).

The shifting economic fortunes of communities and whole nations are sufficiently well known today to be a valid basis for the regular reappraisal of the foundations of social prosperity. The industrial rise of East Asia, for example, or the shifting fortunes of nation and subregions, such as Silicon Valley in the developed world, have served to underscore a set of critical factors that favor success in this new economic environment. While there is much still to debate, there is no disagreement that the quality of human resources and the capacity of social institutions to foster innovation are at the very center of economic advantage.

While the information revolution has been a catalyst for these shifts in perspective and organization, the most fundamental issue before us is how to better use the abundance of information at our fingertips and how to engage more of the population in the processes of using information to solve problems. As information becomes cheaper, intelligence becomes more dear. Preparation of children for the intelligent use of information is a critical policy goal. Just as critical is the development of organizations that inherently foster continuous learning. This is far easier said than done. Thus, while it is rarely disputed that we have entered a period in human history when the processes of learning themselves will be the focus of persistent attention and innovation, the search initiated by these changes at the levels of the organization, the community and the nation for a more innovative system is in its earliest stage. This search is for what we will label here as the "learning society." It is by necessity a search that must draw into one framework improvements in human development, schooling, and work.

In a learning society, the goal is continuous learning, leading to improved knowledge and problem solving, making for better adaptation to rapid change. Innovation includes creating new knowledge, learning to utilize existing knowledge to solve problems, and diffusing such solutions in the population. A learning society is conscious of and focused on improving the fundamental processes of innovation. The most basic aspect of the Information Age in this regard is what might be termed the democratization of knowledge. Information and knowledge are distributed today far more widely and richly than ever before thanks to computers and related technology. This opens up the possibility of much wider participation in the use of information to solve problems; it does not, however, guarantee this result. Critical to success is (1) the general capacity of a population to use information to create knowledge, that is, to think, to evaluate, to analyze, to communicate, and thus to solve problems, and (2) the encouragement of learning within organizations.

It will help to remind ourselves of just how taken for granted and inappropriate much of our current learning software is. Consider the antique chestnut or truism, "You can't teach an old dog new tricks." Applied to people this hoary notion depreciates the potential for learning in adulthood, makes us skeptical of retraining efforts, and perpetuates a critical assumption of our current system holding that we learn appropriate routines and knowledge in school and then apply what we have learned thereafter throughout our increasingly long lives. Such a static picture is obviously maladaptive in today's world. In the past, when the great majority of work was manual and highly repetitive, such an approach to adulthood was largely congruent with the realities of much of the work available. Such unconscious notions will be persistently challenged in our evolution toward a learning society.

THE LEARNING SOFTWARE OF SCHOOLS

A bit of history about schooling will help. We take school systems for granted today much as we take paying our taxes for granted, yet as recently as the early 19th century public education was quite remarkable. Schools by themselves existed, but the notion of universal public education was a dream held by a visionary minority. The absorption of knowledge through lectures and books was of limited importance to almost any 19th-century population. Where they existed, schools occupied a small part of most children's lives. Put differently, before roughly 1850 schools were very largely for the elite and their practical value existed in preparing a professional and managerial class.

What we think of as knowledge was different too. Consider, for example, that in 1850 Harvard had less than 50,000 books in its library. Today it has 13 million and is faced with the challenge of accommodating an explosion of new sources of knowledge stored digitally. Mastery of an inclusive field or specialization was a plausible goal in 1850. Today knowledge work means operating at nodes in vastly complex fields of interrelationship. A transformation of similar magnitude is likely to occur during the next century as the advance of information technology makes our present learning systems obsolete.

A teacher addressing a class of students is a 4,000-year-old learning system. Examples of this form abound in the ancient world. As a learning system this kind of instruction operates at many levels beside the content of the teacher's presentation. The more the teacher talks, the more the students must learn to sit still and generally be silent (certainly for them more still and silent than is usual). As the authority, the teacher "knows" the subject; he/she is the "master." Desks, writing materials, perhaps a blackboard, and a raised platform for the teacher have described the conventional physical setting of schooling for a very long time. The conventional time periods of education defined when to listen, when to practice, and when seeking relief from these efforts was permitted. The university lecture is perhaps the quintessential example of this ancient form of instruction. Our most revered and advanced institution of learning is also rife with ancient pedagogical legacies. Furthermore, textbooks, instructional movies, TV programs for the classroom, drill books, encyclopedia, and other "aids" all fit this mode very well and are so designed. They substitute one "authority," one "master," for another. The direction information flows is still one way, literally "down." Content is packaged to facilitate digestion. Interaction among learners is peripheral and often actually discouraged as disruptive to the central processes of instruction.

This mode of formally offering and ingesting information is still the dominant practice today in a very wide range of circumstances categorized by such inclusive labels as training, education, instruction, school, course, class and so forth—namely, wherever we formalize learning on the basis of our classic assumptions. Quite patently, we learn in many other ways, most of them taken for granted and not formalized. We learn, for example, by "doing," and "on the job," and "at our mother's knee," and "from our mistakes," and in countless other largely informal, less examined, and only vaguely specified ways. Viewed in this light, learning and education are far from synonymous and it is education that appears narrowly routinized and constrained. Come to think about it, learning and education can be antithetical, as in those instances where educational practice actually undermines curiosity.

Furthermore, even 4,000 years is a short period in the evolution of human culture, something that has been evolving as a result of adaptive learning for hundreds of thousands of years, during most of which there were no classrooms or schools and no school systems—other, that is, than the "school of hard knocks." The set of institutionalized forms and assumptions known as education comes very late indeed in the history of human learning. I mention this because disconnecting our assumptions about education from the larger possibilities of learning is an important step in a general reassessment of how learning in schools might be transformed—transformed as work is being transformed today.

Of course, lectures, texts, and so forth are not the only media of communication in our schools and training programs. Some teachers regularly make room for discussion, exploration, student expression, and other interactive practices, and most wish that they should do more in this vein. We know that even as early as the Hellenic era important variations on the lecture mode had developed, yet it is particularly telling that the Socratic method is still very much more honored in the breach than in practice. We do not have the learning software in place to regularly shift over to a mode of learning quite different from what is standard practice, substituting participation for authority, discussion for digestion, uncertainty for certainty, speculation for compliance, and so forth.

What is particularly notable about the still-dominant classroom arrangement is that students are taught to adopt a rather passive and unconscious approach to the process of learning itself. Their job is to pay close attention and be able to replicate what they are told. The student is essentially seen as an empty vessel to be filled. Teachers, on the other hand, in order to be effective in this mode, must not only be articulate and organized, they must exercise firm authority. Their actions set the tone, and their responsibilities embrace the whole. They are the keepers of time and the managers of space. It is they who understand the ends and are trained in the means to those ends. The teacher controls the process—something, it is assumed, his/her students cannot understand. As such the process of learning rarely brings students together. It does not encourage them to explore problem solving jointly; rather, it views students as separate challenges, each striving or stumbling in his/her own confrontation with the task of meeting certain goals. This kind of classic instructional system rests on an implicit and rarely examined formula. This deeper and largely unconscious kind of cultural thought I will call the "social software" of education. In its institutionalized form in schools it can be quite impervious to change, but viewed in the wider historical context it is hardly predestined or immutable. This is where the changing ways of working today comes in.

THE LEARNING SOFTWARE OF LEAN PRODUCTION

Japanese auto manufacturing gained international attention recently for its efficiency (Womack, Jones, & Roos, 1990). While many innovations in production were involved in what the Japanese did, a fundamental part of the system they invented was the assumption that workers should participate in the innovation process itself. Through the development of learning software at the level of what had been seen before as routine work, management gradually evolved methodologies of thoughtful involvement to a point where it was possible to expect continuous learning on the part of teams of production line workers. The underlying story is of one small change leading to the next, yet the assumptions involved were quite revolutionary.

Fordism

To appreciate just how revolutionary those assumptions were we need to review what is now labeled "Fordism," the way factory work was organized for mass production for most of this century. Without a doubt the dominant ideas governing manufacturing have been those attributed to Henry Ford and others who, in building the modern factory system, rationalized mass production into a marvelously efficient (for the time) set of routines. Their theory as epitomized by the production lines in the auto industry was as follows: standardize every activity, and restrict individual jobs to minimal highly repetitive routines that require little training and less worker judgment. Assign responsibility for improvement and innovation to a staff of plant engineers who scrutinize the routines and replace human work with machine work whenever feasible. Engineers with superior knowledge exercise control over the process and thus over the line workers. It is useful to note that this system itself had replaced a method of production dependent on skilled workers doing more complex tasks. The "craftsmen" of the very early stages of the auto industry had exercised considerable control over their own work and generally were concerned with quality. The assembly line model, however, proved superior in lowering costs when volumes of production expanded, and this superiority led to relatively high wages being paid for relatively unskilled, highly routinized work. The craft aspects were taken out of the job for line workers.[3]

Eventually, the new Japanese production methods revealed key problems with this system. One turned out to be the fact that as Fordism advanced, it took the thinking and learning out of work. Fordism not only eliminated the high costs and variability of the skilled crafts approach, it eliminated problem solving at the level of the average worker. Instructed to simply follow routines, the production worker was no longer responsible for quality or for improvements in the process. As the jobs became dull, so did the workers.

Learning depends on the integration of many capacities. As an adaptive, problem-solving activity it begins with feedback, that is, information describing the problem. With this information we can then define the problem and begin exploring the ingredients of a solution. If a part in an engine is incorrectly made, we learn of the problem via some malfunction. If the ozone layer is deteriorating we learn of this via satellite photos and other measurements. Similarly, in highly routinized and meticulous activities, we learn of problems by close observation and attention to small details such as the sound of vibrations from a tool we are using or the friction generated putting things together. Such feedback can become the stimulus for corrective action or improvement, if attention is encouraged and problem solving authorized. Fordism stifled this kind of learning at the site of production. The possibilities for fine-tuning were lost.

Coupled with restrictions on work negotiated by unions as well as poor labor–management relations, Fordism ultimately led to alienated, undermotivated, and inattentive line workers. It joined them to manager-engineers taught to believe that only they could solve problems, only they had the scientific and technical knowledge needed to design solutions, and only they had the training necessary to make sophisticated analyses. The limitations of less-educated line workers, not their potential as fine-tuners, was what Fordism focused upon. As with the military of the time, there were the officers and the foot soldiers. The ultimate fly in the ointment—namely, that, other things being equal, production systems rest on continually getting the details right—was revealed only when the Japanese approach to worker participation had progressed to the point where Fordism's failure in this regard was painfully apparent. Getting the details right, furthermore, is much more than simply a matter of quality; what it really is about is the capacity to adapt and innovate. That is, as we all know, change requires getting the new details right, and a system attentive to the details can change more successfully more often. An assumption that workers were capable of using information for continuous adaptive change was the fundamental difference between Fordism and what developed in Japanese auto factories.

Only first-line workers are regularly in direct touch with the details. They are or can be the sensory system upon which fine-tuning depends. It is particularly telling in this regard that a managerial goal of Fordism was to use technological advances to "foolproof" the system, to make it "worker-proof," so to speak. The goal was to design production so that the expected carelessness, ignorance, and inattention could not affect the flow or quality of the work. Addressing production in this spirit, that is, in terms of coping with an assumed low common denominator of worker intelligence and commitment, meant that Fordism became a self-fulfilling negative prophecy as time passed. As a learning system it was a disaster. Over time the human element and the adaptive capacities of the line system got worse rather than better.

Job Rotation as a Prototypical Learning System

It is in this context that job rotation on the shop floor becomes so interesting. Long before quality control (QC) circles activities were spreading in Japan as a means of worker participation in formalized problem solving, job rotation among blue-collar workers was laying the groundwork for their advance. What kind of learning system does job rotation in Japan or elsewhere create?

First, the very nature of job rotation requires that work be organized on a team basis. This is a crucial organizational assumption. Job rotation within a team serves to enhance the team's integration. Instead of isolating each job, a sense of the connectedness of each person's work with that of others is enhanced. Flexibility obviously increases as team members can substitute for and help one another. Role boundaries decline; job descriptions broaden. Everyone still has a set of tasks and routines, but they no longer imply or impose limits on communication within the team. Because rotation exposes everyone to the same skills and knowledge, it also ameliorates to a degree the hierarchies of seniority and skill within each team. This makes participation in problem-solving discussions easier. By definition, learning increases for everyone and the team's shared knowledge expands. Just as with the rotation of managers in a large organization, line workers gain an understanding of one another's perspectives and a common grasp of the larger picture.

This common base facilitates communication. As cooperation and shared knowledge increase, team members talk more about their work. They note common problems and, if encouraged, they discuss solutions. A knowledge and communication basis for their participation in shared learning is thus established. Encouraged by managers, they can take the initiative in making certain kinds of improvements. This potential obviously rests heavily on the attitudes of management. So-called bottom–up decision making is hardly guaranteed or simple, so accustomed are we all to authority running top to bottom. The education of foremen is thus a crucial ingredient in moving from Fordism to worker participation. When foremen and supervisors learn to encourage production team initiatives they learn a different definition of authority and control.

To return to our previous discussion of classic classroom instruction, those in authority learn to move away from a position of centrality marked by mastery, accepting instead a position of oversight that also involves encouragement and facilitation. Rather than using information to enhance their power, they come to see their job as being a conduit of information to their subordinates. Rather than emphasizing the superiority of their own experience or intelligence, they come to see their success as dependent on the confidence, intelligence, and teamwork of their subordinates. Obviously, the supervisor's job is fundamentally transformed. From fixing things themselves, they find that they can—in fact, *must*—delegate more. From focusing their energies on immediate problems, they find that they have more latitude to focus outward and to plan ahead.

The rub in the older approach was, among other things, a lack of mutual confidence. Managers had and still have difficulty trusting the ability of the next level down to take initiative and solve problems. Workers have similar problems feeling confident that their supervisors are actually ready to relinquish control. The fact that we have literally been "schooled" in the opposite approach to learning helps explain why such a new approach requires such a considerable change of attitudes and habits. We will return to this point shortly.

Quality Control Circles

Job rotation was but a first step in regularizing team learning at the shop floor level. The next step was the institutionalization of QC circles. The development of this kind of learning software in Japanese manufacturing was a deliberate effort aimed at the ultimate goal of continuous learning throughout the organization.[4]

The spread of QC circles to thousands of companies and millions of workers in Japan in a matter of less than two decades was quite amazing when viewed from abroad. The basic methodologies involved in QC circles began in the 1950s when the essays of quality engineers like W. Edward Deming were translated into Japanese. Deming had always intended his formalized statistical methods for the use of engineers in the analysis of QC problems. His basic intention was the creation of a superior technique for professional use. In Japan, however, engineers thought they could teach Deming's methodology to line workers. The reasons this seemed possible had much to do with the fact that job rotation as a basic form of on-the-job training was already in place. The result after some tinkering and experimentation became known as QC circles. The key force behind the national movement for their implementation was the Japanese Union of Scientists and Engineers, an organization of considerable stature that proved very adept at disseminating the experiences of companies that pioneered QC circles. It is this organization that every year offers the Deming Prize to those companies that evidence extraordinary progress in implementing the continuous learning philosophy.

Through the QC circle movement the formal decision-making and statistical methods Deming had devised spread throughout the workforce, enabling workers to address all kinds of immediate problems in the workplace with reliable analytic tools. The methodology (part social organization, part analytic approach) spread from company to company, from large companies to small companies, from manufacturing to the service sector, and even in some cases to government. The consequences were (1) greater worker involvement, (2) higher morale, and (3) the production of an enormous numbers of suggestions for small improvements in routine work. In the light of Fordism, this represented an extraordinary ferment.

What QC circles added was a formalized methodology to all aspects of problem identification, analysis and solution. This methodology then was made standard within a company's routines. This meant that the potential for first-line worker participation in innovation was secured as part of the organization's culture and basic habits. The QC circle movement meant training workers in problem-solving techniques and strongly encouraging them to spend some hours each month discussing how to improve their shared work. It identified time for such activities and set out various re-ward systems that encouraged teams in the process. It also standardized training for all managers in the necessary shift of managerial perspective to that of encouragement and facilitation.

It is important not to be naive about how this movement proceeded. While presented as a voluntary activity for workers, there is no doubt that QC circle introductions took enormous managerial effort. They were rarely spontaneous. That is, even though they were designed to empower workers and encourage their initiative, these qualities required much coaxing and initial behind-the-scenes manipulation. Managerial leadership and persis-tence were critical. That is, for change to begin to be bottom-up as far as routine work was concerned, it had to begin with a top-down effort that was designed to transform the very nature of routine work itself. Robert Cole (1989), an expert on the organizational implementation of such re-forms, argues that to succeed, companies must have what he aptly describes as a "strategy for learning."

Japanese companies have moved on to new kinds of learning software since the late 1970s. Entire organizations today are engaged in methodi-cally reexamining their basic processes of work according to basic goals like customer service. Known generally as the Total Quality Movement (TQM), these advances rest ultimately on the same fundamental shifts in attitude and practice as those we encountered in job rotation as a basic form of learning software (Shiba et al., 1990). Whether at the team level or division level, the basic shift has been to bring learning into the equation.

Lest the reader conclude that all of this may be fine for the Japanese but it won't happen here, we must note the development of similar approaches in many North American manufacturing companies in the last decade and a half. In fact, the Ford Motor Company is a leader in this regard.

The Basics of Learning Software

Whether inspired by the possibilities of computer networking or by the suc-cess of programs for continuous learning, there is a great deal of conver-gence in the thinking of many organizational learning experts on certain basic participative features of learning in organizations. Building on the simple lessons of job rotation and QC activities, I have developed the fol-lowing list of characteristics that together offer a reasonable outline of the emerging consensus:

1. Learning is a social process occurring within teams and networks. While individual learning is an important contribution, it is not the critical arena of learning. Not only are most problems complex, but the informa-tion needed is typically scattered widely. Furthermore, group deliberation on average leads to better solutions.

2. Learning is generally part of routine work, based in activities cen-

tering on problem identification and solution on the job. Classroom training in more general knowledge can supplement this process, but it cannot replace it. If learning is not encouraged by the work environment, training is easily wasted.

3. Problem solving rests most critically on defining the right issues. This rests on reliable feedback. Both of these depend on the quality and relevance of information. The need to diffuse such information further increases as the participation in learning increases. Information systems need to be evaluated from this perspective.

4. Authority shifts from the center to the periphery. Though easy to say, this shift is extremely difficult to implement since it involves many of management's most basic needs and fears. A fundamental cultural shift is involved, and the difficulties in this can never be overestimated.

5. The basic supervisory function is to sponsor learning. Supervisors should be evaluated as teachers and facilitators.

6. Managerial control becomes largely a matter of "system design." Just as job rotation or TQM are standardized processes governing one kind of learning, so throughout organizations the basis of effective control shifts toward the specification of processes rather than authority. In practice this means greater reliance on peer-based processes, on extensive information distribution, and on adequate feedback. System design is not an organizational chart but a detailed specification of interactive processes.

7. Organizational culture sets the general context of goals, values, and standards within which the activity of system design and redesign occur. Systems that facilitate better communications, more initiative, and greater lateral interaction expand gradually as greater attention to process becomes a cultural norm. That mistakes and problems create opportunities for learning is axiomatic.

8. The overlap of functions and specialties is encouraged as a means of greater information exchange. Whether in project teams or networks or routine task teams, variety becomes a resource.

9. The more available information becomes and the more widely it is diffused, the more critical becomes the editorial function. That is, incorrect or misleading information and information overload become increasingly costly problems. Editing—the means for confirming new knowledge and culling old knowledge—must be a special focus of continuous attention.

10. In learning organizations, peer review processes expand. Their integrity also becomes a topic for learning.

11. A learning organization requires its own accounting system, one that monitors learning processes and outcomes. The means for measuring changes in an organization's knowledge assets needs to be found.

12. The most basic kind of knowledge is that focused on learning processes themselves. Senior management must understand the idea of meta-learning and critically review the organization's learning software.

13. Learning to borrow knowledge from outside is as important as in-

venting it internally. In fact, internal boundaries and external boundaries similarly need to be lowered, almost by definition.

Work and Japanese Schooling

If work organizations are evolving in the directions specified above, the question arises as to how schools should be evolving to prepare students for work in such organizations. Put differently, what kind of skills and work habits will be needed to participate in learning organizations?

We can begin a consideration of the answers to these questions by returning to the case of Japan for what it has to tell us about the relationship of schools to work for it is there that many of the changes in industrial work, appear to have begun.

It is curious that the relatively sophisticated analytic methods set out by Deming in his approach to quality improvement, which were intended for college-educated American engineers, were deemed appropriate for Japanese high school educated blue-collar workers. It is even more interesting that what began in Deming's mind as a QC methodology was transformed in Japan into a means for small groups to participate actively in organizational innovation.

We form our fundamental social patterns in childhood. Learning is no exception. Our most deeply held assumptions are formed early, and thus the learning software of the workplace is inherently conditioned and limited by the way learning habits and attitudes are taught in schools. Put another way, path dependency, in a cultural and developmental sense, is as true of learning software as it is of other social patterns and outcomes. If children are not sufficiently nurtured, they are not ready for school. If schools do not prepare the habits required of adults, the conditions of the workplace are limited.

It is germane that early child care in Japan is excellent by all available measures—infant mortality, health, marriage, stability, income distribution, and family size. One can say without hesitation that by any measure, the proportion of 4- and 5-year-olds "at risk" in Japan is remarkably low by North American standards. Upon this enviable base, schooling proceeds to shape the social patterns that eventually become habits of each generation of new entrants to the labor force.

Learning in groups is very definitely encouraged in elementary schools. From kindergarten on, Japanese teachers put children in small groups for many kinds of discussions, both curriculum-related problems and those having to do with matters such as student conduct and cooperation.[5] Teachers do not take an entirely hands-off approach by any means, but there is a good deal of problem solving in groups. It is assumed that children need to learn how to hold discussions in small groups, including learning to pay attention to such basics as listening to one another, taking turns speaking, encouraging full participation, avoiding quick dismissal of ideas, and delegating subtasks like record keeping. This is part of a conscious effort at teaching the techniques of self-governance very early on, techniques that once learned allow teachers to delegate more responsibility to students.[6] Observers of schools in Japan are typically surprised by the degree students even in first and second grades assume much of the classroom's organizational tasks.

This early attention to small groups and self-ordering routines can be taken to quite sophisticated levels. One foreign visitor to an upper elementary classroom was surprised to find the teacher instituting such subtle rules as one that determines the speaking order among students in the group by how much or little those wishing to speak had said so far (C. C. Lewis, personal communication, 1996). By contrast, when small group processes are introduced among North American workers it has been common that training in how to conduct group discussions is a necessary first step. This skill is not taught in our schools, and thus there is no common set of rules or experience available. We learn to debate and to vote but not how to brainstorm or collectively analyze.[7]

It is worth noting in this regard that in Japanese education there is widespread use of small groups as a means of organizing all kinds of nonacademic activities. Within this tradition one finds a complex set of habitual practices that are also found in the Japanese workplace (Rohlen, 1989). Within the small group, for example, leadership tasks and other roles are rotated on a regular basis (Peak, 1991). Every child, in other words, is used to the idea of job rotation. All have had sufficient experience by sixth grade of changing from one role to another that it is fair to say that job rotation in the workplace comes as no surprise. It is also common in school to ask groups to reflect on the day's work or on an interpersonal problem that had arisen. The groups then discuss their evaluations and are encouraged to come up with ideas for improving the way the class as a whole is conducted.[8] Everyone is thus encouraged to think it is his/her duty to help think about making improvements. The process is inclusive, and the teacher's role is to facilitate it.

Using mistakes as opportunities is never as easy as it sounds in teaching, but Japanese elementary teachers have found an interesting approach that takes the sting out of the process. In their lesson plans they note as many plausible ways of answering a question as possible, and then they seek to elicit from the students as many possible responses (some incorrect) as they can. They do not try to model solely on the correct answer, nor do they stop the deliberative process when the right answer is given, nor are they unconsciously inclined to look to the best students for the right answer. Rather, their goal is getting as many options on the board as possible and then fostering a discussion among the students regarding the merits and demerits of each.[9] There are interesting parallels here with what is taught in brainstorming. The intention in each is to overcome our natural fear of being shown to be wrong. Participating is rewarded; being right often turns out to be a group accomplishment. Setting out many possible answers also sets up a more thorough deliberative process of analysis.

There is also much evidence that the math preparation of average Japanese high school graduates is superior to that typical of North Americans (Stevenson & Stigler, 1992). In particular, this is true of statistical analysis. Moreover, acquiring math skills is viewed as a matter of effort and application rather than as a product of inherent interest or talent. We allow the assertion "I'm no good at math" to go unchallenged far more readily than the Japanese do. Such differences in both education and attitude are further elements of the explanation of why QC circles became successful and popular so quickly in Japan at a level in organizations unthinkable to men like Deming.

The emphasis on small-group activities in Japanese schools raises a deeper philosophical issue that also appears related to this question. Throughout their years of schooling, students are exposed continually to the moral teaching that they must cooperate for the good of the whole. This is a normal lesson to teach in schools anywhere, of course, but it seems to be taught especially intensively and thoroughly in Japan. Examples abound in the literature on Japanese education. The question worth at least asking is whether this training encourages subsequently the assumption that management and workers are in the same company boat, so to speak. The much more individual oriented and rule-based approach to morality as taught in North American schools leaves, it would seem, a different imprint. We are taught to assume that self-interest is the most natural of motives, and this underlies our skepticism about claims for the collective good.[10]

Continuous improvement is a form of perfectionism. Perfectionism allows incremental improvements a place in the larger effort to gain efficiency. It is to just such changes that line workers can contribute. In one supermarket chain that I studied, for example, the topic selected for study by part-time checkout clerks in one store was how to reduce wastage in the string used to tie packages. Such minuscule improvements warrant attention to the degree details are a preoccupation. Improvements of this scale of course can add up, but there must be a belief that they matter. Research on Japanese education indicates an attention to detail in such things as cleanliness, neatness, and orderliness that seems to fit this pattern. In the early years, the focus is less on academic issues and more on neatness as a contributor to cooperative living. In middle and high schools teachers emphasize getting the details right as part of preparing students for university entrance exams.[11]

A point of clarification is needed. There is no evidence whatsoever for the idea that Japanese educators had Japanese work routines in mind when they developed their pedagogical approaches. There is little or no communication between the two worlds, and teachers would be offended if it were asserted that they served the interests of businesses or factory managers.

Rather, the parallels appear due primarily to the arrival of Western democratic influences to a group-oriented society in the postwar Occupation period. Historical parallels abound in the educational and working worlds brought on by defeat and occupation. It is a combination of historical/cultural convergence and some degree of accident that such an innovative and highly productive complement developed.

Yet, the education–work practice complement is real. Japanese companies attempting to transfer their work practices related to learning to their overseas plants have had a very difficult time. In fact, evidence points to their giving up or greatly scaling back their expectations. This, I would argue, is partly due to the lack of preparation in the educational experiences overseas of their workers.

Education Reform

The difficulties Japanese managers have encountered in transferring their practices abroad raises the question whether learning software is culture specific and thus limited geographically. I do not doubt for a moment that the context of learning is cultural in the sense that it is created and shaped by human activity and rests on fundamental assumptions and experiences that are neither biological nor universal. But this hardly means that cultural boundaries need be insurmountable limits. History shows that human society is inherently adaptive and that innovations of all kinds have moved from one society to another once they have proved effective. We learn from what works elsewhere, just as others learn from us. Furthermore, Western companies are very actively developing their own learning software today as they recognize the advantages of collaborative problem solving within the routine frameworks. Many chose to call themselves learning organizations or knowledge-creating companies. What the previous subsection does underscore in this regard is the important link between school and the workplace. In effect, it is in school where we first learn the culture of learning, where we are socialized to a particular learning software.

What is particularly notable as we turn our attention to schooling in North America is the number of pedagogical reforms and experiments that seem pointed in much the same direction as the organizational learning movement is heading. To be sure, the overwhelming truth about classroom teaching today is that it remains very much in line with the classic instructional form discussed earlier. This is equally true of the majority of company training programs. And if we turn to vocational programs, the same dominance of the traditional mode is evident. Yet, the effort to set forth new directions has considerable momentum in the pedagogical field.

First, it is quite common today to find teachers expressing the idea that children should do more learning together. In classrooms across North America teachers are trying to do more with groups. The effort is in its infancy in the sense that most teachers possess little sophistication about how to construct and guide group processes, and many fail to put real academic challenges at the heart of their efforts. Nevertheless, the very popularity of the idea that children can, even should, learn together is a step in a new direction. Until teachers themselves better understand the keys to successful communication and cooperation in groups, however, the potential in this idea is likely to remain largely unrealized.

Second, there is a renewed interest in the classroom as a civic environment in which the aim is to strengthen cooperation and instill a sense of shared engagement and responsibility. The tantalizing goal of many pedagogical innovations—that of "creating a community of learners"—sounds surprisingly like the vision statements of those companies most deeply engaged in perfecting their internal processes of learning.

Third, computers play a role in the new approaches—but, it must be underscored, not as a panacea. Rather, computers are viewed as powerful new tools if, and only if, teachers have a deeply understood strategy for their use that integrates them with more fundamental programs for learning. Put bluntly, computers can be great sources of information, they can greatly enhance interaction among students, they can become tools for creative expression, and they can be more effective sources of feedback, but they can also become vehicles for routine drills that do not encourage understanding and they can be (and are) put to the most mind-numbing purposes.

Nor can computers do more than enable the interactive and networked processes that are the true foundations of learning. It is patently obvious to reformers that simply putting computers in schools does nothing to change the way learning occurs. They can actually be detrimental if what the computer becomes is a distraction or a means to trivializing the process. Horror stories abound in this regard of students using computers to look up irrelevant facts, play games with no content, and communicate among themselves without learning goals or effective feedback. In sum, the challenge of computers is the same long-standing challenge that teachers have faced all along—to teach children to solve academic problems together and thereby to build the fundamental habits of learning that lead to deepening understanding and knowledge without perpetuating the centrality of the teacher's initiative and control.

Many experiments are being conducted across the United States and Canada aimed at fostering collective learning among students through the medium of networked computers. In these efforts, students are organized to share information with one another, present and test hypotheses together, and in various interactive processes jointly develop knowledge. The details of the experiments differ, but the fundamental approach of using networked interactive processes to facilitate problem solving and learning is the same. The labels and terminology of these programs, such terms as "discovery learning," "learning for understanding," and "knowledge construction," reveal the essential assumption that children will truly learn when understanding comes through a process of discovering the answers for themselves. The teacher facilitates this process. The authority content of instruction is reduced. Students communicate with each other to arrive at understanding. These changes in the classic approach obviously parallel the directions taken in many work organizations (see also Scardamalia and Bereiter, Chapter 14, this volume).

Other reforms in education seems related as well. There is a growing interest, for example, in how traditional apprenticeship systems exemplify an alternative to the conventional classroom arrangement. The importance of the social context in shaping learning is thus emphasized. In the case of apprenticeship, for example, there is increasing recognition that learning can occur through participation in work activities, beginning at the periphery and moving toward more skilled participation, a process very different from that of explicit verbal instruction centered on the teacher. That this insight is a relatively fresh one in North American education is a reflection of the continuing hold the classic instructional approach has had over the field.

Just as in organizations, these new directions, however appealing in theory, encounter many barriers. Teachers have to adjust their behavior and change basic assumptions about their role and their responsibilities. They have to move in directions very similar to those demanded of middle managers in learning organizations, and (like them) they are asked to do this within a framework of expectations that can be very unforgiving. Discovery processes take time and cannot be controlled in the same manner as when authority is regularly the central defining mechanism guaranteeing results within fixed time frames.

Assumptions about children—about their desire to learn and their capacity for self-regulation in peer groups—also has to change in ways similar to shifts required in organizations. The difference between children and adults in this regard may not be as large as we might expect. We conventionally underestimate potential in both instances. On the other hand, unlike senior managers who generally are caught up in the rhetoric of innovation, parents and school boards are likely to be impatient with new approaches, especially if they view them from a traditional perspective.

SUMMARY AND FINAL COMMENTS

The course of human evolution shows that we solve most problems together, sharing, borrowing, and developing ideas. So basic is this that, like language itself, we take the collective nature of learning for granted and focus instead on individual creativity. Yet behind an Albert Einstein or a Thomas Alva Edison stand thousands of other contributions and social arrangements that have set the stage for their breakthroughs. In a similar fashion, the crucial task of applying new knowledge to an ever-widening realm of uses involves very wide participation within a population. The other side of this coin is that the greatest barriers to learning are also social, namely, shared habits of mind and practice that are no longer suitable or which discourage exploration and innovation. Placed in the context of human history, learning systems assume a central and critical role in the overall adaptive dynamic.

The implications of this point is that there is more to the development of a learning society than the improvement of child care and early education. There is more to it than the education and training of individuals as we typically conceive of the effort. Our learning software itself is in need of fundamental change. Protecting and nurturing infants, preventing unnecessary wastage in human potential, and preparing children for participation as adults all serve to set the stage for subsequent participation in work and community organizations. If the trends in the workplace continue, then we are confronted with the fact that we are certain to encounter enormous human and economic costs if we fail to prepare children in a manner that fits the world they will inherit as adults.

The new ways of working offer greater opportunities to more people for creative participation in the workplace, but only those prepared to problem solve cooperatively will be able to respond to this opportunity. More sobering is the fact that the new, more innovative and participatory approaches to learning will not work if the young are not prepared to respond to these opportunities. The importance of early development in this regard cannot be underscored enough, for failures at that critical juncture have the power to disqualify individuals from any participation.

In conclusion, it is useful to step back and ask a few more basic questions, ones that stem from the fact that we are discussing a new, still tentative, and somewhat idealized direction for change and reform. There is no guarantee that the trends in education discussed in this chapter will hold sway in the future. I have described them from the perspective of a friend, but they also have enemies. Perhaps the most lethal is a satisfaction with the status quo, one that implies that what worked to generate the truly magnificent achievements of this century will be good enough to guarantee success in the next. Why fix what isn't broken? Why change our institutional designs and assumptions about learning? Reasonable questions, one thinks, as long as the 21st century is shaped by the same demands on companies, communities, and nations as shaped the 20th. If the world were static, this argument would have great merit, but the world is changing before our eyes. It is a good bet that it will reward societies that are better at adapting to these changes, meaning that improvements in the institutional encouragement of learning will certainly prove to be of increasing importance.

Furthermore, the idea of a learning organization represents or implies a new social philosophy, one that might be labeled something like a democracy of knowledge. It is worthwhile here to explore what other philosophies challenge it in the arena of popular thought. First, perhaps, is the notion that there are smart people and then there are the rest. The smart people need to be recognized early for their special capacities and given the very best education and opportunities to apply their talents. This view holds that it is they, not the rest, who really innovate and really make a difference. Who can argue that such a perspective is entirely untrue? Clearly, differences of talent exist, and just as clearly high school graduates are not going to perform as well as engineering graduates. Yet, either/or thinking is hardly logical given the range of work and requirements within most organizations. Finding the balance, however, is hardly easy. The effort to create learning organizations, it seems to me, is in fact a search for a more adaptive balance than the one we have inherited from the era of mass production and its analog, mass education.

How the teacher or the manager views the average student or average worker is also a matter of philosophy. It is assumed in the movement to build learning organizations that workers can and want to learn, that they will respond positively to the opportunity to work smart, that they want more responsibility, and that they will take to working in a team-based manner. The very same assumptions about students are at the heart of educational reform. But are these expectations realistic? Admittedly, there is an element of idealism involved. Rather than see this problem as the age-old one of how human nature is defined, it might be more useful to acknowledge that the assumptions inherent in an institutional form, just like the attitudes of teachers and supervisors, have a strong element of self-fulfilling prophecy in the way they shape reality. That is, rather than arguing about human nature as a static essence, it is more constructive to ask what in human nature can be brought forth or encouraged as a means to our best intentions and most challenging goals.

In the dawn of the Information Age, it is quite revealing that the label "learning organization" describes less a reality and more an ambition that is emerging as the requirements of success and the potential for new ways of working are revealing just how conservative our conventional approaches are. We need to remind ourselves that all organizations—factory, school, office, and community—embody profoundly ubiquitous barriers to learning and innovation. We all experience these barriers when we feel the constraints of bureaucracy, red tape, conventional thinking, poor feedback, and the like, but we rarely perceive the depth of the problems involved because we inherently understand organizations as being by nature sources of regulation, specialization, and standardization. The notion of a learning organization is in its most fundamental sense one that seeks to bring to conscious attention the way complex organizations inhibit learning. The issue then becomes how to lower the barriers. This goal is truly revolutionary, and nothing illustrates this better than the enormous effort required to change our thinking and ways of organizing ourselves once this ambition is in place.

ACKNOWLEDGMENT

I wish to express my appreciation to the Bank of Montreal and the Canadian Institute for Advanced Research for their generous fellowship support.

NOTES

1. The list of related management books is very extensive. I have included in the references a partial but representative list.
2. A large number of books and articles in the field of management has been published recently on the subject of organizational learning. Among them I have found especially useful J. S. Brown and Duguid (1995), K. B. Clark and Fujimoto (1991), R. Cole (1989), Drucker (1991), the Economist Intelligence Unit (1996), Hayes, Wheelwright, and Clark (1988), Nonaka (1994), Nonaka and Takeuchi (1995), Quinn (1992), Senge (1990), and Shiba, Graham, and Walden (1990).
3. Many books have described this system retrospectively; see, for example, H. C. Katz (1985) and Gordon, Edwards, and Reichet (1982).
4. See R. Cole (1989) for the best general overview of the historical process.
5. C. C. Lewis (1995), Peak (1991), L. J. Kotloff in Rohlen and LeTendre (1996), and many others have described this practice in detail.
6. I have discussed the Japanese teacher's role in shaping a basic pattern that can be observed in work organizations as well as in schools (Rohlen, 1989; see also Rohlen, 1974, 1975, 1983, 1992).
7. This is based on my personal experience as well as what is described in the literature on QC circle introductions in the United States.
8. Known in Japanese as *hansei*, this practice is highlighted by C. C. Lewis (1995).
9. Studies of such teaching in math and science have been conducted extensively by James Stigler in the case of math teaching plans and Ineko Tsuchida in the case of science. See, for example, Stigler and Perry (1988) and Tsuchida (1993).
10. This observation is based in part on the research and comments of C. C. Lewis (1995).
11. Parenthetically, the Japanese high regard for cleanliness, taught assiduously in schools, seems related to the finding that shop floor productivity gains in Japanese manufacturing can be attributed to improvements in the degree of cleanliness maintained by workers.

14

Schools as Knowledge-Building Organizations

Marlene Scardamalia
Carl Bereiter

Although schools are learning organizations in the sense that they promote learning, few would qualify as learning organizations in the larger sense of the term now current in organizational theory (Senge, 1990; see Rohlen, Chapter 13, this volume). Indeed, from an organizational standpoint schools are often seen as bureaucratic institutions particularly resistant to the kind of purposeful change from within that characterizes learning organizations. But what would it mean for schools to become learning organizations? There are two quite different ways of answering that question. One would constitute an overhaul in management and the organization of work in order for schools to do a better job of performing their traditional functions. The other is a much more radical transformation, in which the basic job of the school is altered. Most current school reform, whether it involves new management structures or the introduction of new standards and curricula, is of the first kind. In this chapter we explore the second, more radical, and also harder-to-grasp form of transformation, which we believe is necessary if schools are to realize their potential in a knowledge society.

Traditionally and typically, schools are service organizations. They provide a variety of services, mainly but not exclusively aimed at the promotion of learning in their clients, the students. (In important senses the clients are not only the students but their parents and the larger society as well, but students are the immediate recipients of most services.) Thus, the first kind of transformation mentioned above involves changes much like those that would occur in any service organization that sets about functioning as a learning organization: layers of management are reduced, and the rank-and-file employees (mainly the teachers in this case) are given fuller responsibilities and are more involved in corporate decisions. A great deal of change of this kind is already underway in many places. Site-based management replaces centralized administration, teachers are given a large measure of control over curriculum, choice of educational materials, and so on. All this is with the aim of providing better services to the clients. And as with many modern organizations the clients are being brought into the improvement process as well. In Ontario, for instance, the Royal Commission on Learning recommended that each school be required to establish a school–community council with membership to include parents, students, teachers, and representatives from various other sectors of the community.

The second and more radical kind of transformation may be put in perspective by considering a fundamental question: what kind of education will best prepare students for life in a knowledge society? Typical answers to this question list characteristics that such education should foster: flexibility, creativity, problem-solving ability, technological literacy, information-finding skills, and above all a lifelong readiness to learn. Within the service framework just described, the job of the schools is to turn these into educational objectives and thence into learning activities, assessment criteria, and the like. That is already happening as new curriculum guidelines and performance standards emerge (e.g., New Standards, 1995; Ontario Ministry of Education & Training, 1995). But there is another way of approaching the question, which is to consider what kind of experience offers the best preparation for life in a knowledge society. The obvious answer is experience in a learning organization. The implications of this disarming answer are quite radical, however. For if schools are to constitute the learning organizations in which students gain experience, the role of students must change from that of clients to that of members. This means changing the function of the school from that of service provider to that of a productive enterprise to which the students are contributors. But what is that productive enterprise? To what are the students contributors?

The idea of students as participants, along with teachers and perhaps others, in a collaborative enterprise has been around at least since John Dewey but has been taking a more definite shape over the past decade in various experimental programs. The new approaches are all to some extent based on the model of the scientific research team, which has also served as an inspiration for reforms in industry (T. Peters, 1987) One popular formulation of the idea is "cognitive apprenticeship" (Collins, Brown, & Newman, 1989), which captures the notion of students as junior members of a discipline rather than as recipients of instructional services. The term is not quite apt, however. As a rule, students are not apprentice teachers and school teachers are not practitioners of the disciplines they teach, and so the apprenticeship metaphor does not fit. A. L. Brown and Campione

(1990, 1994) have used the term "fostering communities of learners" to characterize the very impressive approach they have developed. In it, teaching and learning are closely intertwined. In a typical activity, different groups of students research different aspects of a topic and then instruct the members of the other groups. Perhaps the most thoroughgoing application of the research team model is in what we call "collaborative knowledge building" (Bereiter & Scardamalia, 1992; Scardamalia, Bereiter, & Lamon, 1994). This approach rests on a recognition that the construction of knowledge, as it goes on in the learned disciplines and applied sciences, is different from learning although closely related to it. The distinction is obvious in the work of a scientific research team. The team's job is to produce new knowledge. The individual and collective learning that goes on within the group is secondary—a by-product of knowledge production and a contributor to it (Bereiter & Scardamalia, 1996). Some uses of the term "learning" include innovation within it (see Rohlen, Chapter 13, this volume), but common usage can obscure the central theme we emphasize here, the construction of knowledge.

In classrooms that adopt the collaborative knowledge-building approach, the basic job to be done shifts from learning in the conventional sense to the construction of collective knowledge. The nature of the work is essentially the same as that of a professional research group, with the students being the principal doers of the work. Thus, in the ideal case, there is a complete shift from students as clients to students as participants in a learning organization.

Two terms that may be applied to this kind of educational approach are "problem-based learning" (Savery & Duffy, 1995) and "project-based learning" (Blumenfeld et al., 1991). However, both of these terms cover a range of educational approaches of a less radical nature. Problem-based learning often consists of set problems, such as diagnosing a medical case, explaining a demonstrated scientific phenomenon, or planning a trip to Mars. Community knowledge building, by contrast, deals with problems that arise within the community—real phenomena that people are puzzled about, real texts in need of interpretation, and so on. Project-based learning is often focused on the production of tangible products, such as multimedia presentations, whereas the focus in knowledge building is on the knowledge itself, its physical representation being secondary.

On the face of it, it may seem strange to claim that focusing education on knowledge represents a radical transformation; yet educators in our experience invariably recognize it as radical, once they grasp the idea. But grasping the idea is not easy, and it seems to be more difficult for educators than it is for people in knowledge-based businesses, for instance. The reason, it seems, is that in the educational context people tend to think of knowledge exclusively as content residing in people's minds. The conception of knowledge as resource or knowledge as product, as something that can be created and improved, bought and sold, discarded as obsolete, or found to have new uses—this conception is commonsensical to people in knowledge-based businesses. It can coexist with but is not the same as the educators' conception of knowledge as stuff in the mind. The essence of our argument is that children destined to live in a knowledge society need an educational experience that makes this other conception of knowledge a part of their commonsense understanding as well, a concept that gives meaning to the work they do from day to day.

AUTHENTIC KNOWLEDGE BUILDING

The authenticity of students' knowledge-building efforts is crucial to the conception we are trying to develop of schools as learning organizations. In traditional schools students do work. Indeed, interview studies indicate that to most students and to many teachers, doing schoolwork is basically what school is about (Bereiter & Scardamalia, 1989; Doyle, 1983). But the work only has meaning in relation to benefit gained by the worker. Thus it is analogous to the bodybuilding work one may do in a gymnasium. In more child-centered schools, students have more freedom to pursue their own interests and curiosity and thus to take a more active part in their own mental development. But in neither case do the students gain the experience of doing productive work that has value beyond the satisfaction of their own or their teachers' needs. Community knowledge building, by contrast, is aimed at producing something of value to the community—theories, explanations, problem formulations, interpretations, and so on, which become public property that is helpful in understanding the world and functioning intelligently in it. The knowledge that is created may not have much value beyond the local group (we will discuss current efforts to overcome this limitation later), but within that group students are contributors to a common good. Like workers in a modern industry, they are contributing to the knowledge resources of the organization.

But how authentic can student knowledge building be? Aren't the students in reality only pretending to be scientists, historians, mathematicians, or whatever? There are two notable differences between knowledge building as it goes on in schools and as it goes on in professional research groups that prompt such skepticism. A professional research group usually has a specific problem area—AIDS research or the ecology of the Great Barrier Reef, for instance. An elementary school class, however, has the whole world as its problem area. But so did Aristotle. Breadth of scope does not disqualify a research program as scientific or scholarly. *The job of an elementary school class that adopts a knowledge-building approach is to construct an understanding of the world as the students know it.*

The other difference, of course, is that a professional research group is expected to produce knowledge new to the world, to solve problems that have never been solved before, whereas students, with rare exceptions, will only produce knowledge that is new to them. Furthermore, the knowledge constructed by students will mostly be derived from reference books and other secondary sources, less frequently from experimentation and primary data. This does not discredit student knowledge building, however. We will pursue this point at some length, because it requires the revision of several popular notions about science.

Producing knowledge new to the world is an achievement, not a process. A research team might find out that what they took to be an original finding had already been reported by someone else. This would diminish their achievement, but it would not make the work they had done any less scientific, any less authentic. What makes work "scientific" is a matter of continuing controversy and is not a matter to be settled here; but we may at least agree that science is a form of social practice that goes on, with wide variations, in groups recognized as scientific. To the extent that the practices of any group conform to those of recognized research teams, the group may be said to be practicing real science—regardless of its achievements. During the Cultural Revolution in China, many scientists were forced to abandon their research for more than a decade and were also denied access to scientific journals and to communication with foreign researchers. When that terrible experiment in the suppression of inquiry ended and these people went back to their work, they of course had a great deal of catching up to do. It would be some time before they could begin making original contributions to knowledge again, but they did not have to wait that long to start functioning again as real scientists. They could do that as soon as conditions allowed them to resume the social practices that constituted doing science in their culture and discipline. We see school-age students as being in a similar situation, except that they have about 500 years of science to catch up on instead of 15. They can begin functioning as real scientists as soon as they are able to engage in a form of social practice that is authentically scientific, one that is concerned with the solution of recognizably scientific problems in recognizably scientific ways. Analogous arguments can be made about authentic functioning in history, literature, and other disciplines that students may venture into in their knowledge-building efforts.

Many educators of a constructivist persuasion would accept the preceding argument as it applies to experimentation and other "hands-on" activities of students, but they would not extend it to the very large part of student knowledge building that depends on information and ideas drawn from reference books and other authoritative sources. Indeed, they might reject this as not knowledge construction at all but mere receptive learning, or "knowledge transmission," as it is sometimes called. Any theoretically sensible construal of constructivism, however, will recognize that understanding is a constructive process regardless of where the information comes from. In judging whether authentic knowledge building is going on, the question to ask is not whether students are doing experiments as opposed to reading books but whether they are trying to solve knowledge problems. Doing experiments or tramping the bushes collecting plant samples in no way guarantees that they are. Trying to make sense of information about a topic of interest almost always ensures that they are.

Construing knowledge building as the solving of knowledge problems has the advantage that it puts scholars who are advancing the frontiers of knowledge under the same umbrella as students who are engaged in building an understanding based largely on knowledge that has already been set forth. Constructivism's important contribution here is in the recognition that, though the achievement is different, the process is essentially the same. As Sir Karl Popper put it,

> What I suggest is that we can grasp a theory only by trying to reinvent it or to reconstruct it, and by trying out, with the help of our imagination, all the consequences of the theory which seem to us to be interesting and important. . . . One could say that the process of understanding and the process of the actual production or discovery of . . . [theories, etc.] are very much alike. Both are making and matching processes. (Popper & Eccles, 1977, p. 461)

Scientists devote a good deal of time to trying to understand what their colleagues are up to and what they have accomplished (Dunbar, 1993). In doing so, they are reconstructing solutions rather than creating them de novo, just as students who try to understand how we see colors by working their way through a textbook explanation. The inventive and the reconstructive processes are so much alike and merge into one another so smoothly that participants in a lively research meeting would probably be hard put to say where reconstructing left off and working on new ideas of their own began. Similarly, students who are actively trying to solve a knowledge problem will move readily between developing ideas of their own and trying to negotiate a fit between their own ideas and information obtained from an authoritative source.

This dual character of knowledge building comes through in the following interview excerpt. A middle school class was studying the major biomes. The speaker and his classmate, Brian, were trying to determine why trees do not grow in the Arctic tundra:

> "I thought it was because a tree would freeze, but then I realized that a tree probably couldn't freeze. I don't know about that because me and the kid that's working are still kind of writing. But I thought it was probably just because of the water would freeze and now I realize that its not—its definitely not just the water. There's the wind, nutrients, and the permafrost, and the daylight and everything basically plays a factor in it so. . . .
>
> "There's a speaker that came to talk about tundra. And so Brian

got to go to that because he had studied tundra and he asked. And my new learning is all about what he told me and why trees don't grow. Actually, we don't really agree with the speaker on some of the things. . . . He said that the roots weren't very deep. And I figured this didn't make sense because so what if roots aren't deep? Because if the roots are very shallow in the rain forest because there's not any nutrients deep down in the rain forest, so there's not many roots. And then I asked several tundra people. . . . We kind of think that he's partially right, but we don't understand why that would be true. We believe in that there isn't much water there, but we don't understand why it's for the tree, because obviously the tree needs water to grow. But there's not much water in the desert. . . . "

The last remark reflects the fact that the student also consulted students in another group who were studying deserts, in order to find out how trees got along there with little water.

This example illustrates characteristics that distinguish knowledge building from ordinary school learning activity:

1. The student and his classmates exercise a high level of responsibility. What they are responsible for, however, is not a tangible product such as a display or a presentation (although that may come later). They are responsible for achieving advances in their group's knowledge.
2. Although worthwhile learning undoubtedly occurs, learning is not what they are responsible for. Instead, they are accountable for contributing to the solution of problems—in this case, the problem of why trees do not grow in the arctic tundra.
3. The problems they are working on are not practical problems (such as how to survive in the Arctic). They are knowledge problems— mainly problems of explanation.[1]

When we speak of a school functioning as a knowledge-building community, on the model of research teams and other knowledge-building organizations in the adult world, we have in mind a school in which activity of the above kind is the major occupation of the students. Such work need not be limited to the natural sciences, of course. It may venture into all curricular areas; but always the focus is on the solution of genuine problems of understanding.

THE NEED FOR A NEW DISCOURSE MEDIUM

The centrality of discourse to knowledge creation has come to be recognized throughout the sociology and philosophy of knowledge (Harré &

Gillett, 1994). It reveals itself in the variety of discourse forms, ranging from hallway conversations and brown-bag lunches to peer-reviewed archival journals, that make up the fabric of communication within every discipline. By contrast, knowledge-related discourse in schools tends to be spotty, ephemeral, severely time bound, and almost unavoidably dominated by the teacher, who acts as the hub through which communication passes (Cazden, 1986). Computer network technology, however, provides possibilities for more decentralized forms of discourse that have more of the knowledge building capabilities of discourse in the disciplines. CSILE (Computer Supported Intentional Learning Environments) was developed with a view to realizing these possibilities.

CSILE was not intended to replace either teacher-led or small-group discussion. Both of these have a place in any classroom. Rather, CSILE was designed to complement these in ways that further promote community knowledge building. CSILE is an asynchronous discourse medium, which means that participants do not have to be engaged at the same time, as they do in an oral discussion or in a telephone conversation. In this way it is like e-mail. But, unlike e-mail, it does not consist of person-to-person messages. Instead, it consists of contributions to a community database, which resides on a server and is accessible to everyone in the network. Thus, the knowledge represented by notes in the database is preserved and continually available for search, retrieval, comment, and revision. The database as a whole serves to objectify the advancing knowledge of the group.

Knowledge Forum™ is a second-generation CSILE product that includes Views, which provide high-level graphical organizers for notes and allow notes to be linked to any organizational framework; Rise-above notes that encourage summarization and allow notes to supersede other notes; customizable Scaffolds to support discourse (e.g., theory-building discourse such as "My Theory," "I Need to Understand," or "New Information"); and Reference features that create automatic bibliographies and allow quick access to cited on-line information. For a fuller description, see Scardamalia and Bereiter, 1996 (or visit the CSILE Web site at http://csile.oise.on.ca).

As is true of any medium, much depends on how it is used. In the course of a decade of classroom experimentation, practices have been developed that make good use of CSILE's distinctive supports for knowledge building. We may refer to these practices as collectively constituting a *knowledge-building pedagogy*. Keeping in mind that the objective is not to replace one kind of practice by another but to add missing elements and redress imbalances, we may characterize knowledge-building pedagogy by means of a series of contrasts with conventional practices:

- *Problem focus versus topic focus.* Traditional schoolwork, of both the didactic and the project-based variety, deals with knowledge organized around topics. Unless the topics happen to be of high intrinsic interest, they are likely to result in low motivation, low transferability, and rapid forgetting (Bereiter, 1992). Problem-based learning (Savery & Duffy, 1995) has developed as antidote to these difficulties. Knowledge-building pedagogy is a distinctive variant of problem-based learning, emphasizing problems of understanding and explanation rather than decision problems, as is more often the case when problem-based learning is used in professional education. A problem focus is supported in several ways. A special field on each note encourages users to identify the problem they are addressing, and if a note builds on another, it inherits the problem statement of the parent note, thus aiding coherence and focus. Students enter new problem statements, and can view related problems identified by others. Scaffolds also help to frame the field of discourse, encouraging students to produce "I Need to Understand" notes that identify knowledge they require in order to advance on their problems.

• *Production of knowledge objects versus media objects.* Knowledge-building pedagogy deals with knowledge rather than with the containers of knowledge. Whereas typical school "projects" involve producing a visible object, such as an illustrated report or (the latest rage) a Web page, Knowledge Forum objects are notes or composites of notes, which others respond to on the basis of their content, not their production values. These text and graphic notes are contributed to Views, which are the high-level visualizations of the work on a particular problem or issue. Notes and Views may be converted into illustrated reports, Web pages, multimedia presentations, and so forth, but they do not need to be converted for their value to be evident.

• *Contribution versus display.* The traditional class "recitation," as well as much of traditional written work, is concerned with students demonstrating what they know (or do not know), whereas in normal life using conversation to display what one knows is egotistical. One is supposed to say things that contribute to the common purpose. Although knowledge display (including its formalization in subject-matter tests) has its place in education, knowledge-building pedagogy relegates it to special purposes and places the main emphasis on contributions to the progress of knowledge-building discourse.

• *Theory improvement versus finding answers.* A long-time ideal of learner-centered educational reform has been to have the curriculum driven by children's own questions (Isaacs, 1930; Weber, 1971). However, when children know they are going to have to seek answers to questions, they tend to ask the kinds of straightforward questions that they can readily find answers to in school books, thus defeating the purpose (Scardamalia & Bereiter, 1992). This difficulty can be surmounted by having students first state a problem, then offer a conjecture (hence the "My Theory" Scaffold support in Knowledge Forum), and then undertake to improve upon that conjecture (Scardamalia, Bereiter, Hewitt, & Webb, 1996). Whereas answers are often unattainable, improvement on initial conjectures almost always is. Not only does this result in more experience of success, it also comes much closer to the way scientific advancement actually takes place.

• *Sustained versus single-pass knowledge creation.* Freewheeling classroom discussions are often full of good ideas and questions. However, these are unlikely to be followed up or to lead anywhere unless through the teacher's Socratic guidance. Knowledge Forum also provides a medium for generating abundant ideas and questions, but these are preserved, continually available for further discussion and revision. Analysis of tracking data indicates that significant conceptual change is closely related to students' returning to earlier notes and revising them in the light of classroom comments and new information (Oshima, Scardamalia, & Bereiter, 1996).

• *Public versus person-to-person communication.* Classroom discourse presents anomalies with respect to audience. Oral communication is almost always directed to a single person, usually the teacher. Written composition typically has no intended audience at all, which reduces it to mere exercise (Applebee, 1984). Knowledge-building pedagogy shifts the focus to that which characterizes knowledge work generally: communication that is implicitly directed toward everyone "to whom it may concern."

• *Opportunity for reflection versus 1-second wait time.* A remarkable finding about recitation and teacher-mediated discussion is that teachers typically wait about 1 second for a response before calling on someone else or responding to the question themselves (Rowe, 1974). An asynchronous medium lets students take their time in formulating a contribution. It also reduces the social and emotional barriers that prevent some children from taking part in oral discussions (Lampert, Rittenhouse, & Crumbaugh, 1996).

Although none of these pedagogical shifts is dramatic, in combination they can produce a radical transformation of schooling processes. The students are assuming collective responsibility for the solution of knowledge problems, and the teacher is helping the students grow into that responsibility.

EXAMPLES AND FINDINGS

Table 14.1 provides a sampling of contributions by grade 5 and 6 students to a fairly representative CSILE discussion. A curriculum unit in science or social studies is typically launched by the teacher's framing a very general problem that is central to the relevant discipline. It is then up to the students to formulate the more specific problems that will enable their inquiry to move ahead. The early contributions to a discussion typically consist, as illustrated by the first nine items in Table 14.1, of *conjectures*—usually na-

TABLE 14.1. Contributions of Grade 5/6 Students to Discussion on "How Does the Eye Work?"

- "I think a special set of nerves carries messages from the eye to the brain and back. These messages tell the brain what the eye 'sees.' "
- "I think that the eye works by when the light behind the eye builds up and the light goes through lots of tiny blood vessels and comes out a lens in the front of the eye, that way the lens gives the eye something to see clearer through. I think that when the brain tells the eye to look at something the eye immediately turns to the object."
- "Why two eyes not one eye or three eyes?"
- "Why do people have different coloured eyes—does it affect their eyesight at all or does it just happen by chance?"
- "Why do people see up things right and they see upside-down things on the inside."
- "What are nearsightedness, farsightedness, astigmatism and presbyopia? I would like to know if they are permanent and if not, must they heal naturally? Can they be prevented before they start, or can you be born with one or more of them?"
- "I think that the eye works like this: When the person looks at the picture like a tree the picture turns upside down in the brain but in our eyes it looks like it is not upside down."
- "I think that 20–20 vision is when you can see 20 feet behind and 20 feet in front, and I think that 20–20 vision is the best vision that you can get."
- "The eye provides visual information by changing light waves into nerve impulses that are interpreted in the brain."
- "In a small area, what a person sees is detected by nerve cells. These cells are spread out on the retina, which lines the inside of the eye. There are two types of nerve cells: rods and cones. There are over one hundred million rods in each of your eyes, they detect black and white. There are only seven million cones to detect colour. Each time light hits a cone or rod, they send a nerve signal which goes out of the eye and down the main nerve passage to the brain. At the brain's "sight centre" the impulses are sorted out to create an image. The black and white pictures are combined with the colour pictures, and then the two images from both eyes are combined."
- "I need to understand why people can see in the light but not in the dark?"
- "Cones and rods that send the picture right to the brain, you can see the picture—it does not have to go to the eye."
- "When our eyes open, our central nervous system is exposed which causes our brain to be well prepared for any sudden moves. It will cause our eyes to blink or shut."
- "I think the eye sees more what the brain wants to pay attention to that what enters the eye. So when the eye sees something it is more the brain that is at work to see what it wants to pay attention to."
- "If our lens doesn't change what we see upside down, will our nerves still flip what we see over and would we realize that we are not really upside down?"
- "Last night I learned that when you think you are looking at something, you're not. It is really like bouncing off the object and then the light goes to your eye. That is the reason why you can't see things in the dark. So there is no light to bounce off the object and hit your eye."
- "White light is the light called when it already reached your eyes. When the light gets to the retina the image that you saw is upside down. Then nerves in our eyes sends the message to the back of the brain that is called cortex. In this part of the brain the depth and another thing gets together and colour and shape gets together, then they travel in front of your brain to make the right figure. One third of the brain is for sight."

ive—and *questions*—often quite cogent, like why we have two eyes rather than one or three. The naive conjectures do more than provide a starting point for knowledge advancement. They bring to the fore the students' relevant knowledge, which they are going to have to use in making sense of the new information they encounter and which it is hoped that they will try to reconcile with the new knowledge. (The alternative of leaving one's existing knowledge off to the side and treating the new knowledge as if it applied to a different world appears to be one of the ways in which serious misconceptions take hold; Vosniadou & Brewer, 1987.)

Over the course of the discussion, as new information is brought in from books and from an expert whom students could consult, one can see the students' statements beginning to take on the shape of standard scientific explanations of vision, although oversimplifications and misconceptions still appear. The students are clearly engaged in what we earlier described as reconstruction. They are not simply parroting the authoritative sources. They are reconstructing what they have read or heard so that it makes sense in light of what they already know and reconstructing their prior knowledge in light of the new information. As Popper said, these are "making and matching processes." The following two entries were spaced a day apart, with input from a medical doctor occurring in between. The refinement of understanding that they exhibit is clearly not simply a matter of absorbing what the expert said; it is a matter of incorporating new information into a knowledge-building effort that was already well advanced:

"95.04.04.

Today I learned that the Fovea is sensitive to colour because of the cones. And I also learned that Rods help you to see in the dark. I also learned that there is a yellow spot in the middle of your Fovea, it is called the Macula Lutea. The reason why the Macula Lutea is yellow is probably because red and green cone detectors perhaps reflect yellow."

"95.04.05.

Today I learned that our educated guess (hypotheses) was wrong. It is yellow because inside our retina there are thousands of blood vessels, except near the fovea where the macula Lutea is. There is very little amount of Blood vessels near it and the tissue around it also gives its colour. He also said that the reason why there is a minimal amount of blood vessels in front of our fovea is because they might interfere with the cones that identify colour."

The teacher's role in a discourse like this consists mainly of one-on-one discussions with students about their contributions. Thus, the teacher is not leading or taking responsibility for the knowledge-building effort but is helping individual students shoulder their responsibilities. The technology is virtually indispensable here. It is what enables the teacher to monitor what is happening and provide individual coaching without intruding upon the discourse itself.

In another publication, we examined a CSILE discussion that arose spontaneously in another school and that went on for 3 months, comprising 179 entries (Bereiter, Scardamalia, Cassells, & Hewitt, 1997). Beginning as a personally oriented discussion about growing, it evolved into a scientific inquiry into what regulates bodily growth. Besides pursuing various knowledge sources, the students undertook an empirical study of parent–child correlations in height so as to test whether height was genetically determined. Hakkarainen (1995) has studied a number of CSILE discussions on science topics to ascertain the extent to which they conform to canons of scientific inquiry. His conclusion, buttressed by independent judgments from two philosophers of science, is that the students collectively exhibit a high level of what may properly be called scientific thinking. Hewitt (1995) has traced the changes that took place in one classroom over 3 years as the focus was shifted from personal knowledge accumulation to the collaborative solution of knowledge problems. One of the interesting markers of this shift was an increase in the number of epistemological terms occurring in students' notes. Research in progress by Jan van Aalst (1999) indicates that contributions to knowledge advancement tend to come from students who write a substantial number of notes early that explicate their naive conceptions. In view of the concern that many educators express about student discussions propagating misconceptions, this is a potentially important finding. It makes sense that misconceptions are more likely to be changed if they are brought out into the open rather than remaining hidden from view, as they evidently have been in ordinary school programs.

TEACHING AND LEARNING

A focus on knowledge building does not negate the school's responsibility for individual students' learning. From a learning standpoint, it replaces one indirect means by another. In typical modern schools, learning is an indirect consequence of schoolwork and projects of various sorts. In what we have been describing, individual learning is an indirect consequence of knowledge building. An important reason for distinguishing knowledge building from learning in this context is in order to make sense of that last statement. Such a distinction also makes it evident that there is no incompatibility between a focus on knowledge building and the use of direct teaching. In every organization there are procedures and bodies of information to be learned and skills to be acquired that are necessary for productive work within the organization. Sometimes these can be learned informally as one goes along, but often it is expedient to teach them in a direct manner so as to ensure that everyone learns them and so as to get on with the main work. The same is clearly true in schools, where the things that need to be learned include such basic skills as reading, punctuation, and mental arithmetic.

Some educators act as if a constructivist pedagogy outlaws direct instruction and skill practice, whereas a clear conception of knowledge building as productive work allows the teachers to take a pragmatic approach to learning. They may leave it to come about as a by-product of knowledge building where that proves adequate, but they are ready to move in with more direct approaches as needed. Evaluations of CSILE indicate significant gains in literacy as a by-product of all the reading and writing that go into CSILE-mediated knowledge building (Scardamalia et al., 1992). There are indications that CSILE-based activities can enhance mathematics learning as well (Tiessen, 1996), but we see no way to get around the need for active (though not necessarily didactic) teaching in this area (cf. Lampert et al., 1996). To be avoided is the all-too-common phenomenon of spending 3 years not quite teaching children their multiplication tables.

Teaching in a knowledge-building school is not a simple matter, however: on the one hand, teachers are active participants in the collective effort to build an understanding of the world; on the other, they are professionals charged with the welfare and educational advancement of their students. The two roles are compatible, but only with some adjustment. Teachers report it to be exhilarating and liberating to engage in knowledge building along with their students, and in doing so they help authenticate it as real knowledge building rather than routine exercises or playacting. Yet it cannot be the same for teachers as for students, especially as years go by and problems that are new for the students become familiar to the teacher.

In our experience, the teachers who remain continually fascinated and involved are ones who have a dual interest. They are interested in advancing their understanding of history, geology, biology, cultural anthropology, and so forth; and each year they experience some advances themselves as they work with students on problems in those areas. But they are also interested in understanding the process of understanding itself. The students' efforts (and their own as well) to explain phenomena, to grasp theories, and to overcome naive conceptions are an endless source of insights into that distinctively human phenomenon, the pursuit of understanding.

An interest in understanding how understanding grows does not seem to be a feature of most people's curiosity. It is an acquired interest, and one that teacher education programs ought to be passionately dedicated to developing. Without it, we find, teachers tend to remain detached from students' knowledge-building efforts and to reduce knowledge-building activities to merely another set of schoolwork routines.

EXPANDING THE
KNOWLEDGE-BUILDING COMMUNITY

Up to this point, our discussion has dealt with knowledge-building communities developed within classrooms. This leaves students isolated from other communities that are engaged in building understanding of the world (e.g., from adult scientists) and also from other parts of the education system, such as curriculum planners. The Internet is already being exploited as a way of breaking down the isolation of classrooms, with exchange of e-mail between distant schools, cross-school research projects, and "ask the expert" arrangements with adult volunteers. As an Internet application, Knowledge Forum offers possibilities of forming actual communities of knowledge-building groups in which school classes are a productive part rather than a client population.

We are currently engaged in experiments that link classrooms and teachers to other classrooms and teachers, to science and art museums, students at secondary and university levels, educational researchers, subject-matter specialists, and research scientists. Different groups carry out their own knowledge-building work using Knowledge Forum, but they will be able to visit other databases and observe, comment, add links to notes in other databases, and construct views reflecting their own perspective on issues of mutual interest. Thus, for instance, science museum curators planning an exhibit on vision might visit databases like the one described earlier, where they can identify potential difficulties students will have in understanding demonstrations and can even try out design ideas on the students. The students, in turn, can visit the curators' database and make comments that could affect the design of the exhibit. Another kind of cross-community interaction involves elementary school students and medical school students studying the same health-related problem, with the possible inclusion of researchers engaged with the same problem.

Unlike the many "ask the expert" arrangements that are being tried through e-mail, the knowledge-building approach sticks closer to the idea of a community engaged in solving shared problems. Instead of the experts being cast in the role of question answerer or unpaid teacher, they are free, as are other participants, to find their own roles, to pitch in and help in whatever ways and to whatever extent they wish. Thus, the classroom work on vision discussed earlier could be enhanced by, for instance, giving students access to Chapter 8 in this volume and to the computer-mediated discourse among scientists discussing development of the visual system. The students could insert comments and questions, but these would be addressed to the whole community and would not put pressure on any individual to respond. Max S. Cynader or Barrie Frost or some of their students could in turn visit the elementary school database and get involved in the discussions to whatever extent they wished and in any of the variety of ways that the medium affords.

We have also experimented in a very limited way with breaking down the separation between student discourses and curriculum planning discourses. A database was seeded with the mandated curriculum objectives related to what the students were studying. The students linked their work to appropriate objectives and commented on the relationships, identifying what they saw as additional objectives worth specifying. Although there was no two-way interaction—no curriculum officials were involved—the experiment demonstrated that students could make contributions to curriculum planning as well as providing rich data for anyone investigating curriculum problems. We are, of course, hopeful that at some point officials at a provincial or state level will want to join in and open up their discourse as well—to students, teachers, researchers, and parents.

These efforts are not based on an exalted idea of what students can contribute. Our assumption, rather, is that students are legitimate members of a knowledge society, albeit novices in most respects. The concept of "legitimate peripheral participation" (Lave & Wenger, 1991) thus nicely represents their role. Like newcomers to any cultural practice, they must work gradually into the centers of activity, and they do so by contributing in ways that are within their growing capacities and that are acceptable to the old-timers. Ordinary schooling provides hardly any opportunity for this kind of peripheral participation, and so students graduate into the work world with little sense of how to function in it. When someone is entering a manual occupation, learning may occur rapidly because so much of the activity is open to view. But much of knowledge work is invisible. The approach we are taking is aimed at developing from an early age the social practices that make people responsible participants in the work of a knowledge society.

ACKNOWLEDGMENTS

We are grateful for research support provided by the TeleLearning Network of Centres of Excellence, and thank the Computer-Supported Intentional Learning Environments (CSILE)/Knowledge Building team for contributions to research and development reported here.

NOTE

1. Practical problems and design problems (e.g., producing a computer simulation or designing a space platform) can have considerable educational value, and we do not question their place in school programs. But because of the way the world runs, such student activities are almost invariably a form of play or pretense and so do not meet the criterion of productive knowledge work that has value beyond the worker's own needs.

Part IV

The Ecology
of Child Development:
Lessons for
a Learning Society

In Part IV we build on the analyses in Part III by presenting some strategic perspectives and describing specific initiatives, each of which focuses on the issue of constructing new social alignments to support child development. Although the focus of each is quite specific in terms of the population it serves or the problems it addresses, principles emerge that help elucidate the significance of the changing ecologies of child development and how we might begin to address them.

By focusing on the public health approach to adolescent mental health problems, Chapter 15 by David R. Offord, Helena Chmura Kraemer, Alan E. Kazdin, Peter S. Jensen, Richard Harrington, and J. Samuel Gardner highlights the limitations of, as well as the opportunities for, "compensatory strategies" in child development. It identifies the strategic problems created by the fact of high "relative" risks among relatively small segments of the population, compared with lower relative risks among broader segments of the population (which lead to higher "attributable" risks and thus greater public health impact overall). A strategy for sorting out the best mix of universal, targeted, and clinical interventions in a given community is a challenging task, one which requires effective monitoring of outcomes at the community level.

Focusing on a coordinated community program to enhance child development in poor urban communities, Camil Bouchard illustrates in Chapter 16 the crucial connections between support for child development and promotion of community development. Taken together, Chapters 16 and 17 illustrate ways that the notion of a learning society can be incorporated in the North American context.

In Chapter 17, Alan R. Pence describes efforts to support child development in Aboriginal communities. He deals with the inevitable tensions between expert-driven versus community-driven processes where the experts and the community do not share a common culture. A learning society will need to deal effectively with issues of diversity, and this treatment offers some important object lessons in that regard.

In Chapter 18, Daniel P. Keating returns to the initial question that we posed for ourselves in this volume: how can modern societies best deal with the paradox of great capacity for generating wealth versus growing threats to developmental health? Drawing on the evidence described throughout the volume, he identifies three major themes that may help resolve the paradox both conceptually and practically. First, given what we know about socioeconomic gradients and the innovation dynamic of economies in the emerging Information Age, we can usefully entertain a new conception of the "wealth of nations," one rooted in the developmental health of populations. Second, enhancing developmental health requires a deep understanding of the core dynamics of human development, from biology to society. Third, in a period of rapid change the prospects for societal adaptability depend upon the ability of communities (and nations) to become learning societies. Although we cannot draw a blueprint for designing a learning society because it is a dynamic system, we can specify some key principles that may help to guide its construction.

15

Lowering the Burden of Suffering

MONITORING THE BENEFITS
OF CLINICAL, TARGETED,
AND UNIVERSAL APPROACHES

David R. Offord
Helena Chmura Kraemer
Alan E. Kazdin
Peter S. Jensen
Richard Harrington
J. Samuel Gardner

As we consider how best to address the developmental health of populations, making use of our enhanced understanding of developmental processes and how a learning society might use this framework, we confront the reality that many different approaches have been attempted. In this chapter, we organize what we know about these approaches (clinical, targeted, and universal) to describe their relative strengths and weaknesses. We then take up the issue of how we can decide if the mixture is the right one in any given case. For this task, we explore the notion of community indicators of child developmental outcomes, which allow us to monitor and assess our progress in improving developmental health. The "burden of suffering" is a useful concept for estimating the importance for a society of a condition or disorder, or a group of disorders. The concept is usually described along three dimensions: frequency of the disorder or condition; short-term and long-term morbidity; and costs, both in fiscal and human terms. Presumably, those conditions with a high burden of suffering deserve more attention in terms of dwindling intervention and research resources than do those with a low burden. On all three dimensions, child psychiatric disorder rates extremely high (Institute of Medicine, 1989). There is a need to find the optimal combination of approaches to reduce the burden of suffering that is affordable since the costs of interventions can be enormous, yet are balanced by the cost of the illness itself. What are the possibilities of lowering this burden of suffering? There are three approaches or types of programs that can be employed: clinical, targeted, and universal.

1. *Clinical interventions.* The major characteristic of this type of program is that the family with a child who is perceived to have a disorder seeks help. The family members are seen by some type of clinical service, and this could vary anywhere from an individual practitioner such as a family doctor or child psychiatrist to a specialized mental health service. In the past, the term "tertiary prevention" was used.

2. *Targeted interventions.* The predominant characteristics of these interventions are that children and their families do not seek help, and certain children are singled out for the intervention, not necessarily because they already have a disorder but because they are at high risk for developing one. Children can be identified for targeting in two ways: the identifying characteristics can lie outside the child (e.g., family on social assistance), or the children themselves can have distinguishing characteristics (e.g., mild antisocial behavior). In the report on prevention by the Institute of Medicine, these two types of targeted prevention programs are termed "selective preventive interventions" and "indicated preventive interventions," respectively (P. J. Mrazek & Haggerty, 1994). In the past, the term "secondary prevention" was used.

3. *Universal interventions.* The cardinal characteristics of this type of program are that individual families (and their children) do not seek help and children are not singled out for the intervention. All children in a geographic area or setting (e.g., a school) receive the intervention. There are two types of universal programs: those that focus on particular communities or settings (e.g., a public housing complex), and those that are state- or provincewide or are countrywide. Although the setting itself may be a high-risk one for emotional and behavioral problems in children and adolescents, if the intervention is not targeted at specific children and adolescents but at all children and youth in that location, then the intervention is classified as "universal." In the past, the term "primary prevention" was used.

TRADE-OFFS AMONG CLINICAL, TARGETED, AND UNIVERSAL PROGRAMS

This section discusses the advantages and disadvantages of each of these three approaches.

Clinical

Table 15.1 outlines the advantages and disadvantages of the clinical approach. Clinical programs are the most acceptable to the public and politicians because it is usually apparent that the child has a disorder and needs help. Since clinical programs involve personal contact between the health care provider and the patient, and the health care provider is doing what he/she has been trained to do, both parties are usually highly motivated. Further, clinical programs are efficient in that in the majority of instances the patients present with a relevant disorder or condition.

Clinical programs also have some serious disadvantages, five of which will be discussed here. First, it is difficult to provide adequate coverage of populations. For example, children and families living near a mental health center are more likely to make use of the center's services than are those living much further away who may be in greater need of the service. Second, compliance is a troublesome issue. Among families who begin treatment in mental health services, 40–60% terminate prematurely (Kazdin, 1996). Third, there is the problem of labeling and stigmatization that can result from being seen in a clinical setting. Such labeling may be especially harmful in the case of antisocial behavior because it can lead to an escalation of the antisocial symptoms (Farrington, 1977). Fourth, clinical services are very expensive per child served. Fifth and last, it is difficult with clinical services to ensure equal access, equal participation, and equitable outcomes.

Targeted

Table 15.2 presents the advantages and disadvantages of this approach. As in the clinical program, there can be the presence of a human face with the targeted approach, and this, of course, increases the motivation of both the subject provider and the health provider. Further, along with this personal touch, the intervention can be tailored to the individual. In addition, if the targeting can be done accurately so that the group identified for the inter-

TABLE 15.1. Trade-offs: Clinical

Advantages	Disadvantages
Easiest approach to sell to the public and politicians	Inadequate coverage
	Difficulty with compliance

Human face
    Subject motivation
    Health provider motivation
	Labeling and stigmatization

	Very expensive
Efficient	Difficulty in ensuring equal access, equal participation, and equitable outcomes

TABLE 15.2. Trade-offs: Targeted

Advantages	Disadvantages

Human face
    Subject provider motivation
    Health provider motivation
    Intervention tailored to the
        individual
	Harder approach to sell to the public and politicians
	    Not actual disorder or severity not
	        impressive
	    Difficult to get general support

Potentially efficient	Labeling and stigmatization

Can address problems early on	Difficulties with screening
	        Cost
	        Uptake least among those at
	            greatest risk
	        Boundary problem
	        Risk status unstable
	        Inability to target accurately

	Limited potential for individuals and populations
	    Power to predict future disorder
	        usually very weak
	    A large number of people at small
	        risk may give rise to more cases
	        of disease than the small number
	        who are at high risk

	Tends to ignore the social context as a focus of intervention
	Behaviorally inappropriate

vention has a high likelihood of having the disorder and the group not so identified has a low likelihood of having it, then this can be an efficient approach to preventing the disorder. To have such an accurate identification procedure requires that there are known and strong risk factors for the disorder. Lastly, the targeted approach brings with it the possibility of intervening before symptoms or disorders are well established. This is especially important in conditions such as conduct disorder where the results of treatment are disappointing (Kazdin, 1993).

There are a number of disadvantages to the targeted approach. Compared to clinical services, it is harder to sell to the public and to politicians. The majority of the population that is the focus of the intervention either does not yet have an actual disorder or its severity is not impressive. This makes it difficult to obtain general support for these initiatives. Further, the procedure of targeting individuals brings with it the possibility of labeling and stigmatization. This becomes especially troublesome if the targeting is inaccurate and children, for example, are identified as being at risk for a condition such as learning disorder or antisocial behavior when in fact they are not. A challenge for the targeted approach is to identify accurately the population at risk in such a way that labeling and stigmatization are minimized.

Another potential disadvantage of the targeted approach lies with the screening procedure. First, the procedure itself may be costly. Second, the refusal rate of participation in the collection of the screening data may be highest among those at greatest risk for future disorder (G. Rose, 1985; Rutter, Tizard, & Whitmore, 1970). Third, there is a boundary or threshold issue. At some point, a threshold is set based on the screening data so that those above it screen positive and those below it do not. There will be many subjects around the threshold within this group, and the differences in risk of those who are targeted for the intervention and those who are not may be slight. Fourth, if there is reason to believe that the risk status itself is unstable over time, say, from one year to the next, it may be necessary to consider repeated screenings. For this reason, the type of risk factors that are termed fixed markers (Kraemer et al., 1997) are particularly important for screening. Fifth, there may be an inability to target accurately, as we discuss next.

Table 15.3 presents data for boys and girls on the results of predicting teacher-reported behavioral deviance at age 8 from mother's behavioral ratings at age 3 (J. Stevenson, Richman, & Graham, 1985). Data in row 1 show that of the children who screen positive at age 3 (T1) for behavioral problems, 60% will have behavioral deviance at age 8 (T2) (positive predictive value; PPV), compared to 22% of those who screen negative (1-negative predictive value; 1-NPV). Further, of those with the outcome at T2, only 36% were identified by the screen at T1 (sensitivity; Se), compared to 9% of those not so identified (1-specificity; 1-Sp). Row 2 presents the same data for girls. Here the PPV is 24% (vs. 14%) and the Se has risen to 60% (vs. 44%). Thus, of those girls screening positive at T1, only 1 in 4 (24%) will be reported as having behavioral deviance at T2; and of those with behavioral deviance at T2, 60% of them can be identified at T1.

There are several implications of these results. The ability to accurately distinguish high- from low-risk groups is limited. Generally, as one sets a stricter criterion on the information available, the level of the test (q) goes down, the Se and NPV go up, and the Sp and PPV go down. This describes a certain seesaw effect that can be counteracted only by bringing in new sources of information, that is, new and potent risk factors for the disorder. However, the more information required, the greater will be the screening cost per subject ($S).

Clinicians are often interested only in the PPV. They are concerned about the outcomes without treatment of the disorders of their patients. Thus, the magnitude of the false positive rate becomes of central importance to them. Those interested in population health, on the other hand, must be concerned with both PPV and NPV (or equivalently with Se and Sp). They are interested in the proportion of people with the outcome who can be identified earlier on as being at risk for the outcome (Se), which would enable the clinicians to exercise the opportunity to prevent that outcome. Since a preventive intervention itself carries cost ($P per person), a

TABLE 15.3. Prediction

		Predictor		Outcome							
			Age		Age			Positive	Negative		
			(years)		(years)	Screen	Preva-	predictive	predictive		
	N	Gender	Definition		Definition		+ve	lence T2	value	value	Sensitivity Specificity
(1)	236	Male	Behavioral problem: mother report	3	Behavioral deviance: teacher report	8	17%	28%	60%	78%	36% 91%
(2)	162	Female	Behavioral problem: mother report	3	Behavioral deviance: teacher report	8	47%	19%	24%	86%	60% 56%

Note. Data from J. Stevenson, Richman, and Graham (1985).

298

test with high Se that is likely to identify many false positives (low PPV) will incur unnecessary costs for preventive intervention for many subjects who would not have had the outcome even without such intervention. On the other hand, if one decreases the Se in order to protect against false positives, many subjects who will eventually get the disorder will not be identified early and will go on to require treatment anyway (at $T per person per year).

An additional point to be noted in Table 15.3 is that the same test applied in different clinical populations may have very different sensitivity and specificity. This has been referred to as the "spectrum problem" (Feinstein, 1985) or as the "population specificity of tests" (Kraemer, 1992). Further, mothers of boys tend to underreport future behavioral problems at age 3 (17% vs. 28%) (see row 1), whereas mothers of girls tend to overreport (47% vs. 19%) (see row 2). Accurate screening procedures or effective prevention interventions or treatment interventions may be different for boys and girls. Such considerations also apply to other interacting risk factors. The most appropriate screening, prevention, and treatment options may differ, for example, by gender, age, and socioeconomic status.

Finally, we should also note that the odds ratio between mother report at age 3 and teacher report at age 8 for boys is 5.3, which would be considered very high in comparison to epidemiological applications, but here only 36% of the subjects who are deviant at age 8 are identified as at high risk at age 3 (see Table 15.3, row 1), which would, for prevention purposes, be considered quite low. The potency of a risk factor may be judged very differently for the purpose of application than for the purpose of increasing the knowledge base.

Another disadvantage of an exclusive focus on the targeted approach is that is has limited potential both for individuals and for populations (G. Rose, 1985). There are two reasons for this. The first, as noted above, is that the ability to predict future behaviors is currently very weak. The second reason is that a large number of people at small risk give rise to more cases of a disease or disorder than the small number at high risk. Data from the Ontario Child Health Study, a large ($N = 3,294$) provincewide survey of the mental health of children, 4–16 years of age in Ontario illustrate this point (Offord et al., 1987). Children living in families with an income level under Can.$10,000 are at high risk for one or more psychiatric disorders, with more than one-third of them (36.3%) qualifying as cases. However, only 7.3% of children are in this income category. Thus, economically disadvantaged children account for only 14.5% of the population with psychiatric disorders. On the other hand, children who live in families that are well off financially (Can.$25,000 and above) account for more than half (59%) of the children with psychiatric disorders. The risk for such disorders is much lower in these children than in the poor population, but their large numbers mean that their contribution to the population of disordered children is far greater than that of the poor children.

A further disadvantage of the targeted approach is that it tends to ignore the communitywide social context as a mechanism of change (G. Rose, 1985). The targeted approach focuses on identifying and intervening with those at greatest risk. It centers on detecting risk factors that distinguish the high-risk from the low-risk group. It never considers risk factors that might distinguish one entire population from another. Figure 15.1 illustrates this point. Suppose there are two communities, A and B. In community A, a targeted prevention program is set up where among kindergarten children the top 20% scores on an antisocial behavior checklist are identified as being at risk for conduct disorder. The elements of the intervention program for this at-risk group will be based on knowledge about *causal* risk factors that distinguish this high-risk group from the low-risk group. The only suitable candidates for causal risk factors are those that apply to individuals and their families. Now suppose community A has more than five times the rate of conduct disorder compared to community B. One could argue in this case that the most important issue to address is why community A as a whole has such a high rate of conduct disorder

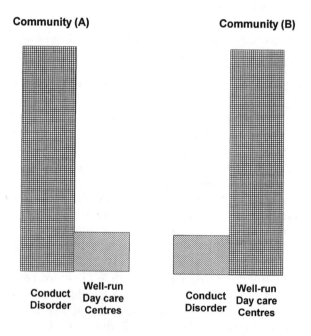

FIGURE 15.1. Contrast of two communities where the hypothesized determinant of the marked difference in the prevalence of conduct disorder in the two settings is in a communitywide characteristic, namely, the different frequencies of well-run day-care centers.

compared to community *B*. The focus in community *A* should not be to attempt to do something about preschool children who are at the extreme of the distribution on antisocial scores, but rather to focus on causal risk factors that distinguish the two communities on the communitywide rate of conduct disorder. Well-run day care centers are given as an example of a causal protective factor that may distinguish these two communities and be related to the markedly different rates of conduct disorder. Thus, efforts to increase day care centers in community *A* might be the primary focus of the communitywide intervention program. In short, the targeted approach never considers as a focus for interventions those causal risk or protective factors that apply to the whole community and are responsible for the disadvantaged status of the children as a group in that community, nor does it ever consider the role of communitywide protective factors (e.g., well-run day care centers).

A final disadvantage of an exclusive focus on the targeted approach is that focusing on changing behavior of a high-risk subgroup will be difficult if the behavior at issue is widespread in the population. The targeted group will have more of it, but almost everyone will have some of it. For example, if one element of the intervention with kindergarten children with high antisocial scores is to reduce physical violence in peer interactions in the classroom, this will be difficult to accomplish if physical violence in even milder forms is widespread among all children in the classroom. It is difficult to change one's behavior when everyone around you is behaving in much the same way. This is an inherent disadvantage of the targeted approach. Indeed, in targeted approaches with adolescents, sometimes youths become worse with the intervention because youths with behavioral problems interact and build peer relationships that promote deviant behavior (e.g., substance abuse; see Dishion & Andrews, 1995).

Universal

Table 15.4 outlines the advantages and disadvantages of the universal approach. Six advantages are noted. First, support from the general public may be easier to obtain for a universal initiative than for a targeted approach because the focus will be on all children or families, not just a selected disadvantaged subgroup. Second, since the intervention is offered to all children in a population, there is no labeling or stigmatization of particular children. Third, in a universal program, there is a greater likelihood of the middle class being one of the recipients, and this increases the chances that the program will be well run. Middle class parents may be more likely than lower class parents to complain about perceived deficiencies in a program for their children—and their complaints are more likely to be acted on. (These three advantages have been mentioned as disadvantages in the case of targeted programs.) Fourth, universal programs can focus intervention efforts on populationwide causal risk factors. Fifth, although such pro-

TABLE 15.4. Trade-offs: Universal

Advantages	Disadvantages
Easier to obtain support from the general public for this approach than for the targeted approach	Hard to sell to public and politicians
No labeling or stigmatization	Impersonal; poor motivation of the subject and the health provider
Middle class demand that the program be well run	Small benefit to individual
Can focus on communitywide contextual factors	Hard to detect an overall effect
	May have the greatest effect on those at lowest risk, thus increasing inequality
Large potential for the population	Unnecessarily expensive
Behaviorally appropriate	Denies the non-high-risk population the opportunity of doing good
	If broader than community level, can undermine community initiatives
	Viewed skeptically by the low-risk population

grams cannot be expected to have a large effect on individuals, they may have a small effect on almost all members of the population that translates into a large effect on the population as a whole. For example, if a universal intervention raises the IQ of each child by an average of 2 points, the gain for each individual child is small but the total gain in IQ from a population perspective would be immense. Sixth, a universal intervention is behaviorally appropriate since, unlike the targeted approach, the target for behavioral change is the whole population, not just high-risk children within it.

The disadvantages of a universal approach are many. It is very difficult to sell to the public and politicians. It may raise concerns about "social engineering" or engender complaints about government interference with personal freedoms or "the family's private business." It is impersonal, and thus it is hard to motivate the subject and the health provider. In addition, there is a small benefit to the individual. In terms of evaluation research, it may be hard to detect reliably an overall beneficial effect of the intervention since the effect sizes will likely be small. A worrisome potential disadvantage of a universal approach alone is that it may have its greatest effects on those at lowest risk. For example, a classwide social skills program that aims to prevent antisocial behavior may in fact have its major effect on reducing the level of antisocial behavior in those children who do not have much of it to begin with, namely, the low-risk children. It may have little or no effect on those children who have the highest current levels of antisocial behavior and are at risk in the future for clinically significant levels of antisocial behavior. In short, the intervention may make nice children even nicer. In the same vein, universal programs aimed at benefiting poor children and their families end up benefiting the middle class to a greater degree (Howe & Longman, 1992; Jones, 1996). Another disadvantage of a universal program is that it may be unnecessarily expensive since the majority of children who are receiving it probably do not need it. If, for example, there is a universal program with the goal of preventing serious antisocial behavior, the at-risk population may be no greater than 20%, so that 8 of 10 children receiving the universal program do not require it.

The last three disadvantages focus on the reactions of the non-high-risk population. A universal program may deny the non-high-risk population the opportunity of helping out with a disadvantaged population. With the universal program in place, the advantaged population feels that there is no need for their efforts since the universal program is perceived as looking after the deficits that they usually address. For example, under ordinary circumstances, members of the middle class may extend themselves to the children of the poor by seeking to ensure that they have full participation in recreational activities. However, if a universal program is in place addressing this issue for all children, then the middle class may retreat from launching any effort in this regard. Along the same line, a universal program brings with it the possibility of undermining community efforts. Members of a community may feel that there is no need for them to take collective responsibility for the children and their families in the community since a universal program is looking after all of this. Lastly, it is possible that in a universal program the low-risk population views the program with skepticism because they realize it is not really needed by their children. The unstated purpose of it is to reach the high-risk population, and this is done under the guise of providing a program for all children.

In summary, clinical, targeted, and universal programs all have advantages and disadvantages. One type of program alone (e.g., clinical) will never be sufficient to lower the burden of suffering from child psychiatric disorders in a meaningful way. What is needed is a combination of all three approaches.

STEPS IN DECIDING THE OPTIMAL MIX OF CLINICAL, TARGETED, AND UNIVERSAL PROGRAMS

There are certain data requirements of interventions that are necessary if rational judgments are to be made about choosing the best mix of clinical, targeted, and universal programs. A detailed discussion of these requirements is outside the scope of this chapter, but they include information on the following issues: the effectiveness of an intervention, that is, the extent to which an intervention does more good than harm to those to whom it is offered (D. L. Sackett, 1980; Tugwell, Bennett, & Sackett, 1985); the extent to which the intervention reaches those who need it (Rossi & Freeman,

1993); the rate of take-up or compliance with the intervention among those who need it; and the cost of the intervention (Department of Clinical Epidemiology & Biostatistics, McMaster University Health Sciences Centre, 1984a; 1984b).

With these prerequisites known, three further steps are involved in deciding on the optimal mix of these three types of programs:

1. Determine the per annum prevalence (p) of the disorder in the absence of any prevention. Determine the per annum cost to a child with the disorder ($T). (This includes treatment cost for those who seek treatment and costs related to consequences of leaving the disorder untreated for those who don't, as well as the costs associated with the consequences of ineffective treatment.)

2. Review what is known about risk factors for the disorder or condition. Are there fixed markers that are easily obtained at low cost per subject that are potent in identifying those likely to get the disorder for use in screening procedures? What screening procedures are available, with what sensitivity (Se), specificity (Sp), and per subject cost ($S)? Consider the possibility of multistage screening, that is, a very low-cost screen with a very high sensitivity used to rule out those subjects very unlikely to get the disorder, with those positive on the initial screen to go on to a higher-cost screen with high sensitivity but with greater specificity to rule out false positives. Only those positive at the second stage would enter the targeted prevention program.

3. Review what is known about causal risk factors for disorder; that is, are there known risk factors that either singly or in combination can be changed, and if changed, can alter the risk of disorder? What prevention programs are available, with what cost per subject ($p) and with what probability of successfully preventing the disorder (c)?

Table 15.5 provides examples of trade-offs resulting from different combinations of clinical, targeted, and universal programs. For every example, two values are fixed: the per annum prevalence of disorder (p) = 20%, and the per annum cost per child with disorder ($T) = $200. The number of children on which calculations are based = 1,000.

In example 1, no screening takes place, there is no prevention program (hence $P = 0$, $c = 0$), and thus the prevalence of disorder = 20%. With a per annum cost per child with disorder of $200 and 200 disordered children, then the cost per child = $40.

The next three examples examine different types of universal programs. In example 2, the cost of the intervention per child ($P) = $8.00 and thus the total cost of the preventive intervention = $8.00 × 1000 = $8,000. The success rate of the preventive intervention (c) is 25%; thus 50 of the 200 cases are prevented. The new prevalence of cases is now (200 − 50)/1,000 = 150/1,000 = 15%. The cost of treating these cases is 150 ×

TABLE 15.5. Examples of Trade-offs among Clinical, Targeted, and Universal Programs

| | | | Input | | | | | | Calculated | |
Example	p	$T	Se	Sp	$S	$P	c	%pop INT	New p	Cost/child
(1)	20%	$200	0%	0%	$0	$0	0%	0%	20%	$40
(2)	20%	$200	100%	0%	$0	$8	25%	100%	15%	$38
(3)	20%	$200	100%	0%	$0	$10	25%	100%	15%	$40
(4)	20%	$200	100%	0%	$0	$8	20%	100%	16%	$40
(5)	20%	$200	75%	94%	$2	$8	25%	20%	16%	$36.10
(6)	20%	$200	75%	94%	$2	$30	25%	20%	16%	$40.00
(7)	20%	$200	100%	80%	$10	$30	50%	25%	10%	$40.80
(8)	20%	$200	100%	80%	$2	$30	50%	25%	10%	$32.80

Note. p, per annum prevalence of disorder; $T, per annum treatment cost per child with disorder; Se, sensitivity of the screen; Sp, specificity of the screen; $S, cost per child of the screen; $P, cost of the intervention per screen-positive child; c, success rate of the preventive intervention; %popINT, percentage of population who received the intervention; New p, the per annum prevalence of disorder after the reduction in cases as a result of the intervention has been taken into account; Cost/child, the total costs of all interventions per child.

305

$200 = \$30,000$. Thus the cost per child of this combined universal and treatment program is $38 per child, a slight savings over the treatment program alone. Examples 3 and 4, also universal programs, illustrate the trade-off between the cost per child of the preventive intervention ($P) and its success rate (*c*). In example 3 compared to 4, $P is higher ($10 vs. $8) but *c* is also higher (25% vs. 20%). Thus, the cost per child in these examples is the same, and identical to that of treatment alone ($40 per child).

Examples 5 to 8 show different trade-offs among Se, Sp, $S, $P, and *c*. Example 8 resulted in the lower cost per child ($32.80). It had 100% Se and a high *c* (50%), the screening wasn't free but was inexpensive ($S = $2); Sp (80%) wasn't the highest and $P ($30) wasn't the lowest, but the balance was effective.

In summary, universal interventions are better than treatment alone, when the condition is quite common (high *p*), the treatment costs ($T) are large, the preventive intervention is relatively inexpensive ($P), and there is a high cure rate (*c*). Universal intervention is better than treatment alone only if $P < \$Tpc$. A targeted program will be most effective when Se and *uc* are high and $S and $P are low. A clinical program is most appropriate when $T, Se, and *c* are low and $S is high. Clearly, detailed knowledge is needed about the effectiveness of intervention programs and their costs so that distinctions can be made among different programs as outlined in Table 15.5.

PRACTICAL IMPLICATIONS

The above discussion leads us to two practical questions:

1. How do we determine the best mix of clinical, targeted, and universal programs for any particular community?
2. How do we monitor whether the mix is working in any particular community?

One way in which a community might begin to answer both of these questions is by developing community-level social reporting efforts and by developing a range of relevant social indicators.

With regard to the first question, ideally a social report would reveal enough about the state of the relevant population so that decisions could be made about what sort of mix of programs would be preferable. For example, take a simplified case involving two distinct communities. In community *A*, it is found out that 5% of the relevant population has some severe form of conduct disorder, with another 5% hovering around the threshold of being considered to have the disorder and 90% having no symptoms of the disorder. In community *B*, the appropriate social reporting reveals that only 1% of the relevant population has some severe form of conduct disorder, with 20% hovering on the threshold and the remaining 79% having no symptoms. Thus in community A it may be decided that emphasis should be placed on clinical programs being in place, given the relatively large percentage of the population suffering from the noted disorder. Conversely, with regard to community B it may be decided that more emphasis should be placed on targeted and/or universal programs that would be more preventive in nature and would help ensure that the 20% on the threshold of conduct disorder do not develop into severe cases of the disorder.

With regard to the second question, regular social reporting on the state of the relevant population may show, in a somewhat primitive fashion, through the ups and downs of the values of various indicators, whether the mix of programs in any community is working to reduce either some particular disorder or the suffering caused by that disorder. The issue of attribution is a problem here. Moreover, the community environment to which individual children and child populations belong are complex systems, and so judgments concerning what is the best *overall* mix of programs affecting many domains are likely to be fraught with difficulty.

By a "social report" is meant any document that discusses what is known about the social conditions of a particular population, community, or society of human beings. It is a report that focuses on an entire population or community, however defined, and is to be contrasted with studies that are based on a clinical population. These latter serve to explore, test, and refine hypotheses, theoretical models, and correlations (see Brusegard, 1979, p. 263, for another way of defining "social report"). The term "indicator" refers to a particular measure or statistic that singly or in combination with other measures serves as a sensitive surrogate measure of an important feature of a population or community. For example, the suicide rate for a particular age group in a specific geographic area for a particular time (or particular time series) might serve as an indicator of the socioemotional health of a population group. Changes in the state of the overall socioemotional health of a population should be mirrored by corresponding changes in the suicide rates for that population, if in fact the latter is a good indicator of the former (see also Carley, 1981, p. 2, and Michalos, 1980, p. 2, for two additional ways of looking at social indicators).

There is a need for an overall conceptual framework that can be used as a template for setting up a social reporting system connected to each domain of children's health and well-being.[1] Such a framework would essentially contain five main components:

1. It would contain an "unpacking" of the central concept. For example, the central concept of "children's mental health" might be broken down into subcategories, with the various known disorders cataloged (e.g., conduct disorder or attention deficit disorder), or a broader, more inclusive

picture might be developed encompassing positive and negative features of mental health.

2. It would contain evidence-based material focusing on the causal influences of each of the identified central conceptual pieces. Thus, the particular risk and protective factors that are known to be causative of conduct disorder would be part of such a conceptual framework (Kraemer et al., 1997).

3. It would contain evidence-based material outlining the various outcomes and developmental pathways that individuals suffering from a particular disorder (or benefiting from a particular protective factor) are likely to experience. Conclusions concerning population-level outcomes would also be worthy of inclusion.

4. It would contain information on what we know works, in terms of the prevention, treatment, and support of a population in relation to the particular disorder. Thus, information on evaluated programs, promising interventions, "Best Practices," etc., should be included in the report and be linked to the information contained in each of the previous three paragraphs.

5. It would contain information of what relevant community resources (i.e., clinical, targeted, and universal programs) are in place. Here the reporting effort would need to inventory the programs, strategies, interventions, facilities, etc., that exist in the community of interest, and categorize them by a variety of resource features, including whether they are clinical, targeted or universal programs (or resources).

Schematically, such a template for a conceptual framework would look something like Figure 15.2. Depending on the contingent feature of data availability, implementing such a framework for a particular concept

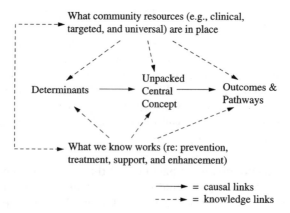

FIGURE 15.2. Basic conceptual framework for community social reporting.

or cluster of concepts would allow for the determination of what mix of programs is needed and later monitoring of how the mix is working, thereby providing some of the basic information needed for making evaluations of the various types of programs in the community and making recommendations on an optimal program mix.

However, the principal limitation in implementing such a conceptual scheme lies in the limited availability of useful data. Apart from engaging in large-scale primary data collection exercises, which are prohibitively expensive for most communities and difficult to continue on an ongoing basis, communities will have to rely on data that can or would be collected by child-caring institutions in the community. These include schools, public health departments, recreation departments, police departments, etc. These institutions may have to alter the data they collect so that the information can be of more central use in monitoring the health and well-being of children in the community. In any case, social reporting at the community level will not only have to be *useful* but will also have to be *feasible* and *acceptable* so that it can be carried out on an ongoing basis.

DISCUSSION

Because of the high burden of suffering of child psychiatric disorders, clinical interventions alone are unlikely to have marked effects on reducing this burden. The most effective strategy will be to put in place for each condition the optimal combination of clinical, targeted, and universal programs. Research efforts should not only address clinical issues but also focus on discovering causal risk factors for disorder that can lead to accurate screening and effective preventive interventions. At present, we do not have sufficient knowledge on the cost-effectiveness of clinical, targeted, and universal interventions in the child mental health field to decide on an optimal mix of programs.

The strategy to reduce the burden of suffering from child psychiatric disorders should be seen as consisting of a number of concurrent steps. First, effective universal programs should be in place. Targeted programs should follow for those not helped sufficiently by the universal programs. The screening could be done in stages, beginning with screens that are inexpensive and have a high sensitivity. These can be followed by screens that, while maintaining a high sensitivity, have increasing levels of specificity and perhaps are more expensive. At each stage, more intensive interventions could be launched. Finally, for those unaffected by the targeted programs, clinical services would be available. Such a strategy has four major advantages. First, it acknowledges the need to reduce the size of the population seeking clinical services. Second, there might be multiplier effects. For instance, a targeted approach might work better for high-risk children if the environment is facilitating due to a universal program. For example, helping high-risk children to avoid accepting illegal drugs when they are offered might be more effective when it is done in conjunction with community policing efforts to reduce availability. Third, the strategy reinforces the need to monitor the level of child psychiatric disorders on a population basis. A systematic approach to social or community monitoring through the strategic use of indicators is essential. Fourth, it makes clear that one-step prevention programs are as unrealistic as are clinical programs as a blueprint to reduce the frequency of child psychiatric disorders. An optimal mix of universal, targeted, and clinical programs is needed. The nature of the combination will change as knowledge accumulates, and there will always be trade-offs among these three approaches.

ACKNOWLEDGMENTS

This work was supported by funds from the Research Network on Psychopathology and Development of the John D. and Catherine T. MacArthur Foundation. David R. Offord was also supported by a National Health Scientist Award, Health Canada, and by the Canadian Institute for Advanced Research, where he is a Fellow in the Human Development Program.

NOTE

1. See, among many others, Innes, (1990) on the need for conceptual frameworks to guide indicator design. For a Canadian perspective on this issue, see Willms and Gilbert (1990).

16

The Community as a Participative Learning Environment

THE CASE OF CENTRAIDE OF GREATER MONTRÉAL *1,2,3 GO!* PROJECT

Camil Bouchard

Researchers have gained crucial knowledge about the diverse ecological configurations of variables contributing to the development of the child. But we still know little about how to encourage the emergence of a culture devoted to the well-being of young children. This culture might be seen as the theory of community members regarding what is best for their children. This theory would in part be anchored in the representations held by the community of a successful child and of a successful adult. These representations are the product of a never-ending process that is fed by experiences, models, information, and social rules. How a community goes about sharing these representations, identifying priorities, and acting upon them in order to promote the well-being of its children is still a matter of empirical study. *1,2,3 GO!* is an experimental project whereby five neighborhoods and one village of the Greater Montréal area are invited to invest their resources in the well-being of children from birth to 3 years of age. The communities are invited to organize themselves and to identify consensual priorities around this goal. Mobilization of the population, cooperation among the various resources, reaching out to the families most in need, involving parents as partners, and offering high-quality support for the participants are overarching principles of the project. Discussion of the project *1,2,3 GO!* will highlight what is believed to be the most important factors that will contribute to the successful implementation of the project. The research processes and challenges are also examined.

DESCRIPTION OF THE PROJECT

Research in the field of child physical abuse and neglect tells us that one of the most important protective factors is the family's immediate social environment. As compared with poor high-risk neigborhoods, poor low-risk neighborhoods present a better social picture: families' social support networks are bigger and more diversified; there are fewer single-parent families; neighbors are less suspicious of each other; residential stability is higher; immigration is lower; and neighbors perceive their environment as safer, less polluted, and a better place to raise a child (Chamberland, Bouchard, & Beaudry, 1986; Coulton, Korbin, Su, & Chow, 1995; Garbarino & Kostelny, 1992; Garbarino & Sherman, 1980; Zuravin, 1989; Zuravin & Taylor, 1987). Coulton et al. (1995) illustrate that some of these same variables are linked to drug and delinquency problems. Controlling for family conditions, Klebanov, Brooks-Gunn, and Duncan (1994) also showed that neighborhood poverty was associated with a less stimulating home and with less maternal warmth.

These observations lead to the hypothesis that child abuse prevention and promotion of children's well-being may profit from building stronger, more cohesive, more accountable, and more problem-solving-oriented communities. J. R. Evans (1996), referring to Putnam's and Yankelovich's work on social capital, strongly argues in favor of strengthening our communities by gaining their commitment around a shared goal. This is the approach that has been borrowed by the project *1,2,3 GO!*

OBJECTIVES AND PRINCIPLES OF *1,2,3 GO!*

1,2,3 GO! is a demonstration project whereby some communities of the Greater Montréal area are selected and invited to mobilize whatever resources are needed, be they material, intellectual, social, or political, in order to develop and sustain an environment concerned with the well-being and the development of its 0- to 3-year-old children. The project aims at improving the chances of children living in poor areas of Greater Montréal by providing them and their parents with more stimulating, supportive, and dedicated local environments. The communities are invited to identify and share priorities and to organize themselves around these common goals.

Although there is a specific concern with enrolling those communities in which children experience higher risks, the overall objective is more in line with a health or well-being promotion approach than with a prevention or remedial approach. As such it relies on three main general strategies: enhancement of individual competencies, institutional/environmental changes, and mass influence (Renaud, Dufour, & O'Loughlin, 1997). It is also worth noting that *1,2,3 GO!* rests on the postulate that communities can and ought to empower themselves around the issue of the development and the well-being of their children. This community action approach is presented as a main principle component of the Ottawa Health Promotion Charter (World Health Organization, 1986). The project is thus concerned with child development, parental support, and community participation.

Six working principles (guidelines) were identified and presented to the participating communities:

1. *Mobilization of the various actors.* The initiative aims at involving a large coalition of citizens in each of the communities so that a vast array of the local population comes to share this concern about the well-being of young children. The mobilization of the population is expected from the very first planning phase of the project (the writing of an action plan) so as to ensure that the priorities of the project are supported by a large community consensus.

2. *Collaboration among local institutions, services, and citizens.* Both to avoid unproductive duplication of efforts and useless competition, financial support is offered when the communities have demonstrated their capacity to work in a collaborative manner. This can take time! (Annie E. Casey Foundation, 1995). Volunteer organizations, health and social governmental services, recreational and local police services, school services, and business organizations are expected to work together in defining, launching, and sustaining a common project.

3. *Reaching out to all children and families.* Special attention is given to reaching those families who would not otherwise spontaneously show up to community activities or social services. Community action plans are expected to specify various ways by which all families are given the opportunity to take part in the project.

4. *Addressing the children directly.* The literature clearly demonstrates the positive impact of programs of high intensity and of projects relying on a rigorous curriculum or approach. The communities' action plans are expected to address this issue and to design projects or activities that will involve children directly.

5. *Parent participation.* There are some positive indications as to the benefits that may be expected from involving parents in the design, the management, and the carrying out of the projects. The impact would seem to be positive for the child, for the other members of the family, and for the parents themselves. Parent participation is also expected to benefit the social network and the whole community.

6. *High-quality interventions.* The knowledge, training, enthusiasm, and involvement of the staff and community members in the projects are necessary components of their success. Adequate support from the leaders of the projects, on-the-job training, access to ad hoc consultations, and efficient means of communication among communities workers and between communities and the project staff are key elements in ensuring high-quality interventions.

MAKING IT WORK

1,2,3 GO! has been initiated by Centraide (United Way) of Greater Montréal. It involves the contribution of three full-time staff members and hundreds of volunteers. A Program Committee (staff and volunteers) has been at work since the very beginning (1993) and has been responsible for designing the overall initiative and for selecting and inviting the communities to participate in the project. Its main task is to support the work of the director of the project and of the three Centraide staff members involved in the day-to-day operations. The Partners Committee is a larger body; it gathers 25 leaders of Greater Montréal in the areas of health and social services, youth protection services, recreational and police services, school services, child care organizations, workers unions, churches, business organizations, and volunteer organizations. The mission of these partners is to facilitate the implementation of the local projects and to promote a strong regional commitment to the initiative and to the well-being of children. A Supporter Committee has also been created. It is led by the former chief executive officer of one of the largest business consortiums of Montréal and is responsible for financing the initiative. Three other bodies are at work in the project. First, a network of consultants in which experts of various fields have agreed to give free consultation time to the communities and to help organize various activities around issues such as child safety, nutrition, language, and social and emotional development, as well as community organization and development. This provides the project with high-quality partners but also widens the support of the initiative to experts and to institutions not directly linked to *1,2,3 GO!* Second, the research team responsible for evaluating the implementation and the impact of *1,2,3 GO!* The team has been mainly concerned during the first months of implementation with consulting community actors and with the project promoters so as to develop a research protocol that reflects the concerns of the participants.[1] Finally, each community relies on the work of a Local Steering Committee, which in fact comprises representatives of local organizations and citizens volunteering in the project. Each of these committee hires a permanent coordinator. The Local Steering Committee has the responsibility for developing an Action Plan and for its implementation.

1,2,3 GO! IN ACTION

In late spring 1995, five urban communities were invited to participate to the project. These communities were chosen according to the following criteria: a high percentage of very-low-income families; a high percentage of preschoolers in the population; an active community life and collaborative networking; and an ethnic composition reflecting the demographic picture of the Greater Montréal area. A sixth community, a village located south of

Montréal, was invited to join *1,2,3 GO!*, as Centraide of Greater Montréal serves both the immediate metropolitan area and more remote rural areas south and north of the city. This offers the opportunity to test the viability of such a project in comparing urban and rural environments where the notion of community may not evoke the same territorial or cultural entities. Each of the urban communities has around 750 children 0–3 years of age; some 300 children of this age live in the rural community.

These six communities were each offered seed money in order to produce an Action Plan that would first describe the community, its problems, its resources, and its assets and would also identify the priorities of the project as selected by the local population. Here are some indicators of what has been accomplished in these communities since then:

• Of the 631 persons invited to the local presentations of the project by the Program Committee in the spring of 1995, 230 showed up.
• Of these, more than 130 persons have been steadily and very actively involved in trying to identify the best ways to implement the project. An impressive web of partners has been at work in each of the neighborhoods, people who have come from a broad array of domains, institutions, services, and organizations. Participation in the Local Steering Committees ranges from 12 to 35 persons.
• Strong signs of collaboration are showing up in the neighborhoods among actors that would otherwise have ignored each other before their involvement in the project, along with signs of some tension among well-established cultural groups or services providers.
• Around 300 parents and numerous other interested individuals have been actively involved in identifying priorities upon which to draw the various community activities or programs. These persons were consulted during special gatherings organized by the local steering committees, through focus groups or individual interviews held in people's homes or in the parks, through questionnaires distributed to parents at their homes or in child care services, and through questionnaires or interviews held with various practitioners or key informants. Parents occupy very active and powerful roles in at least three of the participating communities.
• Five of the six communities have already presented their Action Plan to the Program Committee and to the Centraide Board. *Sufficient and appropriate nutrition of children* has been identified as the top priority in two of these neighborhoods. A second priority is the concern for *cleaner and safer alleys, streets, and play environments* for young children and their parents. A third priority is to ensure *easier access to stimulating environments* for the child: problems with public transportation and with the scarcity of resources are emphasized, as well as the need for developing an integrated service and play center for young children and their parents in the immediate locality. In the rural community, language development has been targeted and has triggered the implementation of a very large project.

Mobilization of the whole community around the idea of a *better world for their children* has been targeted by two communities. Finally, *concerns about family income* have inspired special projects in two of the neighborhoods under the leadership of employment service members who wish to offer opportunities to parents of very young children in their programs.

- In each of these neighborhoods a detailed and well-structured agenda of activities has already been approved by the communities for the next 2 years. Financial support has been awarded to these communities for the coming year.

- One last community is struggling in its attempts to reach a consensus and to write an Action Plan. In this community, there is large diversity of ethnicities already organized around powerful consortia (i.e., interest groups).

THEORETICAL FOUNDATIONS OF *1,2,3 GO!*

The Hierarchical–Organizational Model

In several ways, *1,2,3 GO!* is not original and has much in common with many North American early intervention programs that have been developed in the last 30 years. Most of these programs rest implicitly or explicitly on a *hierarchical–organizational model* of child development. This model posits that normal development is composed of a series of interlocking social, emotional, cognitive, and social-cognitive competencies. When one competence occurs at one level, it allows environmental adaptation and prepares for future competence. Normal development is marked by the integration of earlier competencies into later modes of functioning. It follows then that "early adaptation tends to promote later adaptation and integration" (Cicchetti, 1989, p. 379).[2] From this conceptual model, it follows that intervention should preferably occur as early as possible in the life of the child, and prevention is preferable to remedial strategies. Several types of early intervention models have emerged during the last several decades. Some are child focused; others are more parent focused. In some of the best-known programs, only one or two areas of child development are considered; for example, the Perry Preschool Project (Scheinwart, Barnes, & Weikart, 1993) and the first versions of the North Carolina Abecedarian project (C. T. Ramey, Bryant, Campbell, Sparling, & Wasik, 1990) were mainly concerned with social-cognitive development and were delivered through a traditional professional-to-parent type of approach. In some other well-known projects such as Head Start, the approach is more comprehensive and included concerns with child health, and the program is defined and delivered by a local consortium of lay and professional people. Here parents and citizens play a crucial role in the agenda.

The Ecological–Transactional Model

1,2,3 GO! relates more to the Head Start model. It emphasizes the importance of involving parents and citizens in the project and of adopting a wide perspective in establishing the priorities of intervention. But it also departs from previous early intervention projects in that it explicitly posits the goal of helping the communities to create or reinforce the expression of an environment (both local and global) that will promote the well-being of children. This particular goal relates to an *ecological–transactional model* whereby child development is not only the product of the interactions between the child's characteristics and the characteristics of the immediate environment but must also be understood as emerging from a series of indirect interactions between the child and more distal environments through the influence of more proximal elements. In other words, establishing or reinforcing a local culture concerned with the well-being of children should provide more learning and developmental opportunities for each child within his/her immediate environment (e.g., through families and child care services, which would in turn find better support in the community). The challenge of projects such as *1,2,3 GO!* is to tackle at the same time both the micro-level systems and the exo- and macro-level systems that indirectly but nevertheless profoundly affect the well-being of the child (Bronfenbrenner, 1979; Garbarino, 1982). For example, one suggestion might be that in a well-informed community culture, supermarkets or large drugstores would offer free child care and free delivery for those families with children under 3 years old. This seemingly benign innovation might, however, have an important impact on many poor families' capacity to buy at the best prices the appropriate food or health products for their young children. Otherwise, such families often must rely on the nearest small shop, where prices are usually higher and choices more restricted.

The Ecological–Cultural Model

The design of *1,2,3 GO!* has also espoused the postulate that child development and child-rearing practices of families and communities are heavily influenced by a set of cultural demands that vary from one ethnic group and one social group to the other. We posited above that normal development is composed of a series of interlocking social, emotional, cognitive, and social-cognitive competencies; we are also reminded by anthropologists that "competencies—cognitive, linguistic, social–emotional, and practical—are cultural requirements which parents and other child-rearing agents are obligated to inculcate to children" (Ogbu, 1981, p. 417). Parents prepare their children for exercising tasks required of adults as they are prescribed in their community. The nature of these tasks and the type of adults capable of fulfilling them are influenced by the *effective environment,* that is, by the opportunity structure—the economic resources available to the group. Parents, caregivers, and other proximate adults develop a theory of what constitutes a successful adult that is coherent with this effective environment and thus a theory of child rearing, which in turn influences the selection of suitable child-rearing techniques or strategies.

1,2,3 GO! is implemented in very-low-income areas. Many of these communities are also inhabited by diverse cultural groups. It is our hypothesis that not only child-rearing values and techniques are culture specific but also the views of people about the role of the community and institutions in their family life and about their own participation in designing and launching a project dealing with the issue of the well-being of children are also profoundly affected by their cultural background.[3] Overall, we feel that a project which seeks to reinforce a culture sensitive to children's well-being cannot ignore the cultural specificities of the various groups involved. These cultural nuances involve questions as to what precisely is a healthy and well-developed child, what are suitable or appropriate actions to be taken in a community Action Plan, and indeed what constitutes a community properly dedicated to safeguarding its children.

The Community Systems and Community Development Models

1,2,3 GO! is an experiment in trying to empower communities in building up a secure, warm, supportive, and generous environment in which their children and parents can flourish. As such, the project relies very much on the voluntary participation and collaboration of local groups, organizations, and services (both governmental and voluntary) "to improve the physical, the social and the economical conditions of the communities" (Florin & Wandersman, 1990, p. 45). Community and individual empowerment has recently been linked to citizen participation as empowerment is conceived as "a mechanism by which people, organizations and communities gain mastery over their affairs" (Florin & Wandersman, 1990). Those two concepts of individual/community empowerment and of community development are at the core of the project. One of the big challenges is to try to find an appropriate balance between the contribution of local organizations and citizens and of the various external actors involved in delivering the project; it is also a challenge to adhere to and maintain a nondeficit orientation (Halpern, 1990).[4] It is believed that citizen participation will foster or reinforce a sense of community within the participating neighborhood, which in turn will increase its stability and viability (Prestby, Wandersman, Florin, Rich, & Chavis, 1990). In a similar project conducted in Ontario (Better Beginnings, Better Futures Prevention Project; see Pancer & Cameron, 1994) it is reported that in addition to the development of a sense of community, citizen's involvement enhanced self-confidence and self-esteem of the participants, helped them to establish social contacts, gave them some respite from worries about their children, helped them to get closer to services and institutions, and assisted them in improving their skills and in finding jobs. Participants also felt they had improved their parental image.

   1,2,3 GO! has also been inspired by a community systems model (Shields, 1993). The emphasis is both on environmental and service enhancement, as, for example, there is a strong commitment to sustain any community efforts aimed at improving local life conditions for children and parents and at improving the existing network of health, social, and educational services. Communities are also specifically invited to consider both social and economic dimensions in their Action Plan. This is of course easier said than done, but there are some signs that at least in two neighborhoods economic agents have been challenged to join the participants. The rethinking of existing resources is under way in at least two communities, which also represents a characteristic of a community system approach. For example, *1,2,3 GO!* has created tight relationships with a perinatal project and with a local Healthy City organization in an effort to create a more synergetic organizational environment. Finally, there is also a strong commitment to transfer whatever practical and theoretical learning is acquired during this experiment to policy people. This is one of the mandates of the research team.

1,2,3 GO! UNDER (PARTICIPATIVE) EVALUATION

During the first year of operation, the research team has completed a study aimed at defining the overall research design to be applied during the next 5 years. The team has elected to borrow from a participative-research approach (Fetterman, Kaftarian, & Wandersman, 1995; Guba & Lincoln, 1990). Interviews have been conducted with the promoters of the project, with the members of the program committee, and with the permanent staff members. Focus groups have been held with members of the local steering committees so as to identify the main research concerns to be attended to in the research design. From this exercise the team has conceived a research plan that utilizes both qualitative anthropological methods (Yin, 1994) and quantitative methods. At the organizational level, each community has created an Evaluation Task Group that is in continuous interaction with a research coordination body. This interactive approach will be maintained in all phases of the research. In terms of content, the research will document processes of implementation and impacts of the project both at the community development level (e.g., mobilization, collaboration, reaching out, organization, and individual empowerment) and at the child development level (e.g., parent social integration, parental attitudes and competencies, parental self-efficacy, changes in community settings, policy and services, and changes in children's intellectual, emotional, and social dimensions).

The research team is going to face several challenges in the next few years, not the least of which being the recruitment of researchers capable of accepting the lengthy and sometimes thorny interactions with parents and local organizers in a participatory study. Another problem regards the choice and utilization of child and family impact measures that will have to be sensitive enough to small behavior changes and should be tuned to a promotional approach rather than a deficit approach. A final worry is worth unveiling here: through community-level impacts are already notice-able and will probably be easier to document, the same is certainly not true concerning the child- and family-level changes. It remains to be demon-strated that a community-based approach borrowing from a health promo-tion perspective and from an empowerment perspective will generate enough intensive and specific interventions sufficient to trigger significant changes in the social and psychological status of children (Stagner & Duran, 1997). Many factors could hinder such changes, including the ex-treme residential mobility of poor families, the turnover among members of the Local Steering Committees, the lack of continuity and intensity in the proposed activities, and the lack of training and support for local leaders and practitioners.

CONCLUSION

In very many ways the epistemological foundations of *1,2,3 GO!* refer to the notion of a learning society (Chapters 12 and 13, this volume) or of a knowledge-building environment (Chapter 14, this volume). This experi-mental project asks for collaborative learning, for sharing the available in-formation, for allowing improvements through trial and errors, for chal-lenging the unknown, for meshing the expertise with (perhaps) a more candid or experiential community-based knowledge. Theoretically, at least, it relies more on exploration than on confirmation, more on knowledge de-velopment than on knowledge prescription. In its research component, it borrows heavily from a participatory approach (Green et al., 1995) whereby the various actors of the project contribute to the nature and la-beling of the questions and are given opportunities to learn from the re-search process and outcomes. In this perspective, the evaluation of the pro-ject is designed so as to feed the communities with information capable of improving their approaches, their actions, and their knowledge. This is ex-plicitly acknowledged as a priority (not exclusive though) over contributing to the development of objective or scientific knowledge and, as such, it il-lustrates the inescapable tension between a societal participatory approach and a more objectivist expert approach in both the action and research di-mensions.

NOTES

1. The McConnell Family Foundation has offered seed money to *1,2,3 GO!* in order to help the research team in the planning of the research design.
2. This notion of competence is central, but its representation and its expression may vary in time and space.
3. Special attention has been given to secure the presence of members of the various cultural groups from the very beginning of the project. In one multicultural community this was found to be an almost impossible task, the tensions being quite high between some of the groups. The project still stands on very shaky grounds partly because of this problem. In other communities, the presence of parents from low-income families in an otherwise homogeneous consortium has turned out to be a very constructive and productive asset in establishing the project.
4. People in the communities may show some ambivalence toward relying on expertise, on the one hand, and the desire to master their own agenda, on the other. Avoiding an inclination to foster a sense of dependency on the staff program may represent quite a challenge in some of the communities, as it is also hard for some professionals to refrain from pushing their own agenda, a theme developed further in Chapter 17 of this volume.

17

"It Takes a Village . . . ," *and New Roads to Get There*

Alan R. Pence

Using the analogy of a journey, this chapter describes the author's experiences in working with several aboriginal communities in developing and implementing a unique approach to postsecondary education in early childhood care and development. Those experiences, spanning 10 years and involving seven different tribal organizations, provide an inclusionary model of community participation in the training process that reinforces community responsibility for and involvement in the well-being of children, families, and communities.

The approach described complements community development and educational efforts described in other chapters in this volume, linking them through an interactive process of knowledge generation at the community level. Such inclusionary educational practices are deemed essential if community-sensitive services are to be realized. The processes and understandings of the Aboriginal Generative Curriculum projects share certain similarities with postmodernist movements in philosophy, education, and child development. Characteristics of those movements, and the common ground they share with the generative curriculum approach, will be briefly considered in the concluding section.

DESCRIPTION OF THE INITIAL PROJECT

An Invitation to Participate

> It will be the children who inherit the struggle to retain
> and enhance the peoples' culture, language and history;

who continue the quest for economic progress for a
better quality of life; and who move forward with a
strengthened resolve to plan their own destiny.
— MEADOW LAKE TRIBAL COUNCIL (1989)

Although a central activity of this project concerns postsecondary education, its origins are not in a university or college but in a northern Canada Tribal Council composed of nine First Nations communities.[1] Following the creation of the Tribal Council in the early 1980s, it pursued a variety of economic initiatives. Some of these succeeded and some floundered, but through the process the Council came to the position that "if we wanted to develop economically, we first had to develop our human resources" (V. Bachiu, personal communication at Meadow Lake, Saskatchewan, 1989).

In 1988 the Council recognized, through a recently announced federal child care research and development fund, the opportunity to pursue a key facet of its human resources development agenda: "a child care program developed, administered and operated by [our] own people is a vital contribution to [our] vision of sustainable growth and development" (Meadow Lake Tribal Council, 1989). In order to meet the objectives, the Council needed to establish a relationship with a postsecondary institution that would support the nine communities' vision for their children.

The Council's search led to inquiries to a number of colleges and universities in several provinces. The response from the selected institutions was that they did indeed have an aboriginal child care training program, and they sent along a copy of the curriculum materials. As these curricula were reviewed, the following question was posed: "What of us—our people and our communities—is in here?" In virtually all cases, there was no information specific to their communities. There might be some information about Cree peoples or Dene, but there could be bits of Mohawk, Haida, or Micmac as well. The Council members continued their search for a curriculum that would reflect "themselves": their communities, their values, their ways of being in the world, as well as other peoples' perspectives on the world.

One of the places the Council contacted was my office at the School of Child and Youth Care, University of Victoria, British Columbia. In contrast to some of their other contacts, my response to the query was that we did not have an Aboriginal Child and Youth Care Program, nor did I believe we had the internal expertise to create one. Nevertheless, Ray Ahenakew, the Council's Executive Director, wanted to talk further and we set up a meeting for a couple of weeks later when he would be on the west coast.

I entered the meeting bereft of aboriginally specific materials. Executive Director Ahenakew immediately took control of the discussion—spelling out the role he wished me and the University of Victoria to play, describing the needs analysis work that had been undertaken within the communities over the previous 5 years, and evidencing an extraordinarily high commitment to child, youth, and family issues within the constituent communities of the Tribal Council. Clearly, I was not in the driver's seat in this meeting, nor was I being asked to take the wheel at any point in the proposed future. I was to be a passenger, albeit an invited one and one he and the Council felt was critical to the journey they envisioned. The case the director put forward was compelling, and his personal energy was sincere and powerful—I had little idea where these travels would take us nor how we would get there, but the spirit was right and the trip promised to be fascinating!

> In reflecting back on these very early stages of work that would ultimately continue for more than 10 years (as of this writing) and subsequently move to include five other aboriginal projects, I realize that elements that I would come to consider as key in undertaking such initiatives were present from the beginning:
>
> 1. The initiative and the vision for the project was the community's.
> 2. The personal chemistry between the proposed partners was strong and respectful.
> 3. Being "empty handed" but "open minded" can be an advantageous starting point.

Guidance Systems

> I remember it so clearly, even though it happened back in 1988. MLTC [Meadow Lakes Tribal Council] Executive Director Ray Ahenakew told us to dream the best possible child care program we could imagine. And so we did.
> —MARY ROSE OPEKOKEW, Child Care Program Director in 1988

The proposal to the Canadian federal government was approved for a 3-year period, commencing September 1990. During that 3-year period the Council and the School of Child and Youth Care (hereafter, for brevity, the University) were committed to a partnership that would see the development, delivery, and evolution of a 2-year, university-level program in early childhood care and development (ECCD). If the model was successful, the founders wished to see it applied in other parts of the country as well. Clearly, to meet this "portability" expectation the model would need to be highly process oriented, providing an "open architecture" capable of incorporating different cultures' and communities' inputs. Other realities also had to be considered in the construction of the new approach: early child-hood licensing accreditation and university academic accountability, to name but two. Given the 1,500-kilometer separation between the Council and the University, even meetings posed significant planning and logistical challenges. The partnership was able to coordinate two major planning meetings in the fall of 1990, and out of those emerged agreement regarding a set of guiding principles for the project. These principles represented the shared vision of the partners—"stars" that would guide us in the absence of a map.

The principles included the following:

- A commitment to maintaining community initiative and involve-ment
- A commitment to principles of empowerment
- A respect for *all* cultural beliefs and values
- An understanding of the child in an ecological context
- Providing a base for a broad scope of training and services for chil-dren and families
- Creation of an education and career ladder for participants

In many respects the principles were in opposition to established educa-tional and professional practices. But the failure in so many cases of those established practices to meet the needs of aboriginal children, families, and communities provided the liberation required to "dream the best possible" and to pursue it through the partnership. In short, we had little to lose and much to gain.

> As we moved to operationalize the partnership a number of additional elements emerged as important in undertaking such projects:
>
> 4. The need for a thorough sharing and discussion of partners' and stakeholders' perspectives and visions.
> 5. The need for consensus on a shared set of principles and objectives.
> 6. The need to respect the autonomy, the knowledge, and the capability of one's fellow travelers, that is, to contribute but not dominate.

Curriculum as Process

> It helps when you ask Elders. . . . Older women are the ones you should ask for advice on how you can help people in your work. It's good that you are taking this course, you will go back and work with your people.

You have to go home to work with your people,
otherwise you will lose your culture.
                    —HARRY BLACKBIRD, Elder, Makwa Sahgaiehcan
                    Address to students

If the views, beliefs, and values of the Council communities were to enter into this curriculum, it could not come through the University. Even if the University were able to receive the information, it could not pass it on appropriately as the message is more than content: it concerns *how* information is presented as much as *what* that information is. The Council identified that the bearers and transmitters of their communities' knowledge were the Elders. The structure of the curriculum would need to provide the opportunity for the Elders' teachings, often in Cree in Dene, to be an integral part of the program.

Louis Opikokew was appointed by the Council as the Elder Coordinator for the project. Louis came to his position from a long history of work in Native Alcohol and Drug Treatment Programs for adults. In his own words, he was skeptical about the child care program, its priority for the communities, and what role he could play:

"To tell you the truth, at first I didn't believe in the child care program. But once I saw what they were doing, it really opened my eyes. . . . [I am] pleased that the program gave the Elders a chance to share their knowledge with a younger generation. The students, for their part, recognizing special wisdom of the Elders, began to consult them on personal as well as course related matters."

The words of the Elders, presented weekly to the students and following traditional protocol, represented one key facet of what the project team came to call the Generative Curriculum Model (GCM). Another key feature might be termed the "Words of the West"—the traditional texts and theories of Euro–Western thought. Both perspectives were treated with respect, consistent with the Council's desire that the students would be able to "walk [and work] in both worlds."

As the curriculum project evolved, the traditional Western educational emphasis on content was supplemented with an equal emphasis on application. Knowledge, without an understanding of how such information can be used and applied, is incomplete. Through the context of community, ever present through physical location as well as direct input from Elders and other community members, the praxis of knowledge and action was, to a large extent, achieved.

As the Generative Curriculum evolved it looked less and less like established, Western, postsecondary education practice. While the partners had been busy on the inside of the vehicle addressing issues and problems as they emerged, the route the car was on had left familiar roads and entered new territory.

Key lessons from this period included the following:

7. Partnerships require putting the other first.
8. Focus on what *you* know and bring to the partnership—do not attempt to become the "expert" in your partner's domain.
9. Bring the world outside into the classroom and the classroom out into the world.
10. Come to understand curriculum and knowledge as living, evolving processes.

First Evaluations: Searching for Curriculum and Finding Community

> We must carefully consider the impact on not only our children today, but seven generations from today.
> —DEBBIE I. JETTE, Elder and Evaluator (1993a, p. 2)

Two and a half years into the 3-year project, evaluations of both the curriculum aspect of the project and the community services component of the project were organized. The curriculum evaluation component employed a coordinator who, in addition to interviewing students and instructors, submitted an overview of the project and several individual courses to specific Canadian-based specialists: a cross-cultural ECCD educator, an aboriginal ECCD educator, an early childhood curriculum writer, and a professional editor. In addition, two eminent cross-cultural education specialists were contracted to review the overall curriculum approach. Comments from all six evaluators were consistently positive. The two overview reviewers commented as follows:

Dr. Kofi Marfo, Ghanaian-born specialist in ECCD:

"I have found the MLTC/SCYC [the School of Child and Youth Care] project to be one of the most innovative and well conceptualized approaches to addressing the educational and personnel preparation needs of cultural minority communities I have come across. The curriculum model acknowledges the limits of the knowledge base the principal investigators bring to the project, while appropriately respecting and honoring the tremendous contributions that elders, students, and community members at large can make to the program." (in Cook, 1993)

Dr. Roland Tharp, winner of the Grawemeyer Award for "significant original ideas with the potential for worldwide impact and improvement" for his work with Hawaiian educators and children:

> "The placing of Elders at the origin of each unit, and the recursive reconcili-
> ation of the Native with the Professional concepts, are both philosophically
> and technically an outstanding exemplar of educational empowerment."
> (in Cook, 1993)

The evaluation comments of Dr. Marfo, Dr. Tharp, and the four other
culture, content, and format reviewers provided strong confirmation of the
process followed and the quality of the materials produced. However, the
evaluation that had the most significant impact on me personally, as a key
participant in the journey initiated 5 years earlier, were the comments of
the First Nations' Elder from Ottawa who evaluated the community aspects of the Project. Through her eyes I became aware that our travels had
truly taken us to a different place—a place called community:

> "The most significant outcome of the Indian Child Care program is the re-
> newed interest and impact of the Elders in the life of the communities. As
> one Elder stated, 'The Elders are the messengers and now play a big role in
> the MLTC. We are an information line, a bridge.' . . . " (Jette, 1993b,
> p. 44).

In reading Jette's evaluation report I began to appreciate that through involving and respecting the participation of "community" in the curriculum
not only is student development enhanced but so too can be the community's development. The Elders and other respected community members
who participated in the Generative Curriculum, and there were more than
40, became participatory conduits between the classroom experience and
the community experience, and they themselves, as participants in both
worlds, became part of the transformational process. Other words that
Jette recorded from the community are like ripples and cross-ripples on a
pond:

> "Elders were a big part of the Indian Child Care Program, coming in on a
> weekly basis. This has carried over into other aspects of life and there has
> been a resurgence of Elder involvement."

> "Elders are once again a respected and needed part of society."

> "Students . . . began to consult them [Elders] on personal as well as course-
> related matters."

> "Before, kids were left out of everything. But now they are coming back.
> This is like it was before." (Jette, 1993b, p. 45)

The evaluation of the community aspects of the Council
project represented a turning point in my understanding of
the GCM. The curriculum evaluation provided confirmation

that our *intended* objectives had been achieved; however, the community evaluation indicated that very significant *unintended* outcomes had also been realized. At that point my understanding of our activities was transformed from "curriculum development work" to "community development." In that context, the tool of postsecondary education took on new significance. However, in order for postsecondary education to be effective as a community development tool, considerable reshaping must take place.

11. Elements of the reshaped tool, as constructed in the GCM, include the following:

- Bringing community into the classroom and the classroom into the community.
- Respecting diverse knowledge bases and seeking to understand their sources.
- Emphasizing the *process* of learning, rather than the imparting of information.
- Understanding all participants as learners and all as teachers.

These were elements of the tool that had been created. But before we could more fully understand its properties, we need to pilot the tool in other communities and understand its impact there as well.

SUBSEQUENT PROJECTS

There is no doubt that the [GCM] program addresses issues long obscured by the historically ineffectual attempts of mainstream postsecondary institutions to address the needs of First Nations students. The question now becomes not "should the program continue?" but "what can be done to make it better?"
—A. KEMBLE, Coastal Project Evaluator (1994, p. 2)

The Coastal Project

The evaluation of the original project provided strong confirmation of the value of the approach in the Council communities, but could the model be successfully employed in other environments? The original funding had been predicated on that "portability." The opportunity to test the approach in a very different cultural environment, the Coast Salish people of the Canadian west coast, came in September 1993.

The Coastal Project represented a three-way partnership consisting of the University, the Coastal Council, and a local college program. While in the original project the University had been asked to assume responsibility for both development and delivery, in the Coastal Project the local college would deliver the curriculum under the guidance of the University, and both would work in partnership with the Coastal Council.

The Coastal Project also had many twists and turns on the way to completion, but evaluations conducted at two different points during the program echoed many of the findings from the original project, and similar "ripple impacts" were noted by the Coastal Project evaluator (Riggan & Kemble, 1994).

Midway through the project, one student noted, "This program has a different feeling and atmosphere from mainstream programs." At the conclusion of the full 2 years of the program, another student noted, "I really wish the third and fourth years were Coast-Salish based. This was a great experience for me." A third student commented, "As a native program it has greatly impacted on my need to pursue my native heritage in a more aggressive manner. . . . It has made a difference in my work with native youth."

A nonnative instructor commented on how the experience of listening to the Elders present each week had led her to question her own relationships with "Elders" within her own family and resolve to change that relationship. And perhaps most significant was the impact on the college system itself. College administrators, at the conclusion of the Coastal Project, spoke about how the Elder coordinator approach, with strong involvement by local Elders, had been adopted by other, sometimes long-standing aboriginal programs they operated. The evaluator noted, "The involvement of the Elders has now become pervasive. . . . The profile of First Nations people on campus has changed. The demographics of students, staff and faculty positions has shifted to more accurately reflect the representation of native people . . . " She concluded her second evaluation with this statement: "The CYCL [Child and Youth Care Laddering] program has already made a major impact. The students who have been a part of it will never be the same, nor will the community in which they live" (Kemble, 1995, p. 20).

Additional Communities

A third and fourth community initiated the Generative Curriculum in 1995 and 1996. Again, each of these communities represented different tribal organizations great distances from the first two communities. While no formal evaluations have yet been conducted at either of these sites, informal observation, as well as instructor and student feedback, suggests both strong "internal" (student and class) impact and significant ripple impact externally. Funds have recently been received (in 1998) to undertake an evaluation across the seven sites that either have utilized or are utilizing the GCM.

> The subsequent GCM projects provide support for the adaptability of a process-driven approach to postsecondary education. Other learning from the subsequent projects included the following:
>
> 12. The importance of a very close liaison and mutual feeling of respect among the partners.
> 13. Elder participation is a critical component that should be present from the outset.
> 14. Unanticipated impacts remain a significant element in each project.

Reflections on Experiences with the General Curriculum Model

The preceding case study of the GCM complements and extends this volume's conceptual framework on human development. As will be discussed in the following section, there is a growing awareness throughout North America that if we are to be effective in our promotion of developmental health we must also be supportive of family and community well-being. Doing "more, better" while pursuing a paradigm of "doing to" rather than "doing with" is not the answer.

Community-focused interventions, such as those currently being undertaken in the province of Québec by Camil Bouchard and his colleagues (see Chapter 16, this volume), share a similar conceptual and theoretical base with the First Nations' GCM projects. As with Bouchard, the ecological work of Urie Bronfenbrenner (1979) and his colleagues at Cornell played a major role in the conceptualization of the original Council project. Indeed, the initial definition of "empowerment" utilized in the GCM came from Cochran, Allen, Barr, Dean, and Greene (1989–1992) with the Cornell Empowerment Project. Also, following in part from Bronfenbrenner's early work but also building on a strong tradition within anthropology, has been the work of individuals such as Super and Harkness (1986) and Weisner and colleagues (see Weisner, 1984). The sensitivity of these researchers to "eco-cultural niches" provided important direction to the project in its early period.

While published work on "the learning society" was not a part of the late 1980s early 1990s conceptualization of the GCM, the definition employed by Rohlen (Chapter 13, this volume) resonates with the work of the GCM within First Nations communities: "In a learning society, the goal is continuous learning, leading to improved knowledge and problem solving. . . . Innovation involves creating new knowledge, learning to utilize knowledge to solve problems, and diffusing such solutions in the population." What is critical in the learning society and in GCM First Nations communities is respectful and broad *inclusion* in solving common problems through unique and innovative approaches (see Moss & Pence, 1994).

As noted by Scardamalia and Bereiter (Chapter 14, this volume), "The idea of students as participants, along with teachers and perhaps others, in a collaborative enterprise has been around at least since John Dewey"; nevertheless, the examples of this collaborative approach employed at a community level remain relatively few and far between. Scardamalia and Bereiter's "collaborative knowledge building," while an essential characteristic of the GCM, is relatively rare within the education and professionalization practices of child and family service professionals. Insofar as it is these individuals who are expected to play a major role in including "community" in the well-being equation, the next section will turn to the question of "community" in the provision of child and family services and obstacles on the way to reaching "the village."

ARRIVING AT COMMUNITY: FEATURES OF AN IDEASCAPE

> "It takes a village to raise a child."
> —Generally credited as an African proverb, this quotation is pervasive in 1990s North American society and is the title of a 1996 book by U.S. First Lady Hillary Rodham Clinton. A nice sound byte, but can we get there from here?

The earlier description of Generative Curriculum projects has implications far beyond the several First Nations discussed. At a time when the words quoted above—"It takes a village . . . "—have taken on a mantralike quality across much of North America, we must seriously question if our services to children and families can get "there" from "here." I rather doubt they can—at least not without a fundamental shift in our understanding and in the practices of social services training and professionalization. Both practices mitigate against working with and through communities. What is required for such a shift to take place is not a romanticized return to *Gemeinschaft* or a pining for a "world we have lost," but an active and respectful engagement in cooperative planning with the communities of which we are a part today. By that I mean we must learn to "do with," not "do to," those with whom we live. Professionals and experts must be prepared to be knowledgeable, supportive, and involved coparticipants engaged with communities as listeners as well as speakers, followers as well as leaders. As coparticipants, professionals must become comfortable with the indeterminancy and power sharing that coconstruction requires.

The training for and provision of social services in North America still follows an academic and professional heritage based on principles of immutable "Truth" and restricted access to that Truth. The traditions of the Enlightenment and of logical positivism are but more recent manifestations of an understanding of "knowledge," "truth," and "authority" that have deep roots in Western society, including not only political but religious institutions as well. Certainly not limited to Western society, the essence of such structures is that knowledge is a scarce and specific commodity—a few people have it in "sufficient" quality and quantity, and many do not. Within such a conceptualization of knowledge, exclusionary, as opposed to inclusionary, principles and priorities apply. Both tertiary educational systems and our professionalization practices are exclusionary in nature, whereas the road to "the village" is necessarily inclusionary. Indeed, we cannot get "there" from "here," at least not on the roads we currently travel.

Yet, ironically, while the tenets of professionalism still promote the need for "professional autonomy, self regulation, a specific formal education, and a clientele which recognizes the authority of the profession" (Kelly, 1990, p. 168), the social science bedrock upon which such restrictive and exclusionary principles were based has crumbled. "The epistemology of logical positivism has proven to be untenable. The firm conviction that the world was simply 'out there' waiting to be discovered and described has been exposed as a convenient fiction" (Schwandt, 1996, p. 58). The aftershocks of this Cartesian collapse still reverberate throughout the worlds of science and social science, while in the *social services* these events are often misinterpreted as part of a revolutionary toppling of one power system, opening the way for its replacement by some faction of those formerly dispossessed (a familiar cycle in history). Untransformed in this social services' "revolution" is the core principle that "right answers" do exist—they are just the property of the formerly disenfranchised, who now hold power as the wheel of history turns. Such cycles are not what the GCM is about; it is not the specter of radical relativism wherein "anything goes" and "experts" can be dismissed. The terms "expert" and "professional" must, however, be problematized and their modernist roots exposed and reconstructed in collaboration with those impacted by their practice.

The condition of "Cartesian anxiety" (Bernstein, 1983), created by the collapse of "objective knowledge," is considered resoluble through what Schwandt (1996) calls "practical philosophy," the practice of which is complementary to that described above in the Generative Curriculum process:

> "First, inquirers seek to establish a dialogical relationship of openness with participants in the inquiry. . . .
>
> "Second, inquirers view the participants in the inquiry as themselves engaged in performing a practical art. . . .

"Third, the aim of such inquiry is not to replace practitioners' commonsense knowledge of their respective and joint practices with allegedly more sophisticated, theoretical, scientific knowledge but to encourage practitioners to critically reflect on and reappraise their commonsense knowledge. . . .

"Finally, . . . we retain the Enlightenment insight regarding the importance of self-clarity . . . but we seek to adopt a better or more critically defensible notion of what this entails. . . . " (Schwandt, 1996, pp. 63–64)

A more "practical" approach to understanding and generating community appropriate knowledge has begun to evolve in some areas of child and family related social sciences, although such literature continues to represent a minority of published work.

One such area of research that has been slow to achieve major recognition, despite a fairly long history of activity, is cross-cultural psychology. Through the increasingly prominent work of Majority World[2] child developmentalists, including Kagitcibasi (1996), Nsamenang (1992), and Sinha (1983), to name but three, the degree to which Western perspectives and beliefs of universal patterns of development have dominated our understandings, despite evidence to the contrary, is becoming increasingly apparent. Jahoda and Dasen (1986) deplored the fact that "theories and findings in developmental psychology originating in the First World tend to be disseminated to the Third World as gospel truth" (p. 413). The recent movement of cultural psychology from the periphery of interest to a more central position of recognition in the world of child development can be seen as supportive of efforts, such as the GCM, to respectfully copresent indigenous beliefs and values regarding children and their development alongside Minority World beliefs with the intent of achieving a practical understanding through a dialogical process.

Recent work in early childhood care and development is also moving to redefine the "limits of universals" in understanding quality caregiving. Working separately, but arriving at a similar position, are recent publications by Woodhead (1996) and Moss and Pence (1994). Woodhead argues that quality is "contextual," while Moss and Pence argue that a definition of "quality" must be arrived at through an inclusionary process. Both publications run counter to the present majority of ECCD publications addressing "quality care" that tend to adopt a prescriptive approach. Indeed, most of the publications considered to have relevant features for the community ideascape considered in this chapter were "counter" documents at the time of their publication.

A significant pioneer for those working in both cross-cultural child development and alternative perspectives on early childhood care and development is Urie Bronfenbrenner. Bronfenbrenner's 1970s work, in establishing an ecologically sensitive approach to understanding children's development, has provided personal, professional and scientific support for those who shared his frustration with the "science of the strange behavior of children in strange situations with strange adults for the briefest possible periods of time" (1979, p. 19). Both the recent work in reconceptualizing quality early childhood care and the efforts cited to further appreciate the importance of culture in human development owe a great deal to Bronfenbrenner and "the giants upon whose shoulders we stand" (1979, p. xi). Fruition of the work of those giants in creating a more contextually sensitive understanding of child development may at long last be at hand. As Elder, Modell, and Parke (1993) note, "Science's grip on the discipline of psychology has prevented quite the rout of positivism occurring in philosophy and history, but we see a weakening at the edges" (p. 193).

Such a "weakening at the edges" can be seen as a precondition for communities to engage in meaningful dialogue with "experts." If "Truth" is singular and universal, then dissemination, not dialogue, is the way forward. But dissemination has been tried and for many, like the aboriginal peoples of North America, has been found wanting. These communities, and I believe many others, can very legitimately ask, "What of us is in here?" If we, as "experts," are not prepared to engage in dialogue about that point, to learn as well as to profess, then effective community services for children and families will remain beyond rather than within our grasp (Dahlberg, Moss, & Pence, 1999).

CONCLUDING COMMENTS

> As the twentieth century draws to a close, there is little question that we are living through more than the chronological end of an epoch. . . . Time is imbued with symbolic meaning, it is caught in the throes of forces of which we only have a dim understanding at the present. The many "post-isms," like post-humanism, post-structuralism, post-modernism, post-Fordism, post-Keynesianism, and post-histoire, circulating in our intellectual and cultural lives are at one level only expressions of a deeply shared sense that certain aspects of our social, symbolic and political universe have been profoundly and most likely irretrievably transformed.
> —SEYLA BENHABIB (1992, p. 1)

The First Nations of Canada have long lived in a social, symbolic, and political universe that has been profoundly transformed. The quest of certain of these communities to "find their way" in the context of a world that is vastly different than what they have known in the past may provide direction and insight for others. These communities' understanding that old and new must find ways to coexist, each to respectfully inform and learn from the other, may provide a model for development in uncertain times. The road to healthier communities for those First Nations described in this chapter has, by and large, been a commitment to the well-being of their children. Children may represent the accessible "common ground" upon which families, communities, and child developmentalists can support each other in creating a better, stronger, healthier future. It may be that the basis upon which we can realize that "it takes a village to raise a child" is an appreciation that perhaps "it takes a child to raise a village."

NOTES

1. First Nations is a term preferred by many North American Indian communities in Canada. While it has a technical definition, it also serves as a reminder to the "two founding peoples of Canada" (the English and the French) that the First Nations were here before either arrived.
2. The terms "Majority World," instead of Third World or Developing Countries, and "Minority World," instead of First World or Developed Countries, are used in this chapter both to highlight the significant population difference between the minority who live in "Developed Countries" and the significant majority who live in "Developing Countries," and to avoid the Western biases inherent in the terms "developed" and "First."

18

Developmental Health as the Wealth of Nations

Daniel P. Keating

W e began this tour of key issues in contemporary human development with two major claims. The first was that the physical and mental health, well-being, coping, and competence of human populations—which we have termed developmental health—arise in large part as a function of the over-all quality of the social environment, and that the developmental health of populations can be accurately indexed by examining the steepness of its so-cioeconomic gradients. The second major claim was that the origins of these differences can be largely, though not wholly, attributed to the effects of early developmental experiences as they serve to sculpt various aspects of biological function and structure, especially in the neural, neuroen-docrine, and neuroimmune systems. We described this general set of pro-cesses with the term "biological embedding."

We provided evidence for these two claims in Parts I and II of this vol-ume. Additional research is needed, and is under way, to establish more strongly this link between the developmental health of populations and the quality of the environment that shapes the early development of individu-als. But if we rely on the best available evidence, it now seems prudent to examine our social structures and practices with the understanding that this link is well grounded. The urgency of this examination is heightened when we recognize that the investments we make now—or fail to make—will have large and persistent downstream effects on the developmental health of human populations and on the quality of the social environment they will be capable of sustaining.

We proposed in Parts III and IV that a productive societal examination should focus on two key features. The first is the broad capacity of societies to provide the essential supports for developmental health by drawing on existing resources—material, cultural, and social—to generate new approaches under shifting circumstances. This capacity for societal adaptation is particularly crucial during periods of rapid social and technological change, such as the dramatic transformations we currently experience on a global scale. The second key feature is the capacity of communities within societies to take up these challenges effectively, through creative organization of the everyday social practices that touch directly on human development.

We have described these linked elements of societal adaptability as characteristic of a learning society. We have staked a claim that conscious attention to the building of a learning society, which has as a principal goal the fostering of developmental health, is a key to future societal success. This claim arises from coordinated consideration of the four core dynamics of human development we have identified: the developmental health of populations; the biological embedding of early experiences that contribute to individual developmental health; the nature of human social organization, which structures the ways in which supports for developmental health are maintained, renewed, and distributed; and the specific processes of community, family, and other social networks that shape the circumstances within which human development actually transpires.

If one accepts that these dynamics are interconnected in approximately the way we have outlined, additional questions quickly arise regarding the implications of this framework for human development. We can consider two broad sets of implications: for societal functioning and for economic prosperity, which can be taken together to constitute a revised notion of the "wealth of nations."

SOCIETAL ADAPTABILITY

The implications for society are straightforward and arise directly from the interplay of the four core dynamics. Highly adaptable societies will likely be characterized by populations with high levels of developmental health (as we have defined the term to include physical and mental health, competence, and the ability to cope with stress and novelty), which is in turn a function of the society's ability to provide core supports for individual development. A society's flexible use of its resources for this task is substantially driven by its "social software" that creates both opportunities and constraints for learning (e.g., *opportunities* that stem from the value placed on human development; or *opportunities* and *constraints* produced, respectively, by collaborative versus antagonistic social approaches to addressing problems of human development). For a society to adapt effectively, of course, this social software needs to be applied to the contexts in which development is actually shaped—in the family, in the community, in schools, and later in workplaces and the larger society. A learning society can be defined as one that commits to understanding and then acting on these core dynamics of human development.

From our review of the core dynamics of human development, we can draw some general lessons for a learning society:

- The key necessities for supporting healthy child development can be relatively easily identified: income, nutrition, child care, stimulation, love/support, advocacy, and safety.
- Given what we know, our societies have underinvested in development between conception and school age, compared to what we invest thereafter. In fact, our institutional arrangements are (unconsciously) based on the presumption that early development is the least important, not the most.
- Improving the quality of human development requires paying attention to all levels of social aggregation: family, neighborhood, school, civil society, and the national socioeconomic environment.
- Collecting ongoing evidence of systematic variation in cognitive and behavioral development across communities and understanding its determinants is crucial for positive social change.

The litany of ways that Americans, Canadians, and some other modern societies have *not* attended consciously to the developmental needs of children and youth is a familiar one. There has been a net wealth transfer toward older individuals from younger families who are more likely to have young children. Demographic and labor market changes have placed substantial strains on such families, making the organization of stable, high-quality child care a challenge. The mobility of families has also increased, so that extended family supports are less readily available. Community coherence appears to be declining, reducing the chances that communities will take up the slack when families are having difficulty. Increased income inequality raises the specter of steeper socioeconomic gradients, potentially undermining the overall developmental health of populations. These well-known trends undermine our ability to build supportive contexts for human development. Regardless of how strong or how reversible one believes these trends to be, it is clear that learning how to accommodate to these changes effectively is a key challenge for a learning society.

ECONOMIC PROSPERITY

Although the connection between developmental health and economic prosperity appears at first glance to be less direct, our argument is that these effects are equally strong. Many developmentalists view economic analysis of child development in terms of human resources as "dehumanizing," and many free marketeers do not see how human development fits into econometric equations. Consequently, we lack detailed analyses that establish the economic value of well-crafted investments in human development. But the role of human and intellectual capital in the innovation dynamic as it plays out in the current situation is likely to be large, perhaps even dominant.

Some attempts have been made to estimate the costs and benefits of child development investments, using econometric models. When we examine the costs of failing to provide supportive contexts for developmental health—in terms of reduced school performance, increased antisocial behavior, reduced subsequent work participation, and so forth—we see that they are substantial. Conversely, the savings down the road from early interventions that prevent these problems are also quite substantial. Investment in high-quality early child care on a population basis is likely to have a return in terms of such savings that is at least double the original investment (Cleveland & Krashinsky, 1998). If one focuses on the most disadvantaged sector of the population, this return on investment may be much higher, as much as U.S. $7.00 in savings for each dollar invested (Schweinhart et al., 1993).

There is another cost that is much harder to estimate econometrically: the cost to a society in terms of its future potential to be economically innovative and thus to grow its economy. Underinvestment in its human resources by failing to provide supportive contexts for human development, particularly for early child development, is likely to incur these "hidden costs" of lost opportunities for future economic growth. If the growing economies of the future rely heavily on human and intellectual capital, as many contemporary economic models suggest they will, then this underinvestment may represent a major, though largely hidden, cost to society— the cost of talent lost.

DEVELOPMENTAL HEALTH AS THE WEALTH OF NATIONS: INVESTMENT STRATEGIES

If we accept the central role of developmental health to societal adaptability and to economic prosperity—in combination, a more comprehensive definition of the "wealth of nations" for the Information Age—it makes sense to consider some principles that ought to guide our investments. As noted above, such an analysis is likely to make some developmentalists squeamish, owing to a fear that it dehumanizes children and youth and makes them into mere "exploitable economic resources."

But such squeamishness is inconsistent with the goals of a learning society on two grounds. First, developmental health is a desirable good, independent of what individuals choose to do or not to do in the economic sphere. Indeed, the possession of health, competence, and coping skills almost certainly reduces the prospects of exploitation, by increasing both opportunities and the awareness of choice. Second, the belief that as a society we should provide the supports for developmental health because it is the right thing to do, a moral obligation, has not been notably successful in raising societal awareness or commitment to the level of concerted action.

We need a robust understanding of human development dynamics as they operate in society to complement, and when necessary contend with, the understanding of market dynamics as they operate in the economy. That the social forces underlying developmental health may be as crucial to economic prosperity as are market forces is a potent and potentially valuable convergence. If developmental health and economic growth are fundamentally interdependent in the innovation dynamic that characterizes the Information Age, then it behooves learning societies to devise investment strategies that maximize this potential return. In Part III, we explored some general constraints and opportunities that impact on the building of learning societies, and in Part IV we considered several of many possible examples to illustrate some major issues that demand attention when societies are trying to move along this pathway.

The Learning Society as a Learning Organization

It has become commonplace among those who study effective enterprises to speak of learning organizations that have discovered how to create effective institutional memory, collaborative goal seeking, and continuous improvement. Note that all of these occur in a real sense at the group rather than the individual level. A learning society can be usefully regarded as a generalization of the learning organization. Among the themes most valuable to this generalization are that change is a continuous process, that it can be brought to conscious awareness in which goals are made explicit, that it involves the broader society and not just communities of experts, and that collaborative learning is crucial to effective societal adaptation.

The term "learning society" is, however, fraught with the potential for misinterpretations, which we have sought to clarify in our usage (see Part III for a more detailed discussion). Traditional psychological notions often viewed learning as a purely internal set of processes describing the adaptation of the individual to a relatively fixed external environment (the material "to be learned"). In our usage, learning is not restricted solely to the acquisition of knowledge or skill already attained by others (as in, say, an individual "learning to read" or a firm "diffusing its best practices") but also includes activities better described as collaborative knowledge building and innovation (see Scardamalia & Bereiter, Chapter 14, this volume). Similarly, society is viewed in this context not only as a collection of institutions and practices but also as a culturally integrated organization capable of adapting and learning from experience.

This introduces one further potential misconception, which is that collaborative efforts depend on uniformity of goals among the individual members of a group. From this misconception, it is easy to dismiss the notion of an effective learning organization (or learning society) merely by taking note of the prevalence of conflict and competition in human activity. From this view, the only route to effective collaborative learning or action is to impose uniformity from some central source.

The heart of this misconception is the view that competition and cooperation are exclusive states. It can be observed in many well-functioning complex systems that cooperation and competition are linked in a dynamic tension that is essential to the system's functioning. Neural competition at the level of cells and cooperation at the level of systems is one well-documented example from a different sphere. Indeed, an essential component of a learning organization or a learning society is the assurance that valuable information is not lost to the system due to internal conflict, and thus competing views need to be encouraged and heard.

A number of the principles noted below are specific features that fall under the rubric of a learning society. It would be helpful, of course, if we had blueprints or worked-out examples of functioning learning societies in an Information Age, but such is not the case. The most likely route to building learning societies is an iterative one: ask "What would a learning society do in this situation?"; invent or adapt the means to approach the goal; evaluate the outcomes; ask "How can we improve this process to get a better outcome?"; and so on. As in any continuous improvement scheme, the best way to become a learning society is to begin to act as a learning society would act, observe the results, and learn from them.

We conclude by identifying a number of key principles that a learning society would likely find useful for guiding investments in developmental health. But because complex dynamic systems do not generally follow a fixed blueprint, it is important to recognize that the most important principles are the ones that emerge through the practical task of trying to build a learning society.

Invest in the Core Infrastructure

Any enterprise, to be successful, must invest in the infrastructure that is essential to its survival and growth. Enterprises that ignore the building and maintenance of this core infrastructure court disaster in the long term. Given what we know about the resources that are needed to support developmental health in the population, we can readily identify much of the infrastructure that we either have or still need in order to provide those resources.

In many jurisdictions, the recent trend has unfortunately been to reduce investments in this infrastructure in favor of efforts to address deep concerns about fiscal deficits. The difficulty is that the negative effects of underinvestment in developmental health may not be apparent for some

time, which makes it hard to hold governments accountable for these policies within their normal lifespan. This is compounded by the fact that the
core constituency, children and youth, are not participants in the political
process. Devising ways to raise the profile of such investments is an important task for a learning society.

One version of this underinvestment is a current trend toward off-
loading of fiscal obligation through devolution of responsibilities to more
local levels of government without a commensurate transfer of resources to
support developmental health at the local level. This is particularly troublesome in that there are good reasons, as we have already noted (especially in
Part IV), to see the local, community level as an important arena for organizing developmental resources on behalf of children. But imagining that
communities can self-organize to deal with the manifold problems without
adequate resources borders on magical thinking.

In reality, we need not only to protect current investments but to increase them in key sectors. Protecting the investment is not as simple as
maintaining steady state funding for continuing programs. In many cases,
the program-based model has not been effective in actually providing the
necessary developmental resources, and locked-in funding therefore does
not address the actual goal. The resources to be protected and enhanced are
not only physical infrastructure and programs but also the human resources and expertise that represent a major social investment. Increasing
the case loads of child protection professionals, for example, to the point at
which the attrition rate goes up sharply is ultimately counterproductive.

Increasing the investment in developmental health is also necessary. In
particular, the dramatic underinvestment in early childhood reflects the fact
that we have not been adapting well to the changing demographic and labor market realities. This will likely require more than reallocation of social spending. On the one hand, most existing investments in developmental health are seen as essential, and decreasing these investments seems a
clear case of robbing Peter to pay Paul—besides being politically unpalat-
able for most governments. On the other hand, the deficit reduction strategies seem to have succeeded in most jurisdictions, which should generate a
surplus that should sensibly be addressed to key areas which have suffered
from underinvestment. The general point is that we need to move away
from a stance in which spending on developmental health is seen as a benefit to individuals rather than as the social investment in societal adaptability and economic prosperity that it so clearly is.

Network Available Resources and Ingenuity

In addition to better investments, we need a better model for using the resources we do have and for monitoring the outcomes of our efforts, so that
we can make the best use of whatever investments are available. One of the
hallmarks of learning organizations essential to a learning society is the

ability to network the available resources in order to maximize the benefits of our efforts. What we often discover, however, is that the coordination among public and private organizations which provide developmental resources is minimal or absent altogether. This has often been described as the "silo effect," in which each of the organizations—say, education, health, community and social services, juvenile justice, or the voluntary sector—is structured vertically, with a head office of some sort and a bureaucratic structure which ensures that members of the organization look toward the center for resources and for direction. This usually creates barriers to effective cooperation at the local level, where a given child or family confronts a byzantine array of services or activities that are almost impossible to comprehend, much less use effectively.

Again, because of the inherited structure of organizations, this is a difficult barrier to overcome. It is akin to the difficulties faced by enterprises where the marketing function is unconnected to the product development function. When there is little coordination among these functions, the overall success of the organization is diminished. What is required is better strategic thinking that encourages local networks among those who provide developmental resources, whether in the service delivery or the community development sectors.

It is also important to recognize that diverse approaches will be required, which reflect the different local circumstances for the provision of developmental resources. This is a planning process, not unlike community economic development, which entails the participation of many sectors and a realistic accounting of the assets and liabilities of the community with respect to promoting developmental health (see Bouchard, Chapter 16, this volume). Elements of this infrastructure already exist in some areas, but they are rarely inclusive enough to deal with the full range of activities needed to support developmental health. This planning and networking function is essential, because it is clear that there is no master plan which can be designed to fit all circumstances. Moreover, the active participation of the whole community in such activities is itself important in establishing community engagement in design and in monitoring the outcomes of the efforts. One of the most frequent difficulties is that even successful efforts are hard to sustain, because they rely upon a particular individual whose charismatic leadership drives the whole program. Grounding such efforts in the broader community is likely to be a key to long-term benefits.

Focus on the Core Dynamics

Increased investment, even if networked, may be insufficient to enhance developmental health if the investment is poorly targeted. We need look no further for an example than the enormous investments in correctional systems that yield little in the way of public safety or positive redirection of developmental pathways. Conceptually, there are two related ways to address the targeting function. The first is to understand the core dynamics of the system, so that any efforts have the best chance of success. The second is to monitor the outcomes of those efforts closely, so that they become a feedback loop for learning more about how the system functions.

As a starting point in such an analysis, we can identify some key guidelines on the core dynamics that arise from the framework on human development we have been working on:

• Timing is important. Due to critical and sensitive periods in development, directing specific resources in support of developmental health either too early or too late is likely to lead to disappointing results. Generally, the best opportunities occur at points of natural developmental transition—in the first few years of life, at school entry, at the transition to adolescence, and at the transition to adulthood. There is considerable evidence, as we have seen, that early development is the most critical phase and the least supported; investment strategies need to address this.

• Even the best-designed efforts sometimes have unintended negative consequences, and thus it is essential both to anticipate as many systemic consequences as possible and to monitor the progress of the efforts in order to detect problems early on. When problems are detected, it is valuable to figure out, if possible, what element of the system is awry. By changing a key link in the system, it may be possible to divert a vicious cycle into a virtuous one.

• Be alert to external changes that shift the equations. Neither the ways in which we work to support developmental health nor the contexts in which those efforts take place are static. In this sense, no program ever "solves" a problem in developmental health except temporarily. What this suggests is that we need to move away from an exclusive focus on effective programs or services and toward a more inclusive approach in which the focus is on the overall developmental health of the population.

• Invest in research and development on the best ways to achieve gains. Most modern enterprises recognize that R&D investments are essential for growth. The complexity of human development is such that a better grasp of its core dynamics is a long-term prospect, and our ability to achieve this is in part a function of our social commitment to understanding the system.

Monitor the Outcomes

One of the major drawbacks of many well-intentioned prevention or intervention programs is that their impact is not routinely evaluated or monitored and, when it is, the monitoring is often of the process or the assets that have been added, rather than actual developmental outcomes. This would be like an enterprise that monitors everything but its bottom line. In blunt terms, we need to learn how to keep score. This is not only in comparisons between similar communities but also in comparisons within communities across time. We should be routinely asking whether we are doing better this year than last year on reliable indicators of population developmental health, like children's readiness to learn as they enter school, or rates of antisocial behavior or delinquency.

This feedback loop is essential for learning to occur. Without it, we are effectively "flying blind." In other sectors, such as the economy or the environment, we expect to learn the outcomes of our efforts through routinely collected indicators. Such monitoring of developmental health has additional potential benefits when it is instituted on a routine basis. One important benefit is that it enables us to identify communities or regions which are doing particularly well, so that we can begin to specify and diffuse the best practices in support of developmental health that we have discovered.

A few years ago, the Canadian government launched a National Longitudinal Survey of Children and Youth whose goal is to provide the kind of knowledge that we need to have in order to monitor how well the Canadian population is doing by region in terms of a number of outcomes. It's not just for scientific purposes that we should want such information. Given the factors we have noted above, it becomes critically important that we monitor on a continuing basis how children and youth are faring. Not only do we introduce interventions and policies whose goal is to affect their development, but broader changes are happening in a dramatic way, and an uncontrolled way in many circumstances, including changes in demographics, labor markets, families, and communities. In a learning society, we need to monitor routinely the impact of both planned and unplanned changes on children and youth.

A PARTING THOUGHT

For those of us who have had the good fortune to participate in the conversations that launched this project, the experience has been remarkable. By virtue of how contemporary science is organized, each of us participates in numerous networks, both formal and informal, and their value is hard to overstate. The particular character of this network, which encouraged us to take on questions with much greater scope than we normally encounter within our scientific disciplines and to engage these questions with conscious attention to their potential social value, has afforded us a rare opportunity.

The veritable explosion of knowledge about human development, from biology to society, is one of the most exciting arenas of current scientific research. That this knowledge explosion is occurring simultaneously with major technological and social transformations is no coincidence. Sophisticated tools and techniques for investigation, the ability to accumulate and communicate vast amounts of information, and the natural experiments in social organization going on around the globe, all contribute to this growth of knowledge.

Beyond the intellectual excitement, however, is the hope that the new knowledge may create the opportunity for a new approach, one that recognizes developmental health as a central part of the equations for societal adaptability and economic prosperity. As we noted in Chapter 1, this volume, we see this as the beginning, rather than the end, of the conversation. We look forward to carrying this conversation forward, not only among ourselves but together with other groups and individuals who are working toward similar goals.

References

Abelson, W. D., Zigler, E., & DeBlasi, C. L. (1974). Effects of a four-year follow-through program on economically disadvantaged children. *Journal of Educational Psychology, 66,* 756–771.

Achenbach, T. M., Phares, V., & Howell, C. T. (1990). Seven-year outcome of the Vermont intervention program for low-birthweight infants. *Child Development, 61,* 1672–1681.

Adams, M. J. (1990). *Beginning to read: Thinking and learning about print.* Cambridge, MA: MIT Press.

Ader, R. (1981). *Psychoneuroimmunology.* New York: Academic Press.

Ader, R. (1983). Developmental psychoneuroimmunology. *Developmental Psychobiology, 16,* 251–267.

Ader, R., & Friedman, S. G. (1965). Social factors affecting emotionality and resistance to disease in animals: 5. Early separation from the mother and response to transplanted tumor in the rat. *Psychosomatic Medicine, 27,* 119–122.

Adler, N. E., Boyce, T., Chesney, M. A., Cohen, S., Folkman, S., Kahn, R. L., & Syme, S. L. (1994). Socioeconomic status and health: The challenge of the gradient. *American Psychologist, 49*(1), 15–24.

Adolphs, R., Tranel, D., Damasio, H., & Damasio, A. (1994). Impaired recognition of emotion in facial expressions following bilateral damage to the human amygdala. *Nature, 372,* 669–672.

Alexander, K. L., & Entwisle, D. R. (1988). Achievement in the first two years of school: Patterns and processes. *Monographs of the Society for Research in Child Development, 53*(2, Serial No. 218).

Alexander, K. L., Entwisle, D. R., & Horsey, C. S. (1997). From first grade forward: Early foundations of high school dropout. *Sociology of Education, 70*(2), 87–107.

Amato, P. R., & Keith, B. (1991). Parental divorce and adult well-being: A meta-analysis. *Journal of Marriage and the Family, 53,* 43–58.

Anderson, C. S. (1985). The investigation of school climate. In G. R. Austin & H. Garber (Eds.), *Research on exemplary schools* (pp. 97–126). Orlando, FL: Academic Press.

Andrews, S. R., Blumenthal, J. B., Johnson, D. L., Kuhn, A. J., Ferguson, C. J., Lasater, T. M., Malone, P. E., & Wallace, D. B. (1982). The skills of mothering: A study of parent–child development centres. *Monographs of the Society for Research in Child Development, 47*(6, Serial No. 198).

Annie E. Casey Foundation. (1995). *The path of most resistance: Reflections on lessons learned from new futures.* Internal report, 29 pps. Baltimore, MD.

Applebee, A. N. (1984). *Contexts for learning to write: Studies of secondary school instruction.* Norwood, NJ: Ablex.

Associated Press. (1994, October 19). Just like the Ninja Turtles: Networks cancel kids' program after Norwegian girl, 5, is stoned to death. *Montreal Gazette,* p. A14.

Atkinson, A. B., Rainwater, L., & Smeeding, T. M. (1995). *Income distribution in OECD countries: Evidence from the Luxembourg study.* Paris: Organization for Economic Cooperation & Development (OECD).

Axinn, W., Duncan, G., & Thornton, A. (1997). The effects of parental income, wealth and attitudes on children's completed schooling and self-esteem. In G. J. Duncan & J. Brooks-Gunn (Eds.), *Consequences of growing up poor* (pp. 518–540). New York: Russell Sage Foundation Press.

Bambridge, R. (1962). Early experience and sexual behavior in the domestic chicken. *Science, 136,* 259–260.

Barker, D. J. P. (1991). The intrauterine environment and adult cardiovascular disease. In G. R. Bock & J. Whelan (Eds.), *CIBA Foundation Symposium 156: The childhood environment and adult disease* (pp. 3–16). Chichester, UK: Wiley.

Barker, D. J. P. (Ed.). (1992). *Fetal and infant origins of adult disease.* London: British Medical Journal.

Barker, D. J. P. (1994). *Mothers, babies and disease in later life.* London: British Medical Journal.

Barker, D. J. P., Bull, A., Osmond, C., & Simmonds, S. (1990). Fetal and placental size and risk of hypertension in adult life. *British Medical Journal, 301,* 259–262.

Barker, D. J. P., Godfrey, K., Osmond, C., & Bull, A. (1992). The relation of fetal length, ponderal index and head circumference to blood pressure and the risk of hypertension in adult life. *Pediatric and Perinatal Epidemiology, 6,* 35–44.

Barker, D. J. P., & Martyn, C. (1992). The maternal and fetal origins of cardiovascular disease. *Journal of Epidemiology and Community Health, 46,* 8–11.

Barker, D. J. P., Meade, T., Fall, C., Lee, A., Osmond, C., Phipps, K., & Stirling, Y. (1992). Relation of fetal and infant growth to plasma fibrinogen and factor VII concentrations in adult life. *British Medical Journal, 304,* 148–152.

Barker, D. J. P., & Osmond, C. (1986, May 10). Infant mortality, childhood nutrition, and ischaemic heart disease in England and Wales. *Lancet, i,*1077–1081.

Barker, D. J. P., Osmond, C., Golding, J., Kuh, D., & Wadsworth, M. (1989). Growth in utero, blood pressure in childhood and adult life, and mortality from cardiovascular disease. *British Medical Journal, 298,* 564–567.

Barker, D. J. P., Osmond, C., Simmonds, S., & Wield, G. (1993). The relation of small head circumference and thinness at birth to death from cardiovascular disease in adult life. *British Medical Journal, 306,* 422–426.

Barker, D. J. P., Osmond, C., Winter, P., Margetts, B., & Simmonds, S. (1989, September 9). Weight in infancy and death from ischaemic heart disease. *Lancet, ii,* 577–580.

Barnett, W. S. (1995). Long-term effects of early childhood programs on cognitive and social outcomes. *The Future of Children, 5*(3), 25–50.

Barocas, R., Seifer, R., Sameroff, A., Andrews, T., Croft, R., & Ostrow, E. (1991). Social and interpersonal determinants of developmental risk. *Developmental Psychology, 27*(3), 479–488.

Baron, S. W. (1995). Serious offenders. In J. H. Creechan & R. A. Silverman (Eds.), *Canadian delinquency* (pp. 135–147). Scarborough, Ontario, Canada: Prentice Hall.

Bartrop, R. W., Luckhurst, E., Lazarus, L., Kiloh, L. G., & Penny, R. (1977). Depressed lymphocyte function after bereavement. *Lancet, i,* 834–836.

Baumrin, M. (1975, April). Aristotle's empirical nativism. *American Psychologist,* pp. 486–494.

Baydar, N., Brooks-Gunn, J., & Furstenberg, F. F., Jr. (1993). Early warning signs of functional illiteracy: Predictors in childhood and adolescence. *Child Development, 64*(3), 815–829.

Becker, G. (1964). *Human capital.* New York: Columbia University Press.

Becker, G. S. (1991). *A treatise on the family* (2nd ed.). Cambridge, MA: Harvard University Press.

Belsky, J. (1981). Early human experience: A family perspective. *Developmental Psychology, 17*(1), 3–23.

Belsky, J., & Rovine, M. (1987). Temperament and attachment security in the strange situation: An empirical rapprochement. *Child Development, 58,* 787–795.

Benhabib, S. (1992). *Situating the self.* London: Routledge.

Benschop, R. J., Rodriguez-Feurhahn, M., & Schedlowski, M. (1996). Catecholamine-induced leukocytosis: Early observations, current research and future directions. *Brain, Behavior and Immunity, 10,* 77–91.

Berard, J. (1989). Male life histories. *Puerto Rico Health Sciences Journal, 8,* 4758.

Bereiter, C. (1992). Referent-centered and problem-centered knowledge: Elements of an educational epistemology. *Interchange, 24*(4), 337–361.

Bereiter, C., & Engleman, S. (1966). *Teaching the disadvantaged in the preschool.* Englewood Cliffs, NJ: Prentice-Hall.

Bereiter, C., & Scardamalia, M. (1987). *The psychology of written composition.* Hillsdale, NJ: Erlbaum.

Bereiter, C., & Scardamalia, M. (1989). Intentional learning as a goal of instruction. In L. B. Resnick (Ed.), *Knowing, learning, and instruction: Essays in honor of Robert Glaser* (pp. 361–392). Hillsdale, NJ: Erlbaum.

Bereiter, C., & Scardamalia, M. (1992). Two models of classroom learning using a communal database. In S. Dijkstra (Ed.), *Instructional models in computer-based learning environments* (NATO–ASI Series F: Computer and Systems Sciences, pp. 229–241). Berlin: Springer-Verlag.

Bereiter, C., & Scardamalia, M. (1996). Rethinking learning. In D. R. Olson & N. Torrance (Eds.), *Handbook of education and human development: New models of learning, teaching and schooling* (pp. 485–513). Cambridge, MA: Blackwell.

Bereiter, C., Scardamalia, M., Cassells, C., & Hewitt, J. (1997). Postmodernism, knowledge-building, and elementary science. *Elementary School Journal, 97*(4), 329–340.

Berlin, L. J., Brooks-Gunn, J., Spiker, D., & Zaslow, M. J. (1995). Examining observational measures of emotional support and cognitive stimulation in black and white mothers of preschoolers. *Journal of Family Issues, 16*(5), 664–686.

Berman, C. M., Rasmussen, K. L. R., & Suomi, S. J. (1994). Responses of free-ranging rhesus monkeys to a natural form of social separation: 1. Parallels with mother–infant separation in captivity. *Child Development, 65,* 1028–1041.

Berman, C. M., Rasmussen, K. L. R., & Suomi, S. J. (1997). Group size, infant development, and social networks: A natural experiment with free-ranging rhesus monkeys. *Animal Behavior, 53,* 405–421.

Bernstein, R. J. (1983). *Beyond objectivism and relativism*. Philadelphia: University of Pennsylvania Press.

Bielby, W. T. (1981). Models of status attainment. *Research in Social Stratification and Mobility, 1,* 3–26.

Björkqvist, K., Österman, K., & Kaukiainen, A. (1992). The development of direct and indirect aggressive strategies in males and females. In K. Björkqvist & P. Niemelä (Eds.), *Of mice and woman: Aspects of female aggression* (pp. 51–64). Toronto: Academic Press.

Blakemore, C., & Cooper, G. F. (1970). Development of the brain depends on the visual environment. *Nature, 228,* 477–478.

Blank, R. (1993). Why were poverty rates so high in the 1980s? In D. B. Papadimitriou & E. N. Wolff (Eds.), *Poverty and prosperity in the USA in the late twentieth century.* London: Macmillan.

Blank, R., & Card, D. (1993). Poverty, income distribution and growth: Are they still connected? *Brookings Papers on Economic Activity, 2,* 285–339.

Blumenfeld, P. C., Soloway, E., Marx, R. W., Krajcik, J. S., Guzdial, M., & Palincsar, A. (1991). Motivating project-based learning: Sustaining the doing, supporting the learning. *Educational Psychologist, 26,* 369–398.

Bock, R. D., & Mislevy, R. J. (1988). Comprehensive educational assessment for the states: The duplex design. *Educational Evaluation and Policy Analysis, 10*(2), 89–105.

Booth, C. (1889). *Life and labour of the people.* London: Williams & Norgate.

Borjas, G. J. (1995). Ethnicity, neighborhoods, and human-capital externalities. *American Economic Review, 85*(3), 365–390.

Bornstein, M., & Sigman, M. (1986). Continuity in mental development from infancy. *Child Development, 57,* 251–274.

Bowlby, J. (1960). Grief and mourning in infancy and early childhood. *Psychoanalytic Study of the Child, 15,* 9–52.

Bowlby, J. (1969). *Attachment.* New York: Basic Books.

Bowlby, J. (1973). *Separation: Anger and anxiety.* New York: Basic Books.

Boyce, W. T., Jensen, E. W., Cassel, J. C., Collier, A. M., Smith, A. N., & Ramey, C. T. (1977). Influence of life events and family routines and childhood respiratory tract illness. *Pediatrics, 60,* 609–615.

Boysen, S. T., & Berntson, G. G. (1989). Numerical competence in a chimpanzee. *Journal of Comparative Psychology, 103,* 23–31.

Boysen, S. T., & Berntson, G. G. (1995). Responses to quantity: Perceptual versus cognitive mechanisms in chimpanzees. *Journal of Experimental Psychology: Animal behavior processes, 21,* 23–31.

Boysen, S. T., Berntson, G. G., Shayer, T. A., & Hannan, M. B. (1995). Indicating acts during counting by a chimpanzee. *Journal of Comparative Psychology, 109,* 47–51.

Bradley, L., & Bryant, P. (1985). Rhyme and reason in reading and spelling. *International Academy for Research in Learning Disabilities Monograph, 1,* Ann Arbor, MI.

Bradley, R. (1989). HOME measurement of maternal responsiveness. *New Directions for Child Development, 43,* 63–74.

Bradley, R. H. (1995). Home environment and parenting. In M. Bornstein (Ed.), *Handbook of parenting* (pp. 235–262). Hillsdale, NJ: Erlbaum.

Bradley, R. H., Caldwell, B., & Rock, S. (1988). Home environment and school performance: A ten-year follow-up and examination of three models of environmental action. *Child Development, 59*(4), 852–867.

Bradley, R. H., Caldwell, B. M., Rock, S. L., Ramey, C. T., Barnard, K. E., Gray, C., Hammond, M. A., Mitchell, S., Gottfried, A. W., Sigel, L., & Johnson, D. L. (1989). Home environment and cognitive development in the first three years of life: A collaborative study including six sites and three ethnic groups in North America. *Developmental Psychology, 25,* 217–235.

Brazelton, T. B., & Yogman, M. W. (1986). Introduction. In T. B. Brazelton & M. W. Yogman (Eds.), *Affective development in infancy.* Norwood, NJ: Ablex.

Britton, M., Fox, A. J., Goldblatt, P., Jones, D. R., & Rosato, M. (1990). The influence of socio-economic and environmental factors on geographic variations in mortality in OPCS. *Mortality and geography.* London: Her Majesty's Stationery Office.

Bromwick, R. M., & Parmelee, A. H. (1979). An intervention program for pre-term infants. In T. M. Field, A. M. Sostek, S. Goldberg, & H. H. Shuman (Eds.), *Infants born at risk: Behavior and development* (pp. 389–411). New York: SP Medical & Scientific Books.

Bronfenbrenner, U. (1969). *Statement at hearings before the Committee on Ways and Means, House of Representatives,* 91st Congress. Washington, DC: U.S. Government Printing Office.

Bronfenbrenner, U. (1979). *The ecology of human development: Experiments by nature and design.* Cambridge, MA: Harvard University Press.

Bronfenbrenner, U., McClelland, P., Wethington, E., Moen, P., & Ceci, S. J. (1996). *The state of Americans: This generation and the next.* New York: Free Press.

Brookover, W. B., Schweitzer, J. H., Schneider, J. M., Beady, C. H., Flood, P. K., & Wisenbaker, J. M. (1978). Elementary school social climate and school achievement. *American Educational Research Journal, 15*(2), 301–318.

Brooks-Gunn, J. (1995). Children and families in communities: Risk and intervention in the Bronfenbrenner tradition. In P. Moen, G. H. Elder, & K. Lüsher (Eds.), *Examining lives in context: Perspective on the ecology of human development* (pp. 467–519). Washington, DC: American Psychological Association.

Brooks-Gunn, J., Britto, P. R., & Brady, C. (1998). Struggling to make ends meet: Poverty and child development. In M. E. Lamb (Ed.), *Parenting and child development in "nontraditional" families* (pp. 279–304). Mahwah, NJ: Erlbaum.

Brooks-Gunn, J., Brown, B., Duncan, G. J., & Moore, K. A. (1995). Child development in the context of family and community resources: An agenda for national data collection. In National Research Council Institute of Medicine, *Integrating federal statistics on children: Report of a workshop* (pp. 27–97). Washington, DC: National Academy Press.

Brooks-Gunn, J., Denner, J., & Klebanov, P. K. (1995). Families and neighborhoods as contexts for education. In E. Flaxman & A. H. Passow (Eds.), *Changing populations, changing schools: Ninety-fourth Yearbook of the National Society for the Study of Education, Part II* (pp. 233–252). Chicago: National Society for the Study of Education.

Brooks-Gunn, J., & Duncan, G. J. (1997). The effects of poverty on children. *The Future of Children, 7*(2), 55–71.

Brooks-Gunn, J., Duncan, G., & Aber, J. L. (1997). *Neighborhood poverty: Context and consequences in children.* New York: Russell Sage Foundation Press.

Brooks-Gunn, J., Guo, G., & Furstenberg, F. F., Jr. (1993). Who drops out of and who continues beyond high school?: A 20-year follow-up of black urban youth. *Journal of Research on Adolescence, 3*(3), 271–294.

Brooks-Gunn, J., Klebanov, P. K., & Duncan, G. (1996). Ethnic differences in children's intelligence test scores: Role of economic deprivation, home environment, and maternal characteristics. *Child Development, 67,* 396–408.

Brooks-Gunn, J., Klebanov, P. K., & Liaw, F. (1994). The learning, physical and emotional environment in the home in the context of poverty: The Infant Health and Development Program. *Children and Youth Services Review, 17*(1/2), 251–276.

Brooks-Gunn, J., Klebanov, P. K., Liaw, F., & Duncan, G. J. (1995). Toward an understanding of the effects of poverty upon children. In H. E. Fitzgerald, B. M. Lester, & B. Zuckerman (Eds.), *Children of poverty: Research, health, and policy issues* (pp. 3–41). New York: Garland Press.

Brooks-Gunn, J., Klebanov, P. K., Liaw, F., & Spiker, D. (1993). Enhancing the development of low birth weight premature infants: Changes in cognition and behavior over the first three years. *Child Development, 64*(3), 736–753.

Brooks-Gunn, J., Liaw, F., & Klebanov, P. K. (1992). Effects of early intervention on low birth weight preterm infants: What aspects of cognitive functioning are enhanced? *Journal of Pediatrics, 120,* 350–359.

Brooks-Gunn, J., McCarton, C., Casey, P., McCormick, M., Bauer, C., Bernbaum, J., Tyson, J., Swanson, M., Bennett, F., Scott, D., Tonascia, J., & Meinert, C. (1994). Early intervention in low birth weight premature infants: Results through age 5 years from the Infant Health and Development Program. *Journal of the American Medical Association, 272*(16), 1257–1262.

Brooks-Gunn, J., Phelps, E., & Elder, G. H. (1991). Studying lives through time: Secondary data analyses in developmental psychology. *Developmental Psychology, 27*(6), 899–910.

Brown, A. L., & Campione, J. C. (1990). Communities of learning and thinking, or a context by any other name. *Contributions to Human Development, 21,* 108–126.

Brown, A. L., & Campione, J. C. (1994). Guided discovery in a community of learners. In K. McGilly (Ed.), *Classroom lessons: Integrating cognitive theory and classroom practice* (pp. 229–270). Cambridge, MA: MIT Press/Bradford Books.

Brown, J. S., & Duguid, P. (1991). Organizational learning and communities of practice: Toward a unified theory of working, learning, and innovation. *Organizational Science, 2,* 40–57.

Brunjes, P. C. (1994). Unilateral naris closure and olfactory system development. *Brain Research Reviews, 19,* 146–160.

Brusegard, D. (1979). Rethinking national social reports. *Social Indicators Research, 6,* 261–272.

Bryk, A. S., Lee, V. E., & Smith, J. B. (1990). High school organization and its effects on teachers and students: An interpretative summary of the research. In W. H. Clune & J. F. Witte (Eds.), *Choice and control in American education: Vol. 1. The theory of choice and control in education.* London: Falmer Press.

Bryk, A. S., & Raudenbush, S. W. (1992). *Hierarchical linear models for social and behavioral research: Applications and data analysis methods.* Newbury Park, CA: Sage.

Bumpass, L. (1984). Children and marital disruption: A replication and update. *Demography, 21,* 71–82.

Butler, N. R., & Bonham, D. G. (1963). *Perinatal mortality.* Edinburgh: Livingstone.

Cairns, R. B., & Cairns, B. D. (1986). The developmental interactional view of social behavior: Four issues of adolescent aggression. In D. Olweus, J. Black, & M. Radke-Yarrow (Eds.), *Development of antisocial behavior* (pp. 315–342). New York: Academic Press.

Cairns, R. B., & Cairns, B. D. (1994). *Life lines and risks: Pathways of youth in our time.* New York: Cambridge University Press.

Cairns, R. B., Cairns, B. D., Neckerman, H. J., Ferguson, L. L., & Gariépy, J. L. (1989). Growth and aggression: 1. Childhood to early adolescence. *Developmental Psychology, 25,* 320–330.

Campbell, F. A., & Ramey, C. T. (1994). Effects of early intervention on intellectual and academic achievement: A follow-up study of children from low-income families. *Child Development, 65,* 684–698.

Campos, J. J. (1994, Spring). The new functionalism in emotion. *SRCD Newsletter,* pp. 1, 9–14.

Campos, J. J., Mumme, D., Kermoian, R., & Campos, R. (1994). A functionalist perspective on the nature of emotion. *Monographs of the Society for Research in Child Development, 59*(2/3, Serial No. 240), 284–303.

Camras, L. A. (1992). Expressive development and basic emotions. *Cognition and Emotion, 6,* 269–283.

Carley, M. (1981). *Social measurement and social indicators: Issues of policy and theory.* London: Allen & Unwin.

Carter, C. S. (1992). Oxytocin and sexual behavior. *Neuroscience and BioBehavioral Reviews, 16,* 131–144.

Case, R. (1992). *The mind's staircase: Exploring the conceptual underpinings of children's thought and knowledge.* Hillsdale, NJ: Erlbaum.

Case, R., & Griffin, S. (1991). *Rightstart: An early intervention program for insuring that children's first formal learning of arithmetic is grounded in their intuitive knowledge of numbers.* Report to the James S. McDonnell Foundation, St. Louis, MO.

Case, R., Okamoto, Y., Henderson, B., & McKeough, A. (1993). Individual variability and consistency in cognitive development: New evidence for the existence of central conceptual structures. In R. Case & W. Edelstein (Eds.), *The new structuralism in developmental theory and research: Analysis of individual developmental pathways.* Basel: Karger.

Case, R., & Sandieson, R. (1988). A developmental approach to the identification and teaching of central conceptual structures in middle school science and mathematics. In M. Behr & J. Hiebert (Eds.), *Research agenda in mathematics education: Number concepts and operations in the middle grades* (pp. 236–270). Hillsdale, NJ: Erlbaum.

Case, R., Stephenson, K. M., Bleiker, C., & Okamoto, Y. (1996). Central spatial structures and their development. In R. Case & Y. Okamoto (Eds.), The role of central conceptual structures in the development of children's thought. *Monographs of the Society for Research in Child Development, 61*(Serial No. 246), 83–102.

Cazden, C. B. (1986). Classroom discourse. In M. C. Wittrock (Ed.), *Handbook of research on teaching* (pp. 432–463). New York: Macmillan.

Ceci, S. (1990). *On intelligence . . . More or less.* Englewood Cliffs, NJ: Prentice Hall.

Chamberland, C., Bouchard, C., & Beaudry, J. (1986). Les mauvais traitements envers les enfants: Réalités canadienne et américaine. *Revue canadienne des sciences du comportement, 18,* 391–412.

Champoux, M., Byrne, E., Delizio, R., & Suomi, S. J. (1992). Rhesus maternal behavior and rearing history. *Primates, 33,* 251–255.

Chandra, R. K., & Newberne, P. M. (1977). *Nutrition, immunity and infection.* New York: Plenum.

Chase-Lansdale, L., Gordon, R., Brooks-Gunn, J., & Klebanov, P. K. (1997). Neighborhood and family influences on the intellectual and behavioral competence of preschool and early school-age children. In J. Brooks-Gunn, G. J. Duncan, & J. L. Aber (Eds.), *Neighborhood poverty: Context and consequences for children* (Vol. 1, pp. 79–118). New York: Russell Sage Foundation Press.

Chase-Lansdale, P. L., Mott, F. L., Brooks-Gunn, J., & Phillips, D. (1991). Children of the NLSY: A unique research opportunity. *Developmental Psychology, 27*(6), 918–931.

Cherlin, A. (1992). *Marriage, divorce, remarriage.* Cambridge, MA: Harvard University Press.

Cherlin, A. J., Furstenberg, F. F., Jr., Chase-Lansdale, P. L., Kiernan, K. E., Robins, P. K., Morrison, R., & Teitler, J. O. (1990). Longitudinal studies of effects of divorce on children in Great Britain and the United States. *Science, 252*(5011), 1386–1389.

Choquet, M. (1996). La violence des jeunes: Données épidémiologiques. In C. Rey (Ed.), *Les adolescents face à la violence* (pp. 51–63). Paris: Syros.

Cicchetti, D. (1989). How research on child maltreatment has informed the study of child development: Perspectives from developmental psychopathology. In D. Cicchetti & V. Carlson (Eds.), *Child maltreatment: Theory and research on the causes and consequences of child abuse and neglect* (pp. 377–432). New York: Cambridge University Press.

Cicchetti, D., Ackerman, B., & Izard, C. (1995). Emotions and emotion regulation in developmental psychopathology. *Development and Psychopathology, 7*(1), 1–10.

Cicchetti, D., Ganiban, J., & Barnett, D. (1991). Contributions from the study of high-risk populations to understanding the development of emotion regulation. In K. Dodge & J. Garber (Eds.), *The development of emotion regulation and dysregulation* (pp. 15–48). Cambridge, UK: Cambridge University Press.

Cicchetti, D., & Tucker, D. (1994). Development and self-regulatory structures of the mind. *Development and Psychopathology, 6*(4), 533–549.

Cicerelli, V. (1969). *The impact of Head Start: An evaluation of the effects of Head Start on children's cognitive and affective development.* Washington, DC: Westinghouse Learning Corporation.

Citro, C. F., & Michael, R. T. (Eds.). (1995). *Measuring poverty: A new approach.* Washington, DC: National Academy Press.

Clark, K. B., & Fujimoto, T. (1991). *Product development performance: Strategy, organization and management in the world auto industry.* Cambridge, MA: HBS Press.

Clark, T. N., & Lipset, S. M. (1991). Are social classes dying? *International Sociology, 6*(4), 397–410.

Cleveland, G., & Krashinsky, M. (1998). *The benefits and costs of good child care: The economic rationale for public investment in young children: A policy study.*

Toronto: University of Toronto, Centre for Urban and Community Studies, Childcare Resource and Research Unit.

Cochran, M., Allen, J., Barr, D., Dean, C., & Greene, J. (1989–1992). *Cornell Empowerment Project: Networking Bulletins.* Ithaca, NY: Cornell University.

Coe, C. L. (1993). Psychosocial factors and immunity in nonhuman primates: A review. *Psychosomatic Medicine, 55,* 298–308.

Coe, C. L., Ershler, W. B., Champoux, M., & Olson, J. (1992). Psychological factors and immune senescence in the aged primate. *Annals of the New York Academy of Sciences, 650,* 276–282.

Coe, C. L., Lubach, G. R., Ershler, W. B., & Klopp, R. G. (1989). Effect of early rearing on lymphocyte proliferation responses in rhesus monkeys. *Brain Behavior and Immunity, 3,* 47–60.

Coe, C. L., Lubach, G. R., Karaszewski, J., & Ershler, W. B. (1996). Prenatal endocrine activation influences the postnatal development of immunity in the infant monkey. *Brain, Behavior and Immunity, 10,* 221–234.

Cohen, S. (1988). Psychosocial models of the role of social support in the etiology of physical disease. *Health Psychology, 7*(3), 269–297.

Cohen, S., Tyrell, D. A. J., & Smith, A. P. (1991). Psychological stress in humans and susceptibility to the common cold. *New England Journal of Medicine, 325,* 606–612.

Cohen, S., & Williamson, G. (1991). Stress and infectious disease in humans. *Psychological Bulletin, 198,* 5–24.

Cole, R. (1989). *Strategies for learning: Small group activities in American, Japanese and Swedish industry.* Berkeley: University of California Press.

Coleman, J. S. (1988). Social capital in the creation of human capital. *American Journal of Sociology, 94*(Supplement), S95–S120.

Collins, A., Brown, J. S., & Newman, S. E. (1989). Cognitive apprenticeship: Teaching the crafts of reading, writing, and mathematics. In L. B. Resnick (Ed.), *Knowing, learning, and instruction: Essays in honor of Robert Glaser* (pp. 453–494). Hillsdale, NJ: Erlbaum.

Comer, J. P. (1980). *School power.* New York: Free Press.

Comer, J. P. (1988). Educating poor minority children. *Scientific American, 259*(5), 42–48.

Conger, R. D., Conger, K. J., & Elder, G. H. (1997). Family economic hardship and adolescent adjustment: Mediating and moderating processes. In G. J. Duncan & J. Brooks-Gunn (Eds.), *Consequences of growing up poor* (pp. 288–310). New York: Russell Sage Foundation Press.

Conger, R. D., Conger, K. J., Elder, G. H., Jr., Lorenz, F. O., Simons, R., & Whitbeck, L. B. (1992). A family process model of economic hardship and adjustment of early adolescent boys. *Child Development, 63,* 526–541.

Conger, R. D., Conger, K. J., Elder, G. H., Jr., Lorenz, F. O., Simons, R. L., & Whitbeck, L. B. (1993). A family process model of economic stress and adjustment of early adolescent girls. *Developmental Psychology, 29*(2), 206–219.

Conger, R. D., Ge, S., Elder, G. H., Jr., Lorenz, F. O., & Simons, R. L. (1994). Economic stress, coercive family process, and developmental problems of adolescents. *Child Development, 65,* 541–561.

Connell, J. P., Spencer, M. B., & Aber, J. L. (1994). Educational risk and resilience in African-American youth: Context, self, action, and outcomes in school. *Child Development, 65*(2), 493–506.

Cook, P. (1993). *Curriculum Evaluation of the MLTC/SCYC Career Ladder Project.* Unpublished manuscript, School of Child and Youth Care, University of Victoria, Victoria, British Columbia, Canada.

Coopersmith, S. (1967). *Antecedents of self-esteem.* San Francisco: Freeman.

Coulton, C. J. (1996). Effects of neighborhoods on families and children: Implications for services. In. A. J. Kahn & S. B. Kammerman (Eds.), *Children and their families in big cities: Strategies for service reform* (pp. 87–120). New York: Columbia University School of Social Work, Cross-National Studies Program.

Coulton, C. J., Korbin, J. E., Su, M., & Chow, J. (1995). Community level factors and child maltreatment rates. *Child Development, 66,* 1262–1276.

Courts, P. (1991). *Literacy and empowerment.* New York: Bergin & Garvey.

Crane, J. (1991). The epidemic theory of ghettos and neighborhood effects on dropping out and teenage childbearing. *American Journal of Sociology, 96*(5), 1226–1259.

Crary, B., Borysenko, M., Sutherland, C. D., Kutz, I., Borysenko, J. Z., & Benson, H. (1983). Decrease in mitogen responsiveness of mononuclear cells from peripheral blood after epinephrine administration in humans. *Journal of Immunology, 130,* 694–697.

Cummings, M., & Davies, P. (1996). Emotional security as a regulatory process in normal development and the development of psychopathology. *Development and Psychopathology, 8*(1), 123–139.

Currie, J. M. (1997). Choosing among alternative programs for poor children. *Futures of Children, 7*(2), 113–131.

Currie, J. M., & Thomas, D. (1994). *Does head start make a difference?* Unpublished manuscript. National Bureau of Economic Research, Palo Alto, CA.

Cutler, D. M., & Katz, L. F. (1991). Macroeconomic performances and the disadvantaged. *Brookings Papers on Economic Activity, 2,* 1–74.

Cynader, M., Berman, N., & Hein, A. (1976). Recovery of function in cat visual cortex following prolonged deprivation. *Experimental Brain Research, 25,* 139–156.

Cynader, M., Gardner, J., & Douglas, R. (1978). Neural mechanisms underlying stereoscopic depth perception in cat visual cortex. In S. Cool & I. E. L. Smith (Eds.), *Frontiers of visual science* (pp. 373–386). New York: Springer-Verlag.

Cynader, M., & Mitchell, D. E. (1980). Prolonged sensitivity to monocular deprivation in dark-reared cats. *Journal of Neurophysiology, 43,* 1026–1040.

Cynader, M. S., & Regan, D. (1978). Neurones in the cat parastriate cortex sensitive to the direction of motion in three dimensional space. *Journal of Physiology, 274,* 549–569.

Cynader, M. S. (1994). Mechanisms of brain development and their role in health and well-being. *Daedalus, 123,* 155–165.

Dahl, E. (1994). Social equalities in ill-health: The significance of occupational status, education and income results from a Norwegian survey. *Sociology of Health and Illness, 16,* 644–667.

Dahlberg, G., Moss, P., & Pence, A. R. (1999). *Beyond qualities in early childhood education and care: Postmodern perspectives.* London: Falmer Press.

Danziger, S., & Gottschalk, P. (1995). *America unequal.* Cambridge, MA: Harvard University Press.

Dar, Y., & Resh, N. (1986). Classroom intellectual composition and academic achievement. *American Educational Research Journal, 23,* 357–374.

D'Arcy, C. (1994). Education and socioeconomic status as risk factors for dementia: Data from the Canadian Study of Health and Aging. *Neurobiology of Aging, 14,* S40.

Davis, S., & Davidson, B. (1991). *2020 vision.* New York: Simon & Schuster.

DeCasper, A. J., & Fifer, W. P. (1980). Of human bonding: Newborns prefer their mothers' voices. *Science, 208*(4448), 1174–1176.

Dehaene, S., & Changeux, J. (1993). Development of elementary numerical abilities: A neuronal model. *Journal of Cognitive Neuroscience, 5,* 390–407.

Dehaene, S., & Cohen, L. (1995). Towards an anatomical and functional model of number processing. *Mathematical Cognition, 1,* 83–120.

Dennett, D. C. (1995). *Darwin's dangerous idea: Evolution and the meanings of life.* New York: Touchstone/Simon & Schuster.

Department of Clinical Epidemiology & Biostatistics, McMaster University Health Sciences Centre. (1984a). How to read clinical journals: 7. To understand an economic evaluation (Part A). *Canadian Medical Association Journal, 130,* 1428–1433.

Department of Clinical Epidemiology & Biostatistics, McMaster University Health Sciences Centre. (1984b). How to read clinical journals: 7. To understand an economic evaluation (Part B). *Canadian Medical Association Journal, 130,* 1542–1549.

Derryberry, D., & Reed, M. (1996). Regulatory processes and the development of cognitive representations. *Development and Psychopathology, 8*(1), 215–234.

Derryberry, D., & Rothbart, M. (1997). Reactive and effortful processes in the organization of temperament. *Development and Psychopathology, 9*(4), 633–652.

Dhabhar, F. S., Miller, A. H., McEwen, B. S., & Spencer, R. L. (1995). Effects of stress on immune cell distribution: Dynamics and hormonal mechanisms. *Journal of Immunology, 154,* 5511–5527.

Diamond, A. (1991). Frontal lobe involvement in cognitive changes during the first year of life. In K. Gibson, M. Konner, & A. Peterson. (Eds.), *Brain maturation and cognitive development: Comparative and cross-cultural perspectives. Foundations of human behavior* (pp. 127–180). New York: Aldine Press.

Diamond, M. C., Krech, D., & Rosenzweig, M. R. (1964). The effects of an enriched environment on the histology of the rat cerebral cortex. *Comparative Neurology, 123,* 111–119.

Dishion, T. J., & Andrews, D. W. (1995). Preventing escalation in problem behaviors with high-risk young adolescents. *Journal of Consulting and Clinical Psychology, 63,* 538–548.

Dittus, W. P. J. (1979). The evolution of behaviors regulating density and age specific sex ratios in a primate population. *Behavior, 69,* 265–302.

Divorces and Annulments Rates: United States, 1940–90. (1995, March). *Monthly Vital Statistics Report, 43*(9S).

Dobkin, P. L., Tremblay, R. E., Mâsse, L. C., & Vitaro, F. (1995). Individual and peer characteristics in predicting boys' early onset of substance abuse: A seven-year longitudinal study. *Child Development, 66,* 1198–1214.

Dodge, K. A. (1991). Emotion and social information processing. In J. Garber & K. A. Dodge (Eds.), *The development of emotional regulation and dysregulation.* (pp. 159–181). Cambridge: Cambridge University Press.

Donald, M. (1991). *Origins of the modern mind: Three stages in the evolution of culture and cognition.* Cambridge, MA: Harvard University Press.

Doornbos, G., & Kromhout, D. (1990). Educational level and mortality in a 32-year follow-up study of 18-year-old men in the Netherlands. *International Journal of Epidemiology, 19,* 374–379.

Doyle, W. (1983). Academic work. *Review of Educational Research, 53,* 159–199.

Dreeben, R., & Gamoran, A. (1986). Race, instruction, and learning. *American Sociological Review, 51,* 660–669.

Drucker, P. (1998, January–February). The coming of the new organization. *Harvard Business Review.*

Drucker, P. (1991, November–December). The new productivity challenge. *Harvard Business Review,* pp. 69–79.

Drucker, P. (1993). *Post-capitalist society.* New York: HarperCollins.

Drucker, P. (1994, November). The age of social transformation. *Atlantic Monthly,* pp. 53–80.

Dudley, L. (1991). *The word and the sword.* Cambridge, MA: Blackwell.

Dunbar, K. (1992). Why gossip is good for you. *New Scientist, 136,* 28–31.

Dunbar, K. (1993). How scientists really reason: Scientific reasoning in real-world laboratories. In R. J. Sternberg & J. Davidson (Eds.), *The nature of insight.* Cambridge, MA: MIT Press.

Duncan, G. J. (1988). Volatility of family income over the life course. In P. Baltes, D. Featherman, & R. Lerner (Eds.), *Life-span development and behavior* (pp. 317–358). Hillsdale, NJ: Erlbaum.

Duncan, G. J. (1991). The economic environment of children. In. A. C. Huston (Ed.), *Children in poverty: Child development and public policy* (pp. 23–50). New York: Cambridge University Press.

Duncan, G. J., & Brooks-Gunn, J. (Eds.). (1997a). *Consequences of growing up poor.* New York: Russell Sage Foundation Press.

Duncan, G. J., & Brooks-Gunn, J. (1997b). Income effects across the life span: Integration and interpretation. In G. J. Duncan & J. Brooks-Gunn (Eds.), *Consequences of growing up poor* (pp. 596–610). New York: Russell Sage Foundation Press.

Duncan, G. J., Brooks-Gunn, J., & Klebanov, P. K. (1994). Economic deprivation and early-childhood development. *Child Development, 65*(2), 296–318.

Duncan, G. J., & Hill, D. (1989). Assessing the quality of Household Panel Survey data: The case of PSID. *Journal of Business and Economic Statistics, 7*(4), 441–451.

Duncan, G. J., Yeung, W. J., Brooks-Gunn, J., & Smith, J. R. (1998). How much does childhood poverty affect the life chances of children? *American Sociological Review, 63,* 406–423.

Dunham, P., & Dunham, F. (1990). Effects of mother–infant social interactions on infants' subsequent contingency task performance. *Child Development, 61,* 785–793.

Dunn, A. J. (1989). Psychoneuroimmunology for the psychoneuroimmunologist: A review of animal studies of nervous system–immune system interactions. *Psychoneuroendocrinology, 14,* 251–274.

Dunn, J., & Munn, P. (1985). Becoming a family member: Family conflict and the development of social understanding in the second year. *Child Development, 56,* 480–492.

Echols, F. H., McPherson, A. F., & Willms, J. D. (1990). Parental choice in Scotland. *Journal of Education Policy, 5*(3), 207–222.

Echols, F. H., & Willms, J. D. (1995). Reasons for school choice in Scotland. *Journal of Education Policy, 10*(2), 143–156.

Economist Intelligence Unit. (1996). *The learning organization: Managing knowledge for business success.* Benton, NJ: Roland Offset Service.

Eisenberg, N., & Fabes, R. A. (1992). Emotion, regulation, and the development of social competence. In M. S. Clark (Ed.), *Emotion and social behavior* (pp. 119–150). Newbury Park, CA: Sage.

Eisenberg, N., Fabes, R. A., Bernzweig, J., Karbon, M., Poulin, R., & Hanish, L. (1993). The relation of emotionality and regulation to preschoolers' social skills and sociometric status. *Child Development, 64,* 1418–1438.

Eisenberg, N., Fabes, R. A., Murphy, B. C., Karbon, M., Smith, M., & Maszk, P. (1996). The relations of children's dispositional empathy-related responding to their emotionality, regulation, and social functioning. *Developmental Psychology, 32,* 195–209.

Eisenberg, N., Fabes, R., Nyman, M., Bernzweig, J., & Pinuelas, A. (1994). The relations of emotionality and regulation to children's anger-related reactions. *Child Development, 65,* 109–128.

Eisenberg, N., Fabes, R. A., Shepard, S. A., Murphy, B. C., Guthrie, I. K., Jones, S., Friedman, J., Poulin, R., & Maszk, P. (1997). Contemporaneous and longitudinal prediction of children's social functioning from regulation and emotionality. *Child Development, 68,* 642–664.

Elder, G. H. (1979). Historical change in life patterns and personality. In P. B. Baltes & O. G. Brim (Eds.), *Life-span development and behavior* (pp. 117–159). New York: Academic Press.

Elder, G. H., Modell, J., & Parke, R. D. (1993). *Children in time and place: Developmental and historical insights.* Cambridge, UK: Cambridge University Press.

Elliott, D. S. (1994). Serious violent offenders: Onset, developmental course and termination. (The American Society of Criminology 1993 presidential address). *Criminology, 32,* 1–21.

Elo, I. T., & Preston, S. H. (1996). Educational differentials in mortality: United States, 1979–85. *Social Science and Medicine, 42,* 47–57.

Entwisle, D. R., & Alexander, K. L. (1990). Beginning school math competence: Minority and majority comparisons. *Child Development, 61,* 457–471.

Ershler, W. B., Coe, C. L., Gravenstein, S., Klopp, R. G., Meyer, M., & Houser, W. D. (1988). Aging and immunity in nonhuman primates: 1. Effects of age and gender on cellular immune function in rhesus monkeys (*Macaca mulatta*). *American Journal of Primatology, 15,* 181–188.

Evans, D. A., Beckett, L. A., Albert, M. S., Hebert, L. E., Scherr, P. A., Funkenstein, H. H., & Taylor, J. O. (1993). Level of education and change in cognitive function in a community population of older persons. *Applied Educational Psychology, 3*(1), 71–77.

Evans, J. R. (1996, November). *Reconstructing the context for child development.* Paper presented at the Canadian Child Welfare Conference, Ottawa.

Farrington, D. P. (1977). The effects of public labelling. *British Journal of Criminology, 17,* 112–125.

Farrington, D. P. (1987). Early precursors of frequent offending. In J. Q. Wilson & G. C. Loury (Eds.), *From children to citizens: Vol. 3. Families, schools and delinquency prevention* (pp. 27–50). New York: Springer-Verlag.

Farrington, D. P. (1994). Childhood, adolescent, and adult features of violent males.

In L. R. Huesmann (Ed.), *Aggressive behavior: Current perspectives* (pp. 215–240). New York: Plenum.

Feinstein, A. (1985). *Clinical epidemiology: The architecture of clinical research*. Philadelphia: Saunders.

Feldman, J. J., Makuc, D. M., Kleinman, J. C., & Cornoni-Huntley, J. (1989). National trends in educational differentials in mortality. *American Journal of Epidemiology, 129,* 919–933.

Felleman, D. J., & Van Essen, D. C. (1991). Distributed hierarchical processing in the primate cerebral cortex. *Cerebral Cortex, 1*(1), 1–47.

Ferri, E. (1993). *Life at 33: The fifth follow-up of the National Child Development Study.* London: National Children's Bureau.

Fetterman, D. M., Kaftarian, S. J., & Wandersman, A. (1995). *Empowerment evaluation: Knowledge and tools for self-assessment and accountability.* Thousand Oaks, CA: Sage.

Fischer, K. W., & Rose, S. P. (1994). Dynamic development of coordination of components in brain and behavior: A framework for theory and research. In G. Dawson & K. W. Fischer (Eds.), *Human behavior and the developing brain* (pp. 3–66). New York: Guilford Press.

Florin, P., & Wandersman, A. (1990). An introduction to citizen participation, voluntary organizations, and community development: Insights for empowerment through research. *American Journal of Community Psychology, 18,* 41–54.

Forsdahl, A. (1977). Are poor living conditions in childhood and adolescence an important risk factor for arteriosclerotic heart disease? *British Journal of Preventive and Social Medicine, 31,* 91–95.

Fogel, A., & Thelen, E. (1987). The development of early expressive and communicative action: Re-interpreting the evidence from a dynamic systems perspective. *Developmental Psychology, 23,* 747–761.

Fox, N. (1994). The development of emotion regulation: Biological and behavioral considerations. *Monographs of the Society for Research in Child Development, 59*(2/3, Serial No. 240).

Fox, N. A., Schmidt, L. A., Calkins, S. D., Rubin, K. H., & Coplan, R. J. (1996). The role of frontal activation in the regulation and dysregulation of social behavior during the preschool years. *Development and Psychopathology, 8,* 89–102.

Frankel, K., & Bates, J. (1990). Mother–toddler problem solving: Antecedents in attachment, home behavior, and temperament. *Child Development, 61*(3), 810–819.

Fratiglioni, L., Jorm, A. F., Grut, M., Viitanen, M., Homen, K., Ahlbom, A., & Winblad, B. (1993). Predicting dementia from the mini-mental state examination in elderly population: The role of education. *Journal of Clinical Epidemiology, 46*(3), 281–287.

French–American Foundation. (1996, September 30–October 1). *Youth violence: A public health issue for the 21st century.* Paper presented at the Bi-national Symposium on Youth Violence, United Nations, New York.

Fuchs, V. R., & Reklis, D. (1977). Mathematical achievement in eighth grade. *Jobs and Capital, 6*(3), 27–29.

Furstenberg, F. F., Jr., Brooks-Gunn, J., & Morgan, S. P. (1987). *Adolescent mothers in later life.* New York: Cambridge University Press.

Fuson, K. C. (1982). An analysis of the counting-on solution procedure in addition. In T. P. Carpenter, J. M. Moser, & T. A. Romberg (Eds.), *Addition and subtraction: A cognitive perspective* (pp. 67–82). Hillsdale, NJ: Erlbaum.

Gamoran, A. (1991). Schooling and achievement: Additive versus interactive models. In S. W. Raudenbush & J. D. Willms (Eds.), *Schools, classrooms, and pupils: International studies of schooling from a multilevel perspective* (pp. 37–51). San Diego, CA: Academic Press.

Gamoran, A. (1992). The variable effects of high school tracking. *Sociology of Education, 57,* 812–828.

Gamoran, A., Mane, R. D., & Bethke, L. (1998). *Effects of non-maternal child care on inequality in cognitive skills.* Manuscript submitted for publication.

Garbarino, J. (1982). *Children and families in the social environment.* New York: Aldine.

Garbarino, J., & Kostelny, K. (1992). Child maltreatment as a community problem. *Child Abuse and Neglect, 16,* 455–464.

Garbarino, J., & Sherman, D. (1980). High-risk neighborhoods and high-risk families: The human ecology of child maltreatment. *Child Development, 51,* 188–198.

Garber, J., & Dodge, K. (Eds.). (1991). *The development of emotion regulation and dysregulation.* New York: Cambridge University Press.

Garber, H. L., & Heber, R. (1981). The efficacy of early intervention with family rehabilitation. In M. J. Begab, H. C. Haywood, & H. L. Garber (Eds.), *Psychosocial influences in retarded performance: Vol. 2. Strategies for improving competence* (pp. 71–88). Baltimore: University Park Press.

Gardner, H. (1985). *The mind's new science: A history of the cognitive revolution.* New York: Basic Books.

Gardner, R. A., & Gardner, B. T. (1984). A vocabulary test for chimpanzees (*Pan troglodytes*). *Journal of Comparative Psychology, 98,* 381–404.

Gelman, R. (1978). Counting in the preschooler: What does and what does not develop? In R. Siegler (Ed.), *Children's thinking: What develops?* (pp. 213–242). Hillsdale, NJ: Erlbaum.

Gennaro, S., Fehder, W., Nuamah, I. F., Campbell, D. E., & Douglas, S. D. (1997). Caregiving to very low birthweight infants: A model of stress and immune response. *Brain, Behavior, and Immunity, 11,* 201–205.

Gianino, A., & Tronick, E. Z. (1988). The mutual regulation model: Infant self and interactive regulation, coping and defense. In T. Field, P. McCade, & N. Schneiderman (Eds.), *Stress and coping* (pp. 47–68). Hillsdale, NJ: Erlbaum.

Gibson, K. R. (1990). Tool use, imitation, and deception in a captive cebus monkey. In S. T. Parker & K. R. Gibson (Eds.), *Language and intelligence in monkeys and apes: Comparative developmental perspectives.* New York: Cambridge University Press.

Ginsburg, H. P., Choi, E., Loez, L. S., Netley, R., & Chao-Yuan, C. (1992). *Happy birthday to you: The roles of nationality, ethnicity, social class and schooling in the early mathematical thinking of Asian, South American and U.S. children.* Unpublished manuscript, Columbia University.

Ginsburg, H. P., & Russell, R. L. (1981). Social class and racial influences on early mathematical thinking. *Monographs of the Society for Research in Child Development, 46*(Serial No. 193).

Glaser, R., Kennedy, S., Lafuse, W. P., Bonneau, R. H., Speicher, C., Hillhouse, J., & Kiecolt-Glaser, J. K. (1990). Psychological stress-induced modulation of interleukin 2 receptor gene expression and interleukin 2 production in peripheral blood leukocytes. *Archives of General Psychiatry, 47,* 707–712.

Glaser, R., Kiecolt-Glaser, J. K., Malarkey, W. B., & Sheridan, J. F. (1998). The influence of psychological stress on the immune response to vaccines. *Annals of the New York Academy of Sciences 840,* 649–655.

Glaser, R., Kiecolt-Glaser, J. K., Speicher, C. E., & Holliday, J. E. (1985). Stress, loneliness and changes in herpes virus latency. *Journal of Behavioral Medicine, 8,* 249–260.

Gliksman, M. D., Kawachi, I., Hunter, D., Colditz, G. A., Manson, J. E., Stampfer, M. J., Speizer, F. E., Willett, W. C., & Hennekens, C. H. (1995). Childhood socioeconomic status and risk of cardiovascular disease in middle aged U.S. women: A prospective study. *Journal of Epidemiology and Community Health, 49,* 10–15.

Goelman, H., & Pence, A. R. (1988). Children in three types of day care: Daily experiences, quality of care and developmental outcomes. *Early Child Development and Care, 33,* 66–76.

Goelman, H., & Pence, A. R. (1996). *Where are they now? A longitudinal follow-up study of the children from the Victoria daycare project.* Unpublished manuscript, University of British Columbia, Vancouver, Canada.

Goldstein, H. (1995). *Multilevel statistical models* (2nd ed.). New York: Halsted Press.

Goldstone, J. A. (1991). *Revolution and rebellion in the early modern world.* Berkeley: University of California Press.

Gordon, D. M., Edwards, R., & Reichet, M. (1982). *Segmented work, divided workers: The historical transformations of labor in the United States.* Cambridge, UK: Cambridge University Press.

Goren, C. C., Sarty, M., & Wu, P. Y. (1975). Visual following and pattern discrimination of face-like stimuli by newborn infants. *Pediatrics, 56*(4), 544–549.

Gottfredson, M. R., & Hirschi, T. A. (1990). *A general theory of crime.* Stanford, CA: Stanford University Press.

Gottfried, A. E., Gottfried, A. W., & Bathurst, K. (1995). Maternal and dual-earner employment status and parenting. In M. Bornstein (Ed.), *Handbook of parenting: Vol. 2. Biology and ecology of parenting* (pp. 139–160). Mahwah, NJ: Erlbaum.

Gottfried, A. W. (Ed.). (1984). *Home environment and early cognitive development.* New York: Academic Press.

Gottman, J., & Katz, L. (1989). Effects of marital discord on young children's peer interaction and health. *Developmental Psychology, 25*(3), 373–381.

Graber, J. A., & Brooks-Gunn, J. (1996). Transitions and turning points: Navigating the passage from childhood through adolescence. *Developmental Psychology, 32*(4), 768–776.

Graham, J. W., Beller, A. H., & Hernandez, P. M. (1994). The effect of child support on educational attainment. In I. Garfinkel, S. McLanahan, & P. Robins (Eds.), *Child support and child well-being* (pp. 317–346).Washington, DC: Urban Institute Press.

Grant, I., Brown, G. W., Harris, T., McDonald, W. I., Patterson, T., & Trimble, M. (1989). Severely threatening events and marked life difficulties preceding onset or exacerbation of multiple sclerosis. *Journal of Neurology, Neurosurgery and Psychiatry, 53,* 8–13.

Gray, J. (1989). Multilevel models: Issues and problems emerging from their recent application in British studies of school effectiveness. In D. R. Bock (Eds.), *Multi-*

level analyses of educational data (pp. 127–145). Chicago: University of Chicago Press.

Green, L. W., George, M. A., Daniel, M., Frankish, C. J., Herbert, C. J., Bowie, W. R., & O'Neil, M. (1995). *Study of participatory research in health promotion.* Institute of Health Promotion report for the Royal Society of Canada, the University of British Columbia, and the BC Consortium for Health Promotion Research, Vancouver, Canada.

Greene, W. A., & Miller, G. (1958). Psychological factors and reticuloendothelial disease IV. Observations on a group of children and adolescents with leukemias: An interpretation of disease development in terms of the mother–child unit. *Psychosomatic Medicine, 10,* 124–144.

Griffin, S. A., & Case, R. (1996). Evaluating the breadth and depth of training effects, when central conceptual structures are taught. In R. Case & Y. Okamoto (Eds.), The role of central conceptual structures in the development of children's thought. *Monographs of the Society for Research in Child Development, 61* (Serial No. 246), 83–102.

Griffin, S. A., & Case, R. (1997). Rethinking the primary school math curriculum: An approach based on cognitive science. *Issues in Education, 1*(3), 1–49.

Griffin, S. A., Case, R., & Sandieson, R. (1992). Synchrony and asynchrony in the acquisition of children's everyday mathematical knowledge. In R. Case (Ed.), *The mind's staircase: Exploring the conceptual underpinnings of children's thought and knowledge* (pp. 75–98). Hillsdale, NJ: Erlbaum.

Griffin, S. A., Case, R., & Siegler, R. S. (1994). Rightstart: Providing the central conceptual prerequisites for first formal learning of arithmetic to students at risk for school failure. In K. McGilly (Ed.), *Classroom lessons: Integrating cognitive theory and classroom practice* (pp. 1–50). Cambridge, MA: MIT Press/Bradford Books.

Guba, E. G., & Lincoln, Y. (1990). *Fourth generation evaluation.* Beverly Hills, CA, Sage.

Gunnar, M. R., Mangelsdorf, S., Kestenbaum, R., Lang, S., Larson, M., & Andreas, D. (1989). Temperament, attachment and neuroendocrine reactivity: A systemic approach to the study of stress in normal infants. In D. Cicchetti (Ed.), *Process and psychopathology* (pp. 119–138). Cambridge, UK: Cambridge University Press.

Guo, G., Brooks-Gunn, J., & Harris, K. M. (1996). Parental labor-force attachment and grade retention among urban black children. *Sociology of Education, 69,* 217–236.

Haan, M., Kaplan, G. A., & Camacho, T. (1987). Poverty and health: Prospective evidence from the Alameda County Study. *American Journal of Epidemiology, 125,* 989–997.

Haan, M. N., Kaplan, G. A., & Syme, S. L. (1989). Socioeconomic status and health: Old observations and new thoughts. In J. P. Bunker, D. S. Gomby, & B. H. Keher (Eds.), *Pathways to health* (pp. 76–135). Menlo Park, CA: The Henry J. Kaiser Family Foundation.

Haapasalo, J., & Tremblay, R. E. (1994). Physically aggressive boys from ages 6 to 12: Family background, parenting behavior, and prediction of delinquency. *Journal of Consulting Clinical Psychology, 62,* 1044–1052.

Hakkarainen, K. (1995, August). *Collaborative inquiry in the Computer-Supported Intentional Learning Environments (CSILE).* Poster presented at the biennial meeting of the European Association for Research in Learning and Instruction (EARLI), University of Nijmegen, The Netherlands.

Halpern, R. (1990). Community-based intervention. In S. J. Meisels & J. P. Skonkoff (Eds.), *Handbook of early intervention* (pp. 469–499). New York: Cambridge University Press.

Hansen, E. W. (1966). The development of maternal and infant behavior in the rhesus monkey. *Behavior, 27,* 107–149.

Hanson, L. A., Lindquist, B., Hofvander, Y., & Zetterstrom, R. (1985). Breastfeeding as protection against gasteroenteritis and other infections. *Acta Paediatrica Scandinavica, 74,* 641–642.

Hanson, T. L., McLanahan, S., & Thomson, E. (1997). Economic resources, parental practices, and children's well-being. In G. J. Duncan & J. Brooks-Gunn (Eds.), *Consequences of growing up poor* (pp. 190–238). New York: Russell Sage Foundation Press.

Harlow, H. F. (1969). Age-mate or peer affectional system. In D. H. Lehrman, R. A. Hinde, & E. Shaw (Eds.), *Advances in the study of behavior* (pp. 333–383). New York: Academic Press.

Harlow, H. F., & Harlow, M. K. (1965). The affectional systems. In A. M. Schrier, H. F. Harlow, & F. Stollnitz (Eds.), *Behavior of nonhuman primates* (pp. 287–334). New York: Academic Press.

Harlow, H. F., & Lauersdorf, H. E. (1974). Sex differences in passion and play. *Perspectives in Biology and Medicine, 17,* 348–360.

Harré, R., & Gillett, G. (1994). *The discursive mind.* Thousand Oaks, CA: Sage.

Hart, B., & Risley, T. (1995). *Meaningful differences in the everyday lives of young American children.* Baltimore: Paul H. Brookes.

Hart, C., Davey Smith, G., Blane, D., Hole, D., Gillis, C., & Hawthorne, V. (1995). Social mobility, health, and cardiovascular mortality. *Journal of Epidemiology and Community Health, 49,* 552–553.

Harter, S. (1990). Self and identity development. In. S. S. Feldman & G. R. Elliott (Eds.), *At the threshold: The developing adolescent* (pp. 352–287). Cambridge, MA: Harvard University Press.

Harvey, D. (1989). *The condition of postmodernity.* Cambridge, MA: Blackwell.

Hasselmo, M. E., Rolls, E. T., & Baylis, G. C. (1989). The role of expression and identity in the face-selective responses of neurons in the temporal visual cortex of the monkey. *Behavioral Brain Research, 32,* 203–218.

Hauser, R. M., Brown, B., & Prosser, W. (Eds.). (1997). *Indicators of children's well-being.* New York: Russell Sage Foundation Press.

Hauser, R. M., Sewell, W. H., & Warren, J. R. (1994, August). *Education, occupation, and earnings in the long run: Men and women from adolescence to midlife.* Paper presented at the annual meeting of the American Sociological Association, Los Angeles, CA.

Hauser, R. M., & Sweeney, M. (1997). Does poverty in adolescence affect the life chances of high school graduates? In G. Duncan & J. Brooks-Gunn (Eds.), *Consequences of growing up poor* (pp. 541–595). New York: Russell Sage Foundation Press.

Haveman, R., & Wolfe, B. (1995). The determinants of children's attainments: A review of methods and findings. *Journal of Economic Literature, 33,* 1829–1878.

Haveman, R., Wolfe, B., & Spaulding, J. (1991). Childhood events and circumstances influencing high school completion. *Demography, 28*(1), 133–157.

Haveman, R., Wolfe, B., & Wilson, K. (1997). Childhood poverty and adolescent schooling and fertility outcomes: Reduced form and structural estimates. In G. Duncan & J. Brooks-Gunn (Eds.), *Consequences of growing up poor* (pp. 419–460). New York: Russell Sage Foundation Press.

Hay, D. F., & Ross, H. S. (1982). The social nature of early conflict. *Child Development, 53,* 105–113.

Hayes, R. H., Wheelwright, S. C., & Clark, K. (1988). *Dynamic manufacturing: Creating the learning organization.* New York: Free Press.

Hazen, N., & Durrett, M. (1982). Relationship of security of attachment to exploration and cognitive mapping abilities in 2-year-olds. *Developmental Psychology, 18*(5), 751–759.

Heath, A. (1990). Class inequalities in education in the twentieth century. *Journal of the Royal Statistical Society, Series A, 153*(1), 1–16.

Heinroth, O. (1911). Beiträge zur Biologie, namentlich Ethologie und Psychobiologie des Anatiden. *Verhandlungen des Internationalen Ornithologischen Kongresses, V. Kongress, Berlin, 1910,* pp. 589–702.

Heisel, J. S. (1972). Life changes as etiologic factors in juvenile rheumatoid arthritis. *Journal of Psychiatric Research, 16,* 411–420.

Henderson, V., Mieszkowski, P., & Sauvageau, Y. (1978). Peer group effects and educational production functions. *Journal of Public Economics, 10,* 97–106.

Herbert, T. B., & Cohen, S. (1993). Stress and immunity in humans: A meta-analytic review. *Psychosomatic Medicine, 55,* 364–379.

Hernandez, D. J. (1993). *America's children: Resources from family, government and the economy.* New York: Russell Sage Foundation Press.

Hernandez, D. J. (1997). Poverty trends. In G. Duncan & J. Brooks-Gunn (Eds.), *Consequences of growing up poor* (pp. 18–34). New York: Russell Sage Foundation Press.

Hertzman, C. (1994). The lifelong impact of childhood experiences: A population health perspective. *Daedalus, 123*(4), 167–180.

Hertzman, C. (1995). *Environment and health in Central and Eastern Europe.* Washington, DC: World Bank.

Hertzman, C., Kelly, S., & Bobak, M. (Eds.). (1996). *East–west life expectancy gap in Europe: Environmental and non-environmental determinants* (NATO–ASI Series 19(2)). London: Kluwer.

Hertzman, C., & Wiens, M. (1996). Child development and long-term outcomes: A population health perspective and summary of successful interventions. *Social Science and Medicine, 43*(7), 1083–1095.

Hess, E. H. (1964). Imprinting in birds. *Science, 146,* 1128–1139.

Hess, E. H. (1973). *Imprinting: Early experience and the developmental psychobiology of attachment.* New York: Academic Press.

Hetherington, E. M. (1993). An overview of the Virginia longitudinal study of divorce and remarriage with a focus on early adolescence. *Journal of Family Psychology, 7,* 1–18.

Hetherington, E. M., & Clingempeel, W. G. (1992). Coping with marital transitions: A family systems perspective. *Monographs of the Society for Research in Child Development, 57*(2/3, Serial No. 227).

Hewitt, J. (1995). *Progress toward a knowledge-building community.* Unpublished doctoral dissertation, University of Toronto, Toronto, Ontario, Canada.

Higley, J. D., King, S. T., Hasert, M. F., Champoux, M., Suomi, S. J., & Linnoila, M. (1996). Stability of interindividual differences in serotonin function and its relationship to severe aggression and competent social behavior in rhesus macaque females. *Neuropsychopharmacology, 14,* 67–76.

Higley, J. D., Linnoila, M., & Suomi, S. J. (1994). Ethological contributions. In R. T. Ammerman (Ed.), *Handbook of aggressive behavior in psychiatric patients* (pp. 153–167). New York: Raven Press.

Higley, J. D., Mehlman, P. T., Taub, D. M., Higley, S., Fernald, B., Vickers, J., Lindell, S. G., Suomi, S. J., & Linnoila, M. (1996). Excessive mortality in young free-ranging nonhuman primates with low CSF 5-HIAA concentrations. *Archives of General Psychiatry, 53,* 537–543.

Higley, J. D., & Suomi, S. J. (1986). Parental behavior in primates. In W. Sluckin & M. Herbert (Eds.), *Parental behavior* (pp. 152–207). Oxford, UK: Blackwell.

Higley, J. D., & Suomi, S. J. (1989). Temperamental reactivity in nonhuman primates. In G. A. Kohnstamm, J. E. Bates, & M. K. Rothbard (Eds.), *Handbook of temperament in children* (pp. 153–167). New York: Wiley.

Higley, J. D., Suomi, S. J., & Linnoila, M. (1996). A nonhuman primate model of Type II alcoholism? Part 2: Diminished social competence and excessive aggression correlates with low CSF 5-HIAA concentrations. *Alcoholism: Clinical and Experimental Research, 20,* 643–650.

Higley, J. D., Thompson, W. T., Champoux, M., Goldman, D., Hasert, M. F., Kraemer, G. W., Scanlan, J. M., Suomi, S. J., & Linnoila, M. (1993). Paternal and maternal genetic and environmental contributions to CSF monoamine metabolites in rhesus monkeys (*Macaca mulatta*). *Archives of General Psychiatry, 50,* 615–623.

Hill, M. (1992). The panel study of income dynamics. *The Sage series guides to major social science data bases* (Vol. 2). Newbury Park, CA: Sage.

Hinde, R. A. (1962). Some aspects of the imprinting problem. *Symposia of the Zoological Society of London, 8,* 129–138.

Hinde, R. A. (1970). *Animal behavior: A synthesis of ethology and comparative psychology* (2nd ed.). New York: McGraw-Hill.

Hinde, R. A., & Spencer-Booth, Y. (1967). The behavior of socially living rhesus monkeys in their first two and a half years. *Animal Behavior, 15,* 169–196.

Hinde, R. A., & White, L. E. (1974). The dynamics of a relationship: Rhesus monkey ventro–ventro contact. *Journal of Comparative and Physiological Psychology, 86,* 8–23.

Ho, E., & Willms, J. D. (1996). The effects of parental involvement on eighth grade achievement. *Sociology of Education, 69,* 126–141.

Hodgins, S., & Kratzer, L. (1996, October). *Patterns of crime and characteristics of female as compared to male offenders.* Paper presented at the 1996 meeting of the Life History Research Society, London.

Hofstadter, D. R. (1979). *Gödel, Escher, Bach: An eternal golden braid.* New York: Basic Books.

Hogan, D. P., & Kitigawa, E. M. (1985). The impact of social status, family structure, and neighborhood on the fertility of black adolescents. *American Journal of Sociology, 90,* 825–855.

Holden, C. (1996). Small refugees suffer the effects of early neglect. *Science, 274*(15), 1076–1077.

Hope, S., Power, C., & Rodgers, B. (1998). The relationship between parental separation in childhood and problem drinking in adulthood. *Addiction, 93*(4), 505–514.

Horacek, H. J., Ramey, C. T., Campbell, F. A., Hoffman, K. P., & Fletcher, F. H. (1987). Predicting school failure and assessing early intervention with high-risk children. *American Academy of Child Adolescence Psychiatry, 26,* 758–763.

Horn, G. (1990). Neural bases of recognition memory investigated through the analysis of imprinting. *Philosophical Transactions of the Royal Society of London Series B, 329,* 133–142.

Horn, G. (1991). Imprinting and recognition memory: A review of neural mechanisms. In R. J. Andrew (Eds.), *Neural and behavioural plasticity* (pp. 219–261). Oxford, UK: Oxford University Press.

Horn, G. (1995). Imprinting, or in search of the engram along the Fos way. In M. Burrows, T. Matheson, P. L. Newland, & H. Schuppe (Eds.), *Proceedings of the 4th International Congress of Neuroethology* (p. 7). Stuttgart: Thieme.

Howe, N., & Longman, P. (1992, June). The next new deal. *Atlantic Monthly,* pp. 88–99.

Hubel, D. H., Wiesel, T. N., & LeVay, S. (1977). Plasticity of ocular dominance columns in monkey striate cortex. *Philosophical Transactions of the Royal Society of London Series B, 278,* 377–409.

Huesmann, L. R., Eron, L. D., Lefkowitz, M. M., & Walder, L. O. (1984). Stability of aggression over time and generations. *Developmental Psychology, 20,* 1120–1134.

Huttenlocher, J. E., Haight, W., Bryk, A. S., & Seltzer, M. (1988). *Parental speech and early vocabulary development.* Unpublished manuscript, University of Chicago, Department of Education.

Illsley, R., & Baker, D. (1991). Contextual variations in the meaning of health inequality. *Social Science and Medicine, 32,* 359–365.

Infant Health & Development Program. (1990). Enhancing the outcomes of low birthweight premature infants: A multisite randomized trial. *Journal of the American Medical Association, 263*(22), 3035–3042.

Innes, J. (1990). *Knowledge and public policy* (2nd ed.). New Brunswick, NJ: Transaction.

Insel, T. R., & Shapiro, L. E. (1992). Oxytocin receptor distribution reflects social organization in monogamous and polygamous voles. *Proceedings of the National Academy of Sciences of the United States of America, 89,* 5981–5985.

Institute of Medicine. (1989). *Research on children and adolescents with mental, behavioral and developmental disorders: Mobilizing a national initiative.* Washington, DC: National Academy Press.

Ironson, G., Wynings, C., Schneiderman, N., Baum, A., Rodriguez, M., Breenwood, D., Benight, C., Antoni, M., LaPerriere, A., Huang, H.-S., Klimas, N., & Fletcher, M. A. (1997). Post-traumatic stress symptoms, intrusive thoughts, loss, and immune function after Hurricane Andrew. *Psychosomatic Medicine, 50,* 128–141.

Irvine, D. J. (1982, March). *Evaluation of the New York State Experimental Prekindergarten Program.* Paper presented at the annual meeting of the American Educational Research Association, New York, NY.

Irwin, M., Daniels, M., Smith, T. L., Bloom, E., & Weiner, H. (1987). Impaired natural killer cell activity during bereavement. *Brain, Behavior and Immunity, 1,* 98–104.

Isaacs, S. (1930). *Intellectual growth in young children.* London: Routledge.

Ishigami, T. (1919). The influence of psychic acts on the progress of pulmonary tuberculosis. *American Review of Tuberculosis, 2,* 470–484.

Jackson, A., Brooks-Gunn, J., Huang, C., & Glassman, M. (in press). Single mothers in low-wage jobs: Financial strain, parenting, and preschoolers' outcomes. *Child Development.*

Jacobs, T. J., & Charles, E. (1980). Life events and the occurrence of cancer in children. *Psychosomatic Medicine, 42,* 11–24.

Jahoda, G., & Dasen, P. R. (Eds.). (1986). *International Journal of Behavioral Development* [Special issue], 9(4), 413–416.

Jargowsky, P. A., & Bane, M. J. (1991). Ghetto poverty in the United States, 1970–1980. In C. Jencks & P. E. Peterson (Eds.), *The urban underclass* (pp. 235–273). Washington, DC: Brookings Institution.

Jemmott, J. B., & Locke, S. E. (1984). Psychosocial factors, immunologic mediation, and human susceptibility to infectious diseases: How much do we know? *Psychological Bulletin, 78,* 78–108.

Jerison, H. J. (1997). Evolution of the prefrontal cortex. In N. A. Krasnegor, G. R. Lyon, & P. S. Goldman-Rakic (Eds.), *Development of the prefrontal cortex: Evolution, neurobiology, and behavior.* Baltimore, MD: Paul H. Brookes.

Jester, R., & Guinagh, B. J. (1983). The Gordon parent education infant and toddler program. In Lazar Consortium for Longitudinal Studies, *As the twig is bent: Lasting effects of preschool programs* (pp. 103–132). Hillsdale, NJ: Erlbaum.

Jette, D. I. (1993a). *Address to the graduating class, June 25, 1993.* Unpublished manuscript, Meadow Lake Tribal Council, Meadow Lake, Suskatchewan, Canada.

Jette, D. I. (1993b). *Meadow Lake Tribal Council Indian Child Care Program Evaluation.* Unpublished manuscript, Meadow Lake Tribal Council, Meadow Lake, Suskatchewan, Canada.

Johnson, B. R., Voigt, R., Merrill, C. L., & Atema, J. (1991). Across-fiber patterns may contain a sensory code for stimulus intensity. *Brain Research Bulletin, 26,* 327–331.

Johnson, D. L. (1988). Primary prevention of behavior problems in young children: The Houston Parent–Child Development Center. In E. L. Cowen, R. P. Lorion, & J. Ramos-McKay (Eds.), *Fourteen ounces of prevention: A handbook for practitioners* (pp. 44–52). Washington, DC: American Psychological Association.

Johnson, D. L. (1990). The Houston Parent–Child Development Center Project: Dissemination of a viable program for enhancing at-risk families. In R. P. Lorion (Ed.), *Protecting the children: Strategies for optimizing emotional and behavioral development* (pp. 89–108). London: Haworth Press.

Johnson, D. L., & Breckenridge, J. N. (1982). The Houston Parent–Child Development Center and the primary prevention of behavior problems in young children. *American Journal of Community Psychology, 10,* 305–316.

Johnson, D. L., & Walker, T. (1987). Primary prevention of behavior problems in Mexican-American children. *American Journal of Community Psychology, 15,* 375–385.

Johnson, M. H., & Morton, J. (1991). *Biology and cognitive development: The case of face recognition.* Oxford, UK: Blackwell.

Jones, M. B. (1996). Undoing the effects of poverty in children: Non-economic initiatives. In *Post-Symposium Working Papers: Improving the life quality of children: Options and evidence.* Hamilton, Ontario, Canada: Centre for Studies of Children at Risk.

Judge, K. (1995). Income distribution and life expectancy: A critical appraisal. *British Medical Journal, 311,* 1282–1285.

Kagitcibasi, C. (1996). *Family and human development across cultures.* London: Erlbaum.

Kang, D.-H., Coe, C. L., McCarthy, D. O., & Ershler, W. B. (1996). Academic exams significantly impact immune responses, but not lung function in healthy and well-managed asthmatic adolescents. *Brain, Behavior and Immunity, 10,* 164–181.

Kang, D.-H., Coe, C. L., McCarthy, D. O., Jarjour, N. N., Kelly, E. A., Rodriguez, R. R., & Busse, W. B. (1997). Cytokine profiles of simulated blood lymphocytes in asthmatic and healthy adolescents across the school year. *Journal of Interferon and Cytokine Research, 17,* 481–487.

Kaplan, G. A., Pamuk, E., Lynch, J. W., Cohen, R. D., & Balfour, J. L. (1986). Income inequality and mortality in the United States. *British Medical Journal, 312,* 999–1003.

Karasek, R., & Theorell, T. (1990). *Healthy work: Stress, productivity, and the reconstruction of working life.* New York: Basic Books.

Kasl, S. V., Evans, A. S., & Niederman, J. C. (1979). Psychosocial risk factors in the development of infectious mononucleosis. *Psychosomatic Medicine, 41,* 445–466.

Katz, H. C. (1985). *Shifting gears: Changing labor relations in the U.S. automobile industry.* Cambridge, MA: MIT Press.

Katz, L., & Gottman, J. M. (1991). Marital discord and child outcomes: A social psychological approach. In J. Garber & K. Dodge (Eds.), *The development of emotion regulation and dysregulation* (pp. 129–155). Cambridge, UK: Cambridge University Press.

Kawachi, I., Kennedy, B. P., Lochner, K., & Prothrow-Stith, D. (1996). *Social capital, income inequality, and mortality.* Unpublished manuscript. Department of Health and Social Behavior, Harvard School of Public Health, Boston.

Kazdin, A. E. (1993). Treatment of conduct disorder: Progress and directions of psychotherapy research. *Developmental Psychopathology, 5,* 277–310.

Kazdin, A. E. (1996). Dropping out of child psychotherapy: Issues for research and implications for practice. *Journal of Clinical Child Psychology and Psychiatry, 1,* 133–156.

Keating, D. P. (1990). Charting pathways to the development of expertise. *Educational Psychologist, 25,* 243–267.

Keating, D. P. (1995). The learning society in the information age. In S. A. Rosell (Ed.), *Changing maps: Governing in a world of rapid change* (pp. 205–229). Ottawa: Carleton University Press.

Keating, D. P. (1996a). Habits of mind: Developmental diversity in competence and coping. [With commentary and reply by the author.] In D. K. Detterman (Ed.), *Current topics in human intelligence: Vol. 5. The environment* (pp. 31–44). Norwood, NJ: Ablex.

Keating, D. P. (1996b). Habits of mind for a learning society: Educating for human development. In D. R. Olson & N. Torrance (Eds.), *Handbook of education and human development: New models of learning, teaching, and schooling* (pp. 461–481). Oxford, UK: Blackwell.

Keating, D. P. (1998). Human development in the learning society. In A. Hargreaves,

A. Lieberman, M. Fullan, & D. Hopkins (Eds.), *International handbook of educational change* (Pt. 2, pp. 693–709). Dordrecht, The Netherlands: Kluwer.

Keating, D. P., & Mustard, J. F. (1993). Social economic factors and human development. In D. Ross (Ed.), *Family security in insecure times* (Vol. 1, pp. 87–105). Ottawa: National Forum on Family Security.

Keating, D. P., & Mustard, J. F. (1996). The National Longitudinal Survey of Children and Youth: An essential element for building a learning society in Canada. In *Growing up in Canada: National Longitudinal Survey of Children and Youth* (pp. 7–13). Ottawa: Human Resources Development Canada & Statistics Canada.

Keenan, K., & Shaw, D. S. (1994). The development of aggression in toddlers: A study of low-income families. *Journal of Abnormal Child Psychology, 22,* 53–77.

Kellam, S. G., Brown, C. H., Rubin, B. R., & Ensminger, M. E. (1983). Paths leading to teenage psychiatric symptoms and substance use: Developmental epidemiological studies in Woodlawn. In S. B. Guze, F. J. Earls, & J. E. Barrett (Eds.), *Childhood psychopathology and development* (pp. 17–51). New York: Raven Press.

Kelley, K. W. (1985). Stress and immune function: A bibliographic review. *Annales de Recherches Veterinaires, 11*(4), 445–478.

Kelly, C. (1990). Professionalizing child and youth care: An overview. In J. P. Anglin, C. J. Denholm, R. V. Ferguson, & A. R. Pence (Eds.), *Perspectives in professional child and youth care* (pp. 167–176). New York: Haworth Press.

Kemble, A. (1994). *Mid-project assessment of the child and youth care laddering project.* Unpublished manuscript, School of Child and Youth Care, University of Victoria, Victoria, British Columbia, Canada.

Kemble, A. (1995). *Community impact assessment of the Child and Youth Care Laddering Program.* Unpublished manuscript, School of Child and Youth Care, University of Victoria, Victoria, British Columbia, Canada.

Kemeny, M. E., Cohen, F., Zegans, L. A., & Conant, M. A. (1989). Psychological and immunological predictors of genital herpes recurrence. *Psychosomatic Medicine, 51,* 195–208.

Kendrick, K. M., & Baldwin, B. A. (1987). Cells in temporal cortex of conscious sheep can respond preferentially to the sight of faces. *Science, 236,* 448–450.

Kendrick, K. M., Keverne, E. B., Hinton, M. R., & Goode, J. A. (1992). Oxytocin, amino acid and monoamine release in the medial pre-optic area and bed nucleus of stria terminalis of the sheep during parturition and suckling. *Brain Research, 569,* 199–209.

Kerckhoff, A. C. (1986). Effects of ability grouping. *American Sociological Review, 51*(6), 842–858.

Kerckhoff, A. C. (1993). *Diverging pathways: Social structure and career deflections.* New York: Cambridge University Press.

Kerckhoff, A. C. (Ed.). (1996). *Generating social stratification.* Boulder, CO: Westview Press.

Kessen, W. (1979). The American child and other cultural inventions. *American Psychologist, 34*(12), 815–820.

Kessler, M. J. (1989). A history of the rhesus monkey colony on Cayo Santiago. *Puerto Rico Health Sciences Journal, 8,* 1–11.

Kiecolt-Glaser, J. K., Garner, W., Speicher, C., Penn, C. M., Holiday, J., & Glaser, R. (1984). Psychosocial modifiers of immunocompetence in medical students. *Psychosomatic Medicine, 46,* 7–14.

Kiecolt-Glaser, J. K., Glaser, R., Dyer, C., Suttleworth, E., Ogrocki, P., & Speicher, C. E. (1987). Chronic stress and immunity in family caregivers of Alzheimer's disease victims. *Psychosomatic Medicine, 49,* 523–535.

Kiecolt-Glaser, J. K., Glaser, R., Gravenstein, S., Malarkey, W. B., & Sheridan, J. (1996). Chronic stress alters the immune response to influenze virus vaccine in the elderly. *Proceedings of the National Academy of Sciences of the United States of America, 93,* 3043–3047.

Kiecolt-Glaser, J. K., Glaser, R., Williger, D., Stout, J., Mesick, G., Sheppard, S., Ricker, D., Romisher, S. C., Briner, W., Bonnell, G., & Donnerberg, R. (1985). Psychosocial enhancement of immunocompetence in a geriatric population. *Health Psychology, 4,* 25–41.

Kiecolt-Glaser, J. K., Marucha, P. T., Malarkey, W. B., Mercado, A. M., & Glaser, R. (1995). Slowing of wound healing by psychological stress. *Lancet, 346*(8984), 1194–1196.

Killing of child shocks Britain: Brutal slaying sparks anger and soul-searching. (1993, February 18). *Montreal Gazette,* p. B5.

King, J. A. (1994). Meeting educational needs of at-risk students: A cost analysis of three models. *Educational Evaluation and Policy Analysis, 16*(1), 1–19.

Kirkpatrick, B., Carter, C. S., Newman, S. W., & Insel, T. R. (1994). Axon-sparing lesions of the medial nucleus of the amygdala decrease affiliative behaviors in the prairie vole (*Microtus ochrogaster*): Behavioral and anatomical specificity. *Behavioral Neuroscience, 108,* 501–513.

Kittner, S. J., White, L. R., Farmer, M. E., Wolz, M., Kaplan, E., Moes, E., Brody, J. A., & Feinleib, M. (1986). Methodological issues in screening for dementia: The problem of education adjustment. *Journal of Chronic Disease, 39*(3), 163–170.

Klebanov, P. K., Brooks-Gunn, J., Chase-Lansdale, L., & Gordon, R. (1997). The intersection of the neighborhood and home environment and its influence on young children. In J. Brooks-Gunn, G. Duncan, & J. L. Aber (Eds.), *Neighborhood poverty: Context and consequences for children* (Vol. 1, pp. 119–145). New York: Russell Sage Foundation Press.

Klebanov, P. K., Brooks-Gunn, J., & Duncan, G. J. (1994). Does neighborhood and family poverty affect mothers' parenting, mental health, and social support? *Journal of Marriage and the Family, 56*(2), 441–455.

Klebanov, P. K., Brooks-Gunn, J., McCarton, C., & McCormick, M. C. (1998). The contribution of neighborhood and family income upon developmental test scores over the first three years of life. *Child Development, 69*(5), 1420–1436.

Klebanov, P. K., Brooks-Gunn, J., & McCormick, M. C. (1994). Classroom behavior of very low birth weight elementary school children. *Pediatrics, 94*(5), 700–708.

Klerman, G. L., & Izen, J. E. (1977). The effects of bereavement and grief on physical health and general well-being. *Advances in Psychosomatic Medicine, 5,* 63–104.

Klopfer, P. H. (1971). Imprinting: Determining its perceptual basis in ducklings. *Journal of Comparative and Physiological Psychology, 75,* 378–385.

Klopfer, P. H. (1988). Metaphors for development: How important are experiences early in life? *Developmental Psychobiology, 21*(7), 671–678.

Klopfer, P. H. (1996). "Mother love" revisited: On the use of animal models. *American Scientist, 84,* 319–321.

Klopfer, P. H., & Gamble, J. (1966). Maternal "imprinting" in goats: The role of chemical senses. *Zeitschrift für Tierpsychologie, 23,* 588–592.

Klüver, H., & Bucy, P. C. (1939). Preliminary analysis of functions of the temporal lobes in monkeys. *Archives of Neurological Psychiatry, 42,* 979–1000.

Knierim, J. J., & Van Essen, D. C. (1992). Visual cortex: Cartography, connectivity, and concurrent processing. *Current Opinion in Neurobiology, 2*(2), 150–155.

Kochanska, G. (1995). Children's temperament, mother's discipline, and security of attachment: Multiple pathways to emerging internalization. *Child Development, 66*(3), 597–615.

Kochanska, G. (1997). Multiple pathways to conscience for children with different temperaments: From toddlerhood to age 5. *Developmental Psychology, 33(2),* 228–240.

Kochanska, G., Aksan, N., & Koenig, A. L. (1995). A longitudinal study of the roots of preschoolers' conscience: Committed compliance and emerging internalization. *Child Development, 66,* 1752–1769.

Kopp, C. B. (1989). Regulation of distress and negative emotions: A developmental view. *Developmental Psychology, 25*(3), 343–354.

Korenman, S., & Miller, J. E. (1997). Effects of long-term poverty on physical health of children in the National Longitudinal Survey of Youth. In G. Duncan & J. Brooks-Gunn (Eds.), *Consequences of growing up poor* (pp. 70–99). New York: Russell Sage Foundation Press.

Korenman, S., Miller, J. E., & Sjaastad, J. E. (1995). Long-term poverty and child development in the United States: Results from the National Longitudinal Survey of Youth. *Children and Youth Services Review, 17*(1/2), 127–151.

Kotloff, L. J. (1996). And Tomoko wrote this song for us. In T. Rohlen & G. LeTendre (Eds.), *Teaching and learning in Japan* (pp. 98–119). Cambridge, UK: Cambridge University Press.

Kraemer, H. C. (1992). *Evaluating medical tests: Objective and quantitative guidelines.* London: Sage.

Kraemer, H. C., Kazdin, A. E., Offord, D. R., Kessler, R. C., Jensen, P. S., & Kupfer, D. J. (1997). Coming to terms with the terms of risk. *Archives of General Psychiatry, 54,* 337–343.

Kraus, A. S., & Lilienfield, A. M. (1959). Some epidemiological aspects of the high mortality rate in the young widowed group. *Journal of Chronic Disease, 19,* 207–217.

Kunst, A. E., Guerts, J. J. M., & Berg, J. (1992). *International variation in socioeconomic inequalities in self-reported health.* The Hague: Netherlands Central Bureau of Statistics.

Kunst, A. E., & Mackenbach, J. P. (1992). *An international comparison of socioeconomic inequalities in mortality.* Rotterdam: Erasmus University.

Lally, R. J. (1988). More pride, less delinquency: Findings from the ten year follow-up study of the Syracuse University Family Development Research Program. *Zero to Three, 8,* 13–18.

Lally, R. J., Mangione, P. L., & Honig, A. S. (1988). The Syracuse University Family Development Research Program: Long range impact on an early intervention with low-income children and their families. In D. Powell (Ed.), *Parent education as early childhood intervention: Emerging directions in theory, research and practice* (pp. 79–104). Norwood, NJ: Ablex.

Lampert, M., Rittenhouse, P., & Crumbaugh, C. (1996). Agreeing to disagree: Developing sociable mathematical discourse. In D. R. Olson & N. Torrance (Eds.), *Handbook of education and human development: New models of learning, teaching and schooling* (pp. 731–764). Cambridge, MA: Blackwell.

Land, K. C. (1983). Social indicators. *Annual Review of Sociology, 9,* 1–26.

Landmann, R. M., Muller, F. B., Perini, C., Wesp, M., Erne, P., & Buhler, F. R. (1984). Changes of immunoregulatory cells induced by psychological and physical stress: Relationship to plasma catecholamines. *Clinical and Experimental Immunology, 58,* 127–135.

Landry, G. (1996). *Les liens entre les habiletés langagières et les comportements agressifs chez des enfants de 13 mois.* Research report presented to Professor Virginia Douglas, McGill University, Montréal, Québec, Canada.

Langer, J. (1991). Literacy and schooling: A sociocognitive perspective. In E. Hiebert (Ed.), *Literacy for a diverse society* New York: Teachers College Press.

Laudenslager, M. L., Reite, M. R., & Harbeck, R. J. (1982). Suppressed immune response in infant monkeys associated with maternal separation. *Behavioral and Neural Biology, 36,* 40–48.

Lave, J., & Wenger, E. (1991). *Situated learning: Legitimate peripheral participation.* Cambridge, UK: Cambridge University Press.

Lee, V. E., Groninger, R. G., & Smith, J. B. (1994). Parental choice of schools and social stratification in education: The paradox of Detroit. *Educational Evaluation and Policy Analysis, 16*(4), 434–457.

Lee, V. E., & Smith, J. B. (1993). Effects of school restructuring on the achievement and engagement of middle-grade students. *Sociology of Education, 66,* 164–187.

Lemieux, A., Coe, C. L., & Ershler, W. B. (1996). Surgical and psychological stress differentially affect cytolytic responses in the aged female monkey. *Brain, Behavior and Immunity, 10,* 27–43.

Leon, D. A., Davey-Smith, G., Shipley, M., & Strachan, D. (1995). Adult height and mortality in London: Early life, socioeconomic confounding or shrinkage? *Journal of Epidemiology and Community Health, 49,* 5–9.

Leon, M. (1992). The neurobiology of field learning. *Annual Review of Psychology, 43,* 377–398.

Lerner, D. J., Levine, S., Malpeis, S., & Dagostino, R. B. (1994). Job strain and health related quality of life in a national sample. *American Journal of Public Health, 84,* 1580–1585.

Levenstein, P., O'Hara, J., & Madden, J. (1983). The mother–child home program of the verbal interaction project. In Lazar Consortium for Longitudinal Studies, *As the twig is bent: Lasting effects of preschool programs* (pp. 237–264). Hillsdale, NJ: Erlbaum.

Leventhel, T., & Brooks-Gunn, J. (in press). The neighborhood they live in: Effects of neighborhood residence on child and adolescent outcomes. *Psychological Bulletin.*

Levin, H. M. (1987). Accelerated schools for disadvantaged students. *Educational Leadership, 44*(6), 19–21.

Levy, S., Herberman, R., Maluish, A., Schlien, B., & Lippman, M. (1985). Prognostic risk assessment in primary breast cancer by behavioral and immunological parameters. *Health Psychology, 4*(2), 99–113.

Lewis, C. C. (1995). *Educating hearts and minds: Reflections on Japanese preschools and elementary education.* Cambridge, UK: Cambridge University Press.

Lewis, M. (Ed.). (1983). *Origins of intelligence: Infancy and early childhood* (2nd ed.). New York: Plenum.

Lewis, M. D. (1993a). Early socioemotional predictors of cognitive competency at four years. *Developmental Psychology, 29,* 1036–1045.

Lewis, M. D. (1993b). Emotion–cognition interactions in early infant development. *Cognition and Emotion, 7,* 145–170.

Lindburg, D. G. (1971). The rhesus monkey in North India: An ecological and behavioral study. In L. A. Rosenblum (Ed.), *Primate behavior: Developments in field and laboratory research* (Vol. 2, pp. 1–106). New York: Academic Press.

Linver, M. R., Brooks-Gunn, J., & Kohen, D. (1999). *Parenting behavior and mental health as mediators of family poverty effects upon 3-year-olds' and 5-year-olds' development.* Manuscript submitted for publication.

Lipman, E. L., & Offord, D. R. (1997). Psychosocial morbidity among poor children in Ontario. In G. J. Duncan & J. Brooks-Gunn (Eds.), *Consequences of growing up poor* (pp. 239–287). New York: Russell Sage Foundation Press.

Lipsey, M. W. (1992). Juvenile delinquency treatment: A meta-analytic inquiry into the variability of effects. In T. D. Cook, H. Cooper, D. S. Cordray, H. Hartman, L. V. Hedges, R. J. Light, T. A. Louis, & F. Mosteller (Eds.), *Meta-analysis for explanation* (pp. 83–127). New York: Russell Sage Foundation Press.

Lipton, D., Martinson, R., & Wilks, J. (1975). *The effectiveness of correctional treatment: A survey of treatment evaluation studies.* New York: Praeger.

London, B., & Flanagan, W. G. (1976). Comparative urban ecology: A summary of the field. In J. Walton & L. Masotti (Eds.), *The city in comparative perspective* (pp. 41–66). New York: Wiley.

Lord, F. M. (1980). *Applications of item response theory to practical testing problems.* Hillsdale, NJ: Erlbaum.

Lorenz, K. Z. (1935). Der Kumpan in der Umwelt des Vogels: Die Artgenosse als auslösende Moment sozialer Verhaltungswiesen. *Journal für Ornithologie, 83*(137–213; 289–413). Available in English translation as: Companions as factors in the bird's environment. In K. Z. Lorenz (1970). *Studies in animal and human behavior* (R. Martin, Trans., Vol. 1, pp. 101–258). Cambridge, MA: Harvard University Press.

Lorenz, K. Z. (1937). The companion in the bird's world. *Auk, 54,* 245–273.

Lubach, G. R., Coe, C. L., & Ershler, W. B. (1995). Effects of early rearing on immune responses in infant rhesus monkeys. *Brain, Behavior and Immunity, 9,* 31–46.

Lundberg, O. (1993). The impact of childhood living conditions on illness and mortality in adulthood. *Social Science and Medicine, 36,* 1047–1052.

Ma, X., & Willms, J. D. (1995, April). *The effects of school disciplinary climate on eighth grade achievement.* Paper presented at the annual meeting of the American Educational Research Association, San Francisco.

MacDonald, K. (1992). Warmth as a developmental construct: An evolutionary analysis. *Child Development, 63*(4), 753–759.

Madden, N. A., Slavin, R. E., Karweit, N. L., & Livermon, B. J. (1989). Restructuring the urban elementary school. *Educational Leadership, 46*(5), 13–18.

Maddison, D., & Viola, A. (1968). The health of widows in the year following bereavement. *Journal of Psychosomatic Research, 12,* 297–306.

Maier, S. F., & Watkins, R. (1998). Cytokines for psychologists: Implications of bidirectional immune-to-brain communication for understanding behavior, mood and cognition. *Psychological Review, 105*(1), 83–107.

Main, M. (1983). Exploration, play, and cognitive functioning related to mother–infant attachment. *Infant Behavior and Development, 6,* 167–174.

Mainardi, D., Marsan, M., & Pasquali, A. (1965). Causation of sexual preferences of the house mouse: The behaviour of mice reared by parents whose odour was artificially altered. *Atti della Societa Italiana di Scienze Naturali e del Museo Civico di Storia Naturale in Milano, 104,* 323–338.

Manor, O., Matthews, S., & Power, C. (1997). Comparing measures of health inequality. *Social Science and Medicine, 45,* 761–771.

Marmot, M. G. (1986). Social inequalities in mortality: The social environment. In R. G. Wilkinson (Ed.), *Class and health: Research and longitudinal data* (pp. 21–33). London: Tavistock.

Marmot, M. G. (1993). *Explaining socioeconomic differences in sickness absence: The Whitehall II study.* Toronto: Canadian Institute for Advanced Research.

Marmot, M. G., Kogevinas, M., & Elston, M. (1987). Social/economic status and disease. *Annual Review of Public Health, 8,* 111–135.

Marmot, M. G., Rose, G., Shipley, M., & Hamilton, P. J. S. (1987). Employment grade and coronary heart disease in British civil servants. *Journal of Epidemiology and Community Health, 32,* 244–249.

Marmot, M. G., & Shipley, M. J. (1996). Do socioeconomic differences in mortality persist after retirement?: 25 year follow-up of civil servants from the first Whitehall study. *BioMedical Journal, 313*(7066), 1177–1180.

Marmot, M. G., Shipley, M. J., & Rose, G. (1984). Inequalities in death-specific explanations of a general pattern. *Lancet, i,* 1003–1006.

Marmot, M. G., Smith, G., Stansfeld, S., Patel, C., North, F., Head, J., White, L., Brunner, E., & Feeney, A. (1991). Health inequalities among British civil servants: The Whitehall II study. *Lancet, 337,* 1387–1393.

Marsh, J. T., & Rasmussen, A. F. (1960). Response of adrenals, thymus, spleen, and leukocytes to shuttle box and confinement stress. *Proceedings of the Society of Experimental Biology and Medicine, 104,* 180–183.

Martin, S. L., Ramey, C. T., & Ramey, S. (1990). The prevention of intellectual impairment in children of impoverished families: Findings of a randomized trial of educational daycare. *American Journal of Public Health, 80,* 844–847.

Massey, D. S., Condron, G. A., & Denton, N. A. (1987). The effect of residential segregation on Black social and economic well-being. *Social Forces, 66*(1), 29–56.

Matas, L., Arend, R., & Sroufe, L. A. (1978). Continuity of adaptation in the second year: The relationship between quality of attachment and later competence. *Child Development, 49,* 547–556.

Mayer, S. (1997a). *What money can't buy: Family income and children's life chances.* Cambridge, MA: Harvard University Press.

Mayer, S. (1997b). Trends in the economic well-being and life chances of America's children. In G. Duncan & J. Brooks-Gunn (Eds.), *Consequences of growing up poor* (pp. 49–69). New York: Russell Sage Foundation Press.

Mayes, L. C., & Carter, A. S. (1990). Emerging social regulatory capacities as seen in the still-face situation. *Child Development, 61,* 754–763.

McCall, R. B. (1983). A conceptual approach to early mental development. In M. Lewis (Ed.), *Origins of intelligence: Infancy and early childhood* (2nd ed., pp. 107–134). New York: Plenum.

McCarton, C., Brooks-Gunn, J., Wallace, I., Bauer, C., Bennett, F., Bernbaum, J., Broyles, R., Casey, P., McCormick, M., Scott, D., Tyson, J., Tonascia, J., & Meinert, C. (1997). Results at eight years of intervention for low birthweight premature infants: The Infant Health Development Program. *Journal of the American Medical Association, 227*(2), 126–132.

McEwen, B. S., & Stellar, E. (1993). Stress and the individual: Mechanisms leading to disease. *Archives of Internal Medicine, 153,* 2093–2101.

McFarlane, A. J. (1975). Olfaction in the development of social preferences in the human neonate. In *CIBA Foundation Symposium on Parent–Infant Relationship 33* (pp. 103–117). London: CIBA Foundation.

McIntyre, L. (1996). Starting out. In *Growing up in Canada: National Longitudinal Survey of Children and Youth* (pp. 47–56). Ottawa: Human Resources Development Canada & Statistics Canada.

McKeough, A. (1992). Testing for the presence of a central conceptual structure: Use of the transfer paradigm. In R. Case (Ed.), *The mind's staircase: Exploring the conceptual underpinnings of children's thought and knowledge* (pp. 189–206). Hillsdale, NJ: Erlbaum.

McKinnon, W., Weisse, C. S., Reynolds, C. P., & Baum, A. (1989). Chronic stress, leukocyte subpopulations, and humoral response to latent viruses. *Health Psychology, 8,* 389–402.

McLanahan, S. (1997). Parent absence or poverty: Which matters more? In G. Duncan & J. Brooks-Gunn (Eds.), *Consequences of growing up poor* (pp. 35–48). New York: Russell Sage Foundation Press.

McLanahan, S., & Sandefur, G. D. (1994). *Growing up with a single parent: What hurts, what helps?* Cambridge, MA: Harvard University Press.

McLoyd, V. C. (1990). The impact of economic hardship on black families and children: Psychological distress, parenting, and socioemotional development. *Child Development, 61,* 311–346.

McLoyd, V. C., Jayaratne, T. E., Ceballo, R., & Borquez, J. (1994). Unemployment and work interruption among African-American single mothers: Effects on parenting and adolescent socio-emotional functioning. *Child Development, 65,* 562–589.

McPherson, A. F., & Raab, C. D. (1988). *Governing education: A sociology of policy since 1945.* Edinburgh: Edinburgh University Press.

McPherson, A. F., & Willms, J. D. (Eds.). (1986). *Certification, class conflict, religion and community: A socio-historical explanation of the effectiveness of contemporary schools* (Vol. 6). Greenwich, CT: JAI Press.

Meadow Lake Tribal Council [MLTC]. (1989). *MLTC Vision Statement, MLTC Program Report.* Unpublished document, MLTC, Meadow Lake, Saskatchewan, Canada.

Meaney, M., Aitken, D., Bhatnager, S., van Berkel, C., & Sapolsky, R. (1988). Effect of neonatal handling on age-related impairments associated with the hippocampus. *Science, 239,* 766–768.

Mehlman, P. T., Higley, J. D., Faucher, I., Lilly, A. A., Taub, D. M., Vickers, J., Suomi, S. J., & Linnoila, M. (1994). Low cerebrospinal fluid 5-hydroxyindoleacetic acid concentrations are correlated with severe aggression and reduced impulse control in free-ranging primates. *American Journal of Psychiatry, 151,* 1485–1491.

Mehlman, P. T., Higley, J. D., Faucher, I., Lilly, A. A., Taub, D. M., Vickers, J., Suomi, S. J., & Linnoila, M. (1995). CSF 5-HIAA concentrations are correlated with sociality and the timing of emigration in free-ranging primates. *American Journal of Psychiatry, 152,* 901–913.

Meinecke, D. L., & Rakic, P. (1992). Expression of GABA and GABAA receptors by neurons of the subplate zone in developing primate occipital cortex: Evidence for transient local circuits. *Journal of Comparative Neurology, 317,* 91–101.

Merton, R. (1938). Social structure and "anomie." *American Sociological Review, 3,* 672–682.

Meyer, R. J., & Haggerty, R. J. (1962). Streptococcal infections in families: Factors altering individual susceptibility. *Pediatrics, 29,* 539–549.

Michalos, A. (1980). *North American social report.* Dordrecht, The Netherlands: Reidel.

Miller, F. K. (1995). *The relation of attentional, emotional, and social regulation to cognitive competence, from infancy to school entry.* Unpublished master's thesis, Brock University, St. Catharines, Ontario, Canada.

Miller, F. K., Keating, D. P., & Marshment, R. P. (1996, August). *The prediction of preschool cognitive competence from infant attentional, emotional, and social regulation.* Poster presented at the biennial meeting of the International Society for the Study of Behavioral Development, Québec City, Québec, Canada.

Miller, F. K., Keating, D. P. & Marshment, R. P. (1997, April). *Continuity in habits of mind: Emotion, attention, and social self-regulation from infancy to early childhood.* Poster presented at the biennial meeting of the Society for Research in Child Development, Washington, DC.

Miller, F. K., & Marshment, R.(1998, July). *Observed patterns of regulation predict parental reports of internalizing and externalizing behaviors at preschool.* Poster presented at the biennial meeting of the International Society for the Study of Behavioral Development, Berne, Switzerland.

Miller, J. E., & Korenman, S. (1994). Poverty and children's nutrition status in the United States. *American Journal of Epidemiology, 140,* 233–243.

Miller, L. B., & Bizzell, R. (1983). The Louisville Experiment: A comparison of four programs. In Lazar Consortium for Longitudinal Studies *As the twig is bent: Lasting effects of preschool programs* (pp. 171–200). Hillsdale, NJ: Erlbaum.

Mischel, W., Shoda, Y., & Rodriguez, M. L. (1989). Delay of gratification in children. *Science, 244,* 933–938.

Mitchell, D. E., Freeman, R. D., Millodot, M., & Haegerstrom, G. (1973). Meridional amblyopia: Evidence for modification of the human visual system by early visual experience. *Vision Research, 13,* 535–558.

Mitchell, D. E., & Timney, B. (1984). Postnatal development of function in the mammalian visual system. In I. Darian-Smith (Ed.), *Handbook of physiology: The nervous system* (pp. 507–555). Bethesda, MD: American Physiological Society.

Moffitt, T. E. (1993). The neuropsychology of conduct disorder. *Developmental Psychopathology, 5,* 135–151.

Mora, J. M., Amtmann, L. E., & Hoffman, S. J. (1926). Effect of mental and emotional states on the leukocyte count. *Journal of the American Medical Association, 86,* 945–946.

Mortimer, J. A., & Graves, A. B. (1993). Education and other socioeconomic determinants of dementia and Alzheimer's disease. *Neurology, 43,* S39–S44.

Moss, D., & Pence, A. R. (1994). *Valuing quality in early childhood services: New approaches to defining quality.* New York: Teachers College Press.

Mrazek, D. A., Klinnert, M. D., Mrazek, P., & Macey, T. (1991). Early asthma onset: Consideration of parenting issues. *Journal of the American Academy of Child and Adolescent Psychiatry, 30,* 277–282.

Mrazek, P. J., & Haggerty, R. J. (Eds.). (1994). *Reducing risk for mental disorders:*

Frontiers for preventive intervention research. Washington, DC: National Academy Press.

Muir, D. W., & Hains, S. M. (1993). Infant sensitivity to perturbations in adult facial, vocal, tactile, and contingent stimulation during face-to-face interactions. In B. D. Boysson-Bardies, S. de Schonen, P. Jusczyk, P. McNeilage, & J. Morton (Eds.), *Developmental neurocognition: Speech and face processing in the first year of life*. Dordrecht, The Netherlands: Kluwer.

Muir, D. W., Humphrey, D., & Humphrey, G. K. (1994). Patterns and space perception in young infants. *Spatial Vision, 8*, 141–165.

Munck, A., Guyre, P. M., & Holbrook, N. J. (1984). Physiological functions of glucocorticoids in stress and their relation to pharmacological actions. *Endocrine Reviews, 5*, 25–44.

Murnane, R. J., & Pauly, E. W. (1988, March). Lessons from comparing educational and economic indicators. *Phi Delta Kappan, 69*, 509–513.

Naliboff, B. D., Benton, D., Solomon, G. F., Morley, J. E., Fahey, J. L., Bloom, E. T., Makinodan, T., & Gilmore, S. L. (1991). Immunological changes in young and old adults during brief laboratory stress. *Psychosomatic Medicine, 53*, 121–132.

New Standards. (1995). *Performance standards: English language arts, mathematics, science, applied learning*. Rochester, NY: National Center on Education and the Economy.

Nicol, A. U., Brown, M. W., & Horn, G. (1995). Neurophysiological investigations of a recognition memory system for imprinting in the domestic chick. *European Journal of Neuroscience, 7*, 766–776.

Noël, J. M., Leclerc, D., & Strayer, F. F. (1990). Une analyse fonctionnelle du répertoire social des enfants d'âge pré-scolaire en groupe de pairs. *Enfance, 45*, 405–421.

Nolen-Hoeksema, S. (1994). An interactive model for the emergence of gender differences in depression in adolescence. *Journal of Research on Adolescence, 4*(4), 519–534.

Nonaka, I. (1994). A dynamic theory of organizational knowledge creation. *Organizational Science, 5*(1), 14–37.

Nonaka, I., & Takeuchi, H. (1995). *The knowledge-creating company*. New York: Oxford University Press.

North, F. M., Syme, S. L., Feeney, A., Shipley, M., & Marmot, M. (1996). Psychosocial work environment and sickness absence among British civil servants: The Whitehall II study. *American Journal of Public Health, 86*, 332–340.

Novak, M. A., & Suomi, S. J. (1991). Social interaction in nonhuman primates: An underlying theme for primate research. *Laboratory Animal Science, 41*, 308–314.

Nsamenang, A. B. (1992). *Human development in cultural context*. London: Sage.

Nystrom Peck, A. M. (1994). The importance of childhood socioeconomic group for adult health. *Social Science and Medicine, 39*, 553–562.

Nystrom Peck, A. M., & Vagero, D. (1989). Adult body height, self perceived health and mortality in the Swedish population. *Journal of Epidemiology and Community Health, 43*, 380–384.

Offord, D. R., Boyle, M. H., Szatmari, P., Rae-Grant, N. I., Links, P. S., Cadman, D. T., Byles, J. A., Crawford, J. W., Munroe-Blum, H., Byrne, C., Thomas, H., & Woodward, C. A. (1987). Ontario Child Health Study: Six-month prevalence of disorder and rates of service utilization. *Archives of General Psychiatry, 44*, 832–836.

Offord, D. R., Boyle, M. H., Racine, Y. A., Fleming, J. E., Cadman, D. T., Monroe-Blum, H., Byrne, C., Links, P., Lipman, E. L., MacMillan, H. L., Sanford, M. N., Szatmari, P., Thomas, H., & Woodward, C. A. (1992). Outcome, prognosis and risk in a longitudinal follow-up study. *Journal of the American Academy of Child and Adolescent Psychiatry, 31,* 916–923.

Ogbu, J. U. (1981). Origins of human competencies: A cultural–ecological perspective. *Child Development, 52,* 413–429.

Olds, D. L., Henderson, C. R., Chamberlin, R., & Talelbaum, R. (1986). Preventing child abuse and neglect: A randomized trial of nurse home visitation. *Pediatrics, 78,* 65–78.

Ollia, L., & Mayfield, M. (Eds.). (1991). *Emerging literacy.* Toronto: Allyn & Bacon.

Olson, D. R. (1994). *The world on paper: The conceptual and cognitive implications of writing and reading.* Cambridge, UK: Cambridge University Press.

Olson, S. L., Bates, J. E., & Bayles, K. (1984). Mother–infant interaction and the development of individual differences in children's cognitive competence. *Developmental Psychology, 20,* 166–179.

Ontario Ministry of Education & Training. (1995). *The common curriculum: Policies and outcomes, Grades 1–9.* Toronto: Author.

Organization for Economic Cooperation & Development (OECD) & Statistics Canada. (1995). *Literacy, economy, and society: Results of the first international adult literacy survey.* Paris: OECD/Ottawa: Ministry of Industry Canada.

Orshansky, M. (1988). Counting the poor: Another look at the poverty profile. *Social Security Bulletin, 51*(10), 25–51.

Oshima, J., Scardamalia, M., & Bereiter, C. (1996). Collaborative learning processes associated with high and low conceptual progress. *Instructional Science, 24,* 125–155.

Pagani, L., Boulerice, B., & Tremblay, R. E. (1997). The influence of poverty on children's classroom placement and behavior. In J. Brooks-Gunn & G. Duncan (Eds.), *Consequences of growing up poor* (pp. 311–339). New York: Russell Sage Foundation Press.

Pallas, A. (1988). School climate in American high schools. *Teachers College Record, 89,* 541–553.

Palmer, F. H. (1979). Long-term gains from early intervention: Findings from longitudinal studies. In E. Zigler & J. Valentine (Eds.), *Project Head Start: A legacy of the war on poverty.* New York: Free Press.

Palmer, F. H. (1983). The Harlem study: Effects by type of training, age of training and social class. In Lazar Consortium for Longitudinal Studies, *As the twig is bent: Lasting effects of preschool programs* (pp. 201–236). Hillsdale, NJ: Erlbaum.

Pancer, M. S., & Cameron, G. (1994). Resident participation in the Better Beginnings, Better Futures Prevention Project: The impacts of involvement. *Canadian Journal of Community Mental Health, 13,* 197–211.

Panskepp, J. (1992). A critical role for "affective neuroscience" in resolving what is basic about basic emotions. *Psychological Review, 99,* 554–560.

Papert, S. (1993). *The children's machine: Rethinking school in the age of the computer.* New York: Basic Books.

Pappas, G., Queen, S., Hadden, W., & Fisher, G. (1993). The increasing disparity in mortality between socioeconomic groups in the United States, 1960 and 1986. *New England Journal of Medicine, 329,* 103–108.

Parke, R. D., Cassidy, J., Burkes, V., Carson, J. L., & Boyum, L. (1992). Familial contributions to peer competence among young children: The role of interactive and affective processes. In R. Parke & G. Ladd (Eds.), *Family–peer relationships* Hillsdale, NJ: Erlbaum.

Parker, G. (1992). Early environment. In E. S. Paykel (Ed.), *Handbook of affective disorders* (2nd ed., pp. 171–183). New York: Guilford Press.

Pavlidis, N., & Chirigos, M. (1980). Stress-induced impairment of macrophage tumoricidal function. *Psychosomatic Medicine, 42,* 47–54.

Pawelec, G., & Solana, R. (1997). Immunosenescence. *Immunology Today, 18*(11), 514–516.

Peak, L. (1991). *Learning to go to school in Japan: The transition from home to preschool life.* Berkeley: University of California Press.

Perrett, D. I., Rolls, E. T., & Caan, W. (1982). Visual neurons responsive to faces in monkey temporal cortex. *Experimental Brain Research, 47,* 329–342.

Peters, E., & Mullis, N. (1997). The role of the family and sources of income in adolescent achievement. In G. Duncan & J. Brooks-Gunn (Eds.), *Consequences of growing up poor* (pp. 340–381). New York: Russell Sage Foundation Press.

Peters, T. (1987). *Thriving on chaos: Handbook for a management revolution.* New York: Knopf.

Phillips, M., Brooks-Gunn, J., Duncan, G. J., Klebanov, P. K., & Jencks, C. (1998). Family background, parenting practices, and the black–white test score gap. In C. Jencks & M. Phillips (Eds.), *The Black–White test score gap* (pp. 103–145). Washington, DC: Brookings Institute.

Piaget, J. (1970). Piaget's theory. In P. H. Mussen (Ed.), *Carmichael's handbook of child development* (pp. 703–732). New York: Wiley.

Plewis, I. (1991). Using multilevel models to link educational progress with curriculum coverage. In S. W. Raudenbush & J. D. Willms (Eds.), *Schools, classrooms, and pupils: International studies of schooling from a multilevel perspective* (pp. 149–166). San Diego, CA: Academic Press.

Popper, K. R., & Eccles, J. C. (1977). *The self and its brain.* Berlin: Springer-Verlag.

Posner, M. I., & Rothbart, M. K. (1992). Attentional mechanisms and conscious experience. In A. D. Milner & M. D. Rugg (Eds.), *The neuropsychology or consciousness* (pp. 91–111). London, UK: Academic Press.

Power, C., & Bartley, M. (1993). Health and health service use: Sex differences. In E. Ferri (Ed.), *Life at 33: The fifth follow-up of the National Child Development Study* (pp. 134–161). London: Economic and Social Research Council, City University, National Children's Bureau.

Power, C., & Hertzman, C. (1997). Social and biological pathways linking early life and adult disease. In M. Marmot and M. Wadsworth (Eds.), *Fetal and early child environment: Long-term health implications.* London: The Royal Society of Medicine Press.

Power, C., Manor, O., & Fox, A. J. (1991). *Health and class: The early years.* London: Chapman & Hall.

Power, C., & Matthews, S. (1997). Origins of health inequalities in a national population sample. *Lancet, 350,* 1584–1589.

Prestby, J. E., Wandersman, A., Florin, P., Rich, R., & Chavis, D. (1990). Benefits, cost, incentive management and participation in voluntary organizations: A means to understand and promote empowerment. *American Journal of Community Psychology, 18,* 117–151.

Pulkkinen, L., & Tremblay, R. E. (1992). Patterns of boys' social adjustment in two cultures and at different ages: A longitudinal perspective. *International Journal of Behavioural Development, 15,* 527–553.

Putnam, R. D. (1992). *Making democracy work: Civic traditions in modern Italy.* Princeton, NJ: Princeton University Press.

Quetelet, A. (1833). *Research on the propensity for crime at different ages* (2nd ed.). Brussels: Hayez.

Quinn, J. B. (1992). *Intelligent enterprise.* New York: Free Press.

Raffe, D., & Willms, J. D. (1989). School attainment and the labour market. In D. Raffe (Ed.), *Fourteen to eighteen: The changing pattern of schooling in Scotland* (pp. 174–193). Aberdeen, Scotland: Aberdeen University Press.

Ramey, C. T., Bryant, D. M., Campbell, F. A., Sparling, J. J., & Wasik, B. H. (1990). Early intervention for high-risk children: The Carolina Early Intervention Program. *Prevention in Human Services, 7,* 33–57.

Ramey, C. T., & Haskins, R. (1981). The modification of intelligence through early experience. *Intelligence, 5,* 5–19.

Ramey, C. T., & Ramey, S. L. (1992). Early educational intervention with disadvantaged children and low income families: To what effect? *Applied and Preventive Psychology, 1*(3), 131–140.

Ramey, S. L., & Ramey, C. T. (1994). The transition to school: Why the first few years matter for a lifetime. *Phi Delta Kappan, 76*(3), 194–198.

Raudenbush, S. W., & Kasim, R. M. (1998). Cognitive skill and economic inequality: Findings from the national adult literacy survey. *Harvard Educational Review, 68*(1), 33–79.

Raudenbush, S. W., & Willms, J. D. (Eds.). (1991). *Schools, classrooms, and pupils: International studies of schooling from a multilevel perspective.* San Diego, CA: Academic Press.

Raudenbush, S. W., & Willms, J. D. (1995). The estimation of school effects. *Journal of Educational and Behavioural Statistics, 20*(4), 307–335.

Reich, R. B. (1991). *The wealth of nations: Preparing ourselves for the 21st century.* New York: Knopf.

Renaud, L., Dufour, R., & O'Loughlin, J. (1997). Intervenir localement selon les axes de la Charte d'Ottawa: Défi de la promotion de la santé. *Rupture, 4,* 23–34.

Resnick, L. B. (1983). A developmental theory of number understanding. In H. P. Ginsburg (Ed.), *The development of mathematical thinking* (pp. 110–152). New York: Academic Press.

Restoin, A., Montagner, H., Rodriguez, D., Girardot, J. J., Laurent, D., Kontar, F., Ullmann, V., Casagrande, C., & Talpain, B. (1985). Chronologie des comportements de communication et profils de comportement chez le jeune enfant. In R. E. Tremblay, M. A. Provost, & F. F. Strayer (Eds.), *Éthologie et développement de l'enfant* (pp. 93–130). Paris: Éditions Stock/Laurence Pernoud.

Reyes, T. M., & Coe, C. L. (1996). Interleukin-18 differentially affects interleukin-6 and soluble interleukin-6 receptor in the blood and central nervous system of the monkey. *Journal of Neuroimmunology, 66,* 135–141.

Reyes, T. M., & Coe, C. L. (1997). Prenatal manipulations reduce the pro-inflammatory response to a cytokine challenge in juvenile monkeys. *Brain Research, 769,* 29–35.

Riggan, R., & Kemble, A. (1994). *The Cowichan Tribes' Early Childhood Education and Youth Care Career Ladder Project.* Unpublished report to the Centre for

Curriculum and Professional Development, Victoria, British Columbia, Canada.

Riley, M. S., Greeno, J. G., & Heller, J. I. (1983). The development of children's problem solving ability in arithmetic. In H. P. Ginsburg (Ed.), *The development of mathematical thinking*. New York: Academic Press.

Riley, V., Fitzmaurice, M. A., & Spackman, D. H. (1981). Psychoneuroimmunologic factors in neoplasia: Studies in animals. In R. Ader (Ed.), *Psychoneuroimmunology* (pp. 31–102). New York: Academic Press.

Rodgers, B., Power, C., & Hope, S. (1997). Parental divorce and adult psychological distress: Evidence from a national birth cohort: A research note. *Journal of Child Psychology and Psychiatry, 38*(7), 867–872.

Rohlen, T. P. (1974). *For harmony and strength: Japanese white-collar organization in anthropological perspective*. Berkeley: University of California Press.

Rohlen, T. P. (1975). The company work group. In E. Vogel (Ed.), *Modern Japanese organization and decision-making*. Berkeley: University of California Press.

Rohlen, T. P. (1983). *Japanese high schools*. Berkeley: University of California Press.

Rohlen, T. P. (1989). Order in Japanese society: Attachment, authority, and routine. *Journal of Japanese Studies, 15*(1), 5–40.

Rohlen, T. P. (1992). Learning: The mobilization of knowledge in the Japanese political economy. In S. Kumon & H. Rosovsky (Eds.), *The political economy of Japan: Social and cultural dynamics*. Stanford, CA: Stanford University Press.

Rohlen, T. P., & LeTendre, G. (Eds.). (1996). *Teaching and learning in Japan*. Cambridge, UK: Cambridge University Press.

Rose, G. (1985). Sick individuals and sick populations. *International Journal of Epidemiology, 14,* 32–38.

Rose, R. (1995). *New Russia barometer: IV. Survey results* (Studies in Public Policy 250). Glasgow: Centre for the Study of Public Policy, University of Strathclyde.

Rose, R., & Haerpfer, C. (1994). *New democracies barometer: III. Learning from what is happening* (Studies in Public Policy 230). Glasgow: Centre for the Study of Public Policy, University of Strathclyde.

Rosen, K., & Rothbaum, F. (1993). Quality of parental caregiving and security of attachment. *Developmental Psychology, 29*(2), 358–367.

Rosenberg, N., & Birdzell, L. E. (1986). *How the West grew rich: The economic transformation of the industrial world*. New York: Basic Books.

Ross, C. E., & Wu, C. (1995). The links between education and health. *American Sociological Review, 60,* 719–745.

Ross, H. S., & Goldman, B. D. (1977). Infants' sociability toward strangers. *Child Development, 48,* 638–642.

Rossi, P. H., & Freeman, H. E. (1993). *Evaluation: A systematic approach* (5th ed.). Newbury Park, CA: Sage.

Rothbart, M., Posner, M., & Rosicky, J. (1994). Orienting in normal and pathological development. *Development and Psychopathology, 6*(4), 635–652.

Rothbart, M. K., Ziaie, H., & O'Boyle, C. (1992). Self-regulation and emotion in infancy. In N. Eisenberg & R. A. Fabes (Eds.), *Emotion regulation and its early development* (pp. 7–23). San Francisco: Jossey-Bass.

Rowan, B., & Miracle, A. W., Jr. (1983). Systems of ability grouping and the stratification of achievement in elementary schools. *Sociology of Education, 56*(2), 133–144.

Rowe, M. B. (1974). Wait-time and rewards as instructional variables, their influence on language, logic, and fate control: 1. Wait time. *Journal of Research in Science Teaching, 11,* 81–94.

Rubin, K., Coplan, R., Fox, N., & Calkins, S. (1995). Emotionality, emotion regulation, and preschoolers' social adaptation. *Development and Psychopathology, 7*(1), 49–62.

Rubin, K. H., Fein, G. G., & Vandenberg, B. (1983). Play. In P. H. Mussen (Ed.), *Handbook of child psychology* (pp. 693–774). New York: Wiley.

Rubin, K. H., Hymel, S. L., Mills, R., & Rose-Krasnor, L. (1991). Conceptualizing different developmental pathways to and from withdrawal in childhood. In D. Cicchetti & S. L. Toth (Eds.), *Internalizing and externalizing expression of dysfunction.* Hillsdale, NJ: Erlbaum.

Rumberger, R., & Willms, J. D. (1992). The impact of racial and ethnic segregation on the achievement gap in California high schools. *Educational Evaluation and Policy Analysis, 14*(4), 377–396.

Ruppenthal, G. C., Arling, G. L., Harlow, H. F., Sackett, G. P., & Suomi, S. J. (1976). A 10-year perspective of motherless mother monkey behavior. *Journal of Abnormal Psychology, 85,* 341–349.

Ruppenthal, G. C., Harlow, M. K., Eisele, C. D., Harlow, H. F., & Suomi, S. J. (1974). Development of peer interactions of monkeys reared in a nuclear family environment. *Child Development, 45,* 670–682.

Russell, M. J. (1976). Human olfactory communication. *Nature, 260,* 520–522.

Russon, A. E. (1995, June). *Tool use in orangutans returned to the wild.* Paper presented at the annual meeting of the Jean Piaget Society, Berkeley, CA.

Rutter, M. (1994). Continuities, transitions and turning points in development. In M. Rutter & D. F. Hay (Eds.), *Development through life: A handbook for clinicians* Oxford, UK: Blackwell.

Rutter, M., Tizard, J., & Whitmore, K. (1970). *Education, health and behavior.* London: Longman.

Sackett, D. L. (1980). Evaluation of health services. In J. Last (Ed.), *Preventive Medicine and Public Health* (pp. 1800–1823). New York: Appleton-Century-Crofts.

Sackett, G. P. (1966). Monkeys reared in isolation with pictures as visual input: Evidence for an innate learning mechanism. *Science, 154,* 1468–1472.

Sade, D. S. (1967). Determinants of social dominance in a group of free-ranging rhesus monkeys. In S. A. Altmann (Ed.), *Social communication among primates* (pp. 99–114). Chicago: University of Chicago Press.

Salkind, N. J., & Haskins, R. (1982). Negative income tax: The impact on children and low income families. *Journal of Family Issues, 3,* 165–180.

Sameroff, A. J., & Suomi, S. J. (1996). Primates and persons: A comparative developmental understanding of social organization. In R. B. Cairns, G. H. Elder, & E. J. Costello (Eds.), *Developmental science* (pp. 97–120). Cambridge, UK: Cambridge University Press.

Sampson, R. J., & Morenoff, J. (1997). Ecological perspectives on the neighborhood context of urban poverty: Past and present. In J. Brooks-Gunn, G. Duncan, & J. L. Aber (Eds.), *Neighborhood poverty: Context and consequences for children: Vol. 2. Conceptual, methodological, and policy approaches to studying neighborhoods* (pp. 1–23). New York: Russell Sage Foundation Press.

Sampson, R. J. (1995). The community. In J. Q. Wilson & J. Petersilia (Eds.), *Crime* (pp. 196–216). San Francisco: Institute for Contemporary Studies.

Sand, E. A. (1966). *Contribution à l'étude du développement de l'enfant: Aspects médico-sociaux et psychologiques.* Brussels: Éditions de l'Institut de sociologie de l'Université libre de Bruxelles.

Sapolsky, R. M. (1992). *Stress, the aging brain, and the mechanisms of neuron death.* Cambridge, MA: MIT Press.

Savage-Rumbaugh, E. S., Murphy, J., Sevick, R. A., Brakke, K. E., Williams, S. L., & Rumbaugh, D. (1993). Language comprehension in ape and child. *Monographs of the Society for Research in Child Development 58*(Serial No. 233).

Savery, J., & Duffy, T. (1995). Problem-based learning: An instructional model and its constructivist framework. *Educational Technology, 35,* 31–38.

Saxe, G. B., Guberman, R. R., & Gearhart, M. (1987). Social processes in early number development. *Monographs of the Society for Research in Child Development, 52*(Serial No. 216).

Scardamalia, M., & Bereiter, C. (1992). Text-based and knowledge-based questioning by children. *Cognition and Instruction, 9*(3), 177–199.

Scardamalia, M., & Bereiter, C. (1996). Student communities for the advancement of knowledge. *Communications of the ACM, 39*(4), 36–37.

Scardamalia, M., Bereiter, C., Brett, C., Burtis, P. J., Calhoun, C., & Smith Lea, N. (1992). Educational applications of a networked communal database. *Interactive Learning Environments, 2*(1), 45–71.

Scardamalia, M., Bereiter, C., Hewitt, J., & Webb, J. (1996). Constructive learning from texts in biology. In K. M. Fischer & M. Kirby (Eds.), *Relations and biology learning: The acquisition and use of knowledge structures in biology* (pp. 44–64). Berlin: Springer-Verlag.

Scardamalia, M., Bereiter, C., & Lamon, M. (1994). The CSILE project: Trying to bring the classroom into world 3. In K. McGilly (Ed.), *Classroom lessons: Integrating cognitive theory and classroom practice* (pp. 201–228). Cambridge, MA: MIT Press/Bradford Books.

Scarr, S., & Weisberg, R. A. (1978). The influence of "family background" on intellectual attainment. *American Sociological Review, 43,* 674–692.

Schein, M. W. (1963). On the irreversibility of imprinting. *Zeitschrift für Tierpsychologie, 20,* 462–467.

Schein, M. W., & Hale, E. B. (1959). The effect of early social experience on male sexual behaviour of androgen injected turkeys. *Animal Behaviour, 7,* 189–200.

Schleifer, S. J., Keller, S. E., Camerino, M., Thornton, J. C., & Stein, M. (1983). Depression of lymphocyte stimulation following bereavement. *Journal of the American Medical Association, 250,* 374–377.

Schneider, M. L., & Coe, C. L. (1993). Repeated stress during pregnancy impairs neuromotor development of the primate infant. *Journal of Developmental and Behavioral Pediatrics, 14*(2), 81–87.

Schneider, M. L., Coe, C. L., & Lubach, G. R. (1992). Endocrine activation mimics the adverse effects of prenatal stress on the neuromotor development of the primate infant. *Developmental Psychobiology, 25*(6), 427–439.

Schneider-Rosen, K., & Cicchetti, D. (1984). The relationship between affect and cognition in maltreated infants: Quality of attachment and the development of visual self-recognition. *Child Development, 55,* 648–658.

Schultz, T. W. (1963). *The economic value of education.* New York: Columbia University Press.

Schwandt, T. A. (1996). Farewell to criteriology. *Qualitative Inquiry, 3*(1), 58–72.

Schwartz, J. E., Friedman, H. S., Tucker, J. S., Tomlinson-Keasey, C., Wingard, D. L., & Criqui, M. H. (1995). Sociodemographic and psychosocial factors in childhood as predictors of adult mortality. *American Journal of Public Health, 85,* 1237–1245.

Schweinhart, L. J., Barnes, H. V., & Weikart, D. P. (1993). *Significant benefits: The High/Scope Perry Preschool Study through age 27.* Ypsilanti, MI: High/Scope Press.

Schweinhart, L. J., & Weikart, D. P. (1997). Lasting differences: The High/Scope preschool curriculum comparison study through age 23. *Monographs of the High/Scope Education Research Foundation, 12.*

Sedlacek, J. (1964). Further findings on the conditions of formation of temporary connections in chick embryos. *Physiologia Bohemoslovenia, 13,* 411–420.

Seeman, T. E., & McEwen, B. S. (1996). Impact of social environment characteristics on neuroendocrine regulation. *Psychosomatic Medicine, 58,* 459–471.

Senge, P. M. (1990). *The fifth discipline: The art and practice of the learning organization.* New York: Doubleday.

Serbin, L. A., Peters, P. L., McAffer, V. J., & Schwartzman, A. E. (1991). Childhood aggression and withdrawal as predictors of adolescent pregnancy, early parenthood, and environmental risk for the next generation. *Canadian Journal of Behavioral Science, 23,* 318–331.

Serbin, L. A., Schwartzman, A. E., Moskowitz, D. S., & Ledingham, J. E. (1991). Aggressive, withdrawn and aggressive–withdrawn children in adolescence: Into the next generation. In D. Pepler & K. Rubin (Eds.), *The development and treatment of childhood aggression* (pp. 51–70). Hillsdale, NJ: Erlbaum.

Sewell, W. H., Hauser, R. M., & Featherman, D. (Eds.). (1976). *Schooling and achievement in American society.* New York: Academic Press.

Shafrir, U., & Eagle, M. (1995). Response to failure, strategic flexibility and learning. *International Journal of Behavioral Development, 18*(4), 677–700.

Shafrir, U., Ogilvie, M., & Bryson, M. (1990). Attention to errors and learning: Across-task and across-domain analysis of the post-failure reflectivity measure. *Cognitive Development, 5,* 405–425.

Shavit, Y., & Williams, R. A. (1985). Ability grouping and contextual determinants of educational expectations in Israel. *American Sociological Review, 50,* 62–73.

Shaw, C. R., & McKay, H. D. (1942). *Juvenile delinquency and urban areas.* Chicago: University of Chicago Press.

Shaw, D. S., Vondra, J. I., Hommerding, K. D., Keenan, K., & Dunn, M. (1994). Chronic family adversity and early child behavior problems: A longitudinal study of low income families. *Journal of Child Psychology and Psychiatry, 35*(6), 1109–1122.

Shiba, S., Graham, A., & Walden, D. (1990). *The new America, TQM: Four practical revolutions in management.* Portland, OR: Productivity Press.

Shields, C. (1993). *Community systems initiative: An introductory overview.* Internal paper, Laidlaw Foundation, Toronto, Ontario, Canada.

Shipley, M. T., Halloran, F. J., & de la Torre, J. (1985). Surprisingly rich projection from locus coeruleus to the olfactory bulb in rat. *Brain Research, 329,* 294–299.

Shure, M., & Spivack, G. (1982). Interpersonal problem solving in young children: A cognitive approach to prevention. *American Journal of Community Psychology, 10,* 341.

Shure, M. B., & Spivack, G. (1988). Interpersonal cognitive problem solving. In E. L. Cowen, R. P. Lorion, & J. Ramos-McKay (Eds.), *Fourteen ounces of prevention: A handbook for practitioners* (pp. 69–82). Washington, DC: American Psychological Association.

Siegler, R. S. (1996). *Emerging minds: The process of change in children's thinking.* New York: Oxford University Press.

Siegler, R. S., & Robinson, M. (1982). The development of numerical understanding. In H. W. Reese & L. P. Lipsitt (Eds.), *Advances in child development and behavior* (pp. 241–312). New York: Academic Press.

Sinha, D. (1983). Cross-cultural psychology: A view from the Third World. In J. B. Deregowski, S. Dziurawiecj, & R. C. Annis (Eds.), *Expiscations in cross-cultural psychology.* Lisse, The Netherlands: Swets & Zeitlinger.

Slavin, R. E. (1987). Ability grouping and student achievement in elementary schools: A best-evidence synthesis. *Review of Educational Research, 57*(3), 293–336.

Smeeding, T. M., & Gottschalk, P. (1996, May). *The international evidence on income distribution in modern economies: Where do we stand?* Paper presented at the annual meeting of the Population Association of America, New Orleans, LA.

Smith, A. (1952). An inquiry into the nature and causes of the wealth of nations. In R. M. Hutchins (Ed.), *Great books of the Western World: 39. Adam Smith.* Chicago: Encyclopedia Britannica. (Original work published 1776)

Smith, F. V. (1969). *Attachment of the young: Imprinting and other developments.* Edinburgh: Oliver & Boyd.

Smith, H. (1995). *Rethinking America: A new game plan from the American innovators—Schools, businesses, people, work.* New York: Random House.

Smith, J. R., Brooks-Gunn, J., & Klebanov, P. (1997). The consequences of living in poverty for young children's cognitive and verbal ability and early school achievement. In G. J. Duncan & J. Brooks-Gunn (Eds.), *Consequences of growing up poor* (pp. 132–189). New York: Russell Sage Foundation Press.

Smith, M. S., & Bissell, J. (1970). Report analysis: The impact of Head Start. *Harvard Educational Review, 42,* 51–129.

Snow, C. E. (1993). Families as social contexts for literacy development. In C. Daiute (Ed.), *The development of literacy through social interaction* (pp. 11–24). San Francisco: Jossey-Bass.

Snowdon, D. A., Kemper, S. J., Mortimer, J. A., Greiner, L. H., Wekstein, D. R., & Markesbery, W. R. (1996). Linguistic ability in early life and cognitive function and Alzheimer's disease in late life. *Journal of the American Medical Association, 275*(7), 528–532.

Solomon, G. F. (1981). Emotional and personality factors in the onset and course of autoimmune disease, particularly rheumatoid arthritis. In R. Ader (Ed.), *Psychoneuroimmunology* (pp. 159–184). New York: Academic Press.

Solomon, G. F., Fiatarone, M. A., Benton, D., Morley, J. E., Bloom, E., & Makinodan, T. (1988). Psychoimmunologic and endorphin function in the aged. *Annals of the New York Academy of Sciences, 521,* 43–58.

Solomon, G. F., Levine, S., & Kraft, J. K. (1968). Early experience and immunity. *Nature, 220,* 821–822.

Solomon, G. F., Segerstrom, S. C., Grohr, P., Kemeny, M., & Fahey, J. (1997).

Shaking up immunity: Psychological and immunologic changes after a natural disaster. *Psychosomatic Medicine, 59,* 114–127.

Sorensen, A. B., & Hallinan, M. (1984). Effects of race on assignment to ability groups. In P. L. Peterson, L. C. Wilkinson, & M. Hallinan (Eds.), *The social context of education.* New York: Academic Press.

Spalding, D. A. (1873). Instinct, with original observations on young animals. *McMillan's Magazine, 27,* 282–293. Reprinted in *British Journal of Animal Behavior* (1959), *2,* 2–11.

Sroufe, L. A. (1979). Socioemotional development. In J. D. Osofsky (Ed.), *Handbook of infant development* (pp. 462–516). New York: Wiley.

Sroufe, L. A., & Jacobvitz, D. (1989). Diverging pathways, developmental transformations, multiple etiologies and the problem of continuity in development. *Human Development, 32*(3/4), 196–203.

Stagner, M. N., & Duran, A. M. (1997). Comprehensive communities initiative: Principles and lessons. *The Fuure of Children, 7,* 132–140.

Starkey, P. (1992). The early development of numerical reasoning. *Cognition, 43,* 93–126.

Starkey, P., & Klein, A. (1992). Economic and cultural influences on early mathematical development. In F. L. Parker, R. Robinson, S. Sombrano, C. Piotrowski, J. Hagen, S. Randolph, & A. Baker (Eds.), *New directions in child and family research: Shaping Head Start in the 90s.* New York: National Council of Jewish Women.

Statistics Canada. (1996). *Growing up in Canada: National Longitudinal Survey of Children and Youth.* Ottawa: Human Resources Development Canada.

Statistics Canada & Human Resources Development Canada. (1995). *National Longitudinal Survey of Children: Overview of survey instrument for 1994–1995. Data collection cycle 1.* (Statistics Canada Catalogue No. 95-02). Ottawa: Ministry of Industry Canada.

Stattin, H., & Klackenberg-Larsson, I. (1993). Early language and intelligence development and their relationship to future criminal behavior. *Journal of Abnormal Psychology, 102,* 369–378.

Stern, Y., Gurland, B., Tatemichi, T. K., Tang, M. X., Wilder, D., & Mayeux, R. (1994). Influence of education and occupation on the incidence of Alzheimer's disease. *Journal of the American Medical Association, 271,* 1004–1010.

Stevenson, H. W., & Stigler, J. W. (1992). *The learning gap: Why our schools are failing and what we can learn from Japanese and Chinese education.* New York: Summit Books.

Stevenson, J., Richman, N., & Graham, P. (1985). Behavior problems and language abilities at three years and behavioral deviance at eight years. *Journal of Child Psychology and Psychiatry, 26*(2), 215–230.

Strauman, T. J., Lemieux, A. M., & Coe, C. L. (1993). Self-discrepancies and natural killer cell activity: The influence of negative psychological situations on stress physiology. *Journal of Personality and Social Psychology, 6*(5), 1042–1052.

Stigler, J. W., & Perry, M. (1988). Mathematics learning in Japanese, Chinese, and American classrooms. In G. Saxe & M. Gearhart (Eds.), *Children's mathematics.* San Francisco: Jossey-Bass.

Stringer, C., & Gamble, C. (1993). *In search of the Neanderthals: Solving the puzzle of human origins.* London: Thames & Hudson.

Strodtbeck, F. L. (1965). The hidden curriculum in the middle class home. In J. D.

Krumboltz (Ed.), *Learning and the educational process*. Chicago: Rand McNally.

Suen, H. K. (1990). *Principles of test theories*. Hillsdale, NJ: Erlbaum.

Sullivan, R. M., Wilson, D. A., & Leon, M. (1989). Norepinephrine and learning induced plasticity in infant rat olfactory system. *Journal of Neuroscience, 9*(3998–4006).

Summers, A. A., & Wolfe, B. L. (1977). Do schools make a difference? *American Economic Review, 67,* 639–652.

Suomi, S. J. (1979). Peers, play, and primary prevention in primates. In M. W. Kent & J. E. Rolf (Eds.), *Primary prevention in psychopathology* (Vol. 3, pp. 127–149). Hanover, NH: University Press of New England.

Suomi, S. J. (1986). Anxiety-like disorders in young primates. In R. Gittelman (Ed.), *Anxiety disorders of childhood* (pp. 1–23). New York: Guilford Press.

Suomi, S. J. (1987). Genetic and maternal contributions to individual differences in rhesus monkey biobehavioral development. In N. Krasnagor, E. Blass, M. Hofer, & W. Smotherman (Eds.), *Perinatal development: A psychobiological perspective* (pp. 397–420). New York: Academic Press.

Suomi, S. J. (1991a). Up-tight and laid-back monkeys: Individual differences in the response to social challenges. In S. Brauth, W. Hall, & R. Dooling (Eds.), *Plasticity of development* (pp. 27–56). Cambridge, MA: MIT Press.

Suomi, S. J. (1991b). Primate separation models of affective disorders. In J. Madden (Ed.), *Neurobiology of learning, emotion, and affect* (pp. 195–214). New York: Raven Press.

Suomi, S. J. (1995). Influence of Bowlby's attachment theory on research on nonhuman primate biobehavioral development. In S. Goldberg, R. Muir, & J. Kerr (Eds.), *Attachment theory: Social, developmental, and clinical perspectives* (pp. 185–201). Hillsdale, NJ: Analytic Press.

Suomi, S. J. (1997). Early determinants of behavior: Evidence from primate studies. *British Medical Bulletin, 53,* 170–184.

Suomi, S. J. (1999). Conflict and cohesion in rhesus monkey family life. In M. Cox & J. Brooks-Gunn (Eds.), *Conflict and cohesion in families* (pp. 283–299). Mahwah, NJ: Erlbaum.

Suomi, S. J., & Levine, S. (1998). Psychobiology of intergenerational effects of trauma: Evidence from animal studies. In Y. Daniele (Ed.), *International handbook of multigenerational legacies of trauma* (pp. 623–625). New York: Plenum.

Suomi, S. J., Rasmussen, K. L. R., & Higley, J. D. (1992). Primate models of behavioral and physiological change in adolescence. In E. R. McAnarney, R. E. Kriepe, D. P. Orr, & G. D. Comerci (Eds.), *Textbook of adolescent medicine* (pp. 135–139). Philadelphia: Saunders.

Suomi, S. J., & Ripp, C. (1983). A history of motherless mother monkey mothering at the University of Wisconsin Primate Laboratory. In M. Reite & N. Caine (Eds.), *Child abuse: The nonhuman primate data* (pp. 49–77). New York: Liss.

Super, C., & Harkness, S. (1986). The developmental niche: A conceptualization at the interface of child and culture. *International Journal of Behavioral Development, 9,* 545–569.

Sutherland, E. (1939). *Principles of criminology*. Philadelphia: Lippincott.

Tamis-LeMonda, C., & Bornstein, M. (1989). Habituation and maternal encouragement of attention in infancy as predictors of toddler language, play, and representational competence. *Child Development, 60,* 738–751.

Teachman, J. D., Paasch, K. M., Day, R. D., & Carver, K. P. (1997). Poverty during adolescence and subsequent educational attainment. In G. J. Duncan & J. Brooks-Gunn (Eds.), *Consequences of growing up poor* (pp. 382–418). New York: Russell Sage Foundation Press.

Temoshok, L., & Fox, B. H. (1984). Coping styles and other psychological factors related to medical status and to prognosis in patients with cutaneous malignant melanoma. In B. H. Fox & B. H. Newberry (Eds.), *Impact of psychoendocrine systems in cancer and immunity* (pp. 258–287). Lewiston, NY: Hogrefe.

Tennant, C. (1988). Parental loss in childhood. *Archives of General Psychiatry, 45,* 1045–1050.

Thatcher, R. W. (1992). Cyclical cortical reorganization during early childhood. *Brain and Cognition, 20,* 24–50.

Thomas, C. B., Duszynski, K. R., & Shaffer, J. W. (1979). Family attitudes reported in youth as potential predictors of cancer. *Psychosomatic Medicine, 41,* 287–302.

Thompson, R. A. (1990). Emotion and self-regulation. In R. A. Thompson (Ed.), *Socioemotional development.* (pp. 367–467). Lincoln: University of Nebraska Press.

Thompson, R. A. (1994). Emotion regulation: A theme in search of a definition. In N. A. Fox (Ed.), The development of emotion regulation: Biological and behavioral considerations. *Monographs of the Society for Research in Child Development, 59*(2/3, Serial No. 240).

Thompson, R. A., & Calkins, S. (1996). The double-edged sword: Emotional regulation for children at risk. *Development and Psychopathology, 8*(1), 163–182.

Tiessen, E. (1996). *Computer supports for mathematical discourse in elementary school classrooms.* Unpublished doctoral dissertation, University of Toronto, Toronto, Ontario, Canada.

Tomasello, M., Kruger, A. C., & Ratner, H. H. (1993). Cultural learning. *Behavioral and Brain Sciences, 16,* 495–552.

Total Quality Management. (1993). *California Management Review* [Special issue], *35*(3).

Tovée, M. J. (1995). What are faces for? *Current Biology, 5,* 480–482.

Tremblay, R. E., Boulerice, B., Harden, P. W., McDuff, P., Pérusse, D., Pihl, R. O., & Zoccolillo, M. (1996). Do children in Canada become more aggressive as they approach adolescence? In *Growing up in Canada: National Longitudinal Study of Children and Youth* (pp. 127–137). Ottawa: Human Resources Development Canada & Statistics Canada.

Tremblay, R. E., & Craig, W. (1995). Developmental crime prevention. In M. Tonry & D. P. Farrington (Eds.), *Building a safer society: Strategic approaches to crime prevention* (pp. 151–236). Chicago: University of Chicago Press.

Tremblay, R. E., Kurtz, L., Mâsse, L. C., Vitaro, F., & Pihl, R. O. (1995). A bimodal preventive intervention for disruptive kindergarten boys: Its impact through mid-adolescence. *Journal of Consulting and Clinical Psychology, 63,* 560–568.

Tremblay, R. E., Mâsse, B., Perron, D., & LeBlanc, M. (1992). Disruptive behavior, poor school achievement, delinquent behavior, and delinquent personality: Longitudinal analyses. *Journal of Consulting and Clinical Psychology, 60,* 64–72.

Tremblay, R. E., Mâsse, L. C., Pagani, L., & Vitaro, F. (1996). From childhood physical aggression to adolescent maladjustment: The Montréal Prevention Experiment. In R. D. Peters & R. J. McMahon (Eds.), *Preventing childhood disorders, substance abuse and delinquency* (pp. 268–298). Thousand Oaks, CA: Sage.

Tremblay, R. E., McCord, J., Boileau, H., Charlebois, P., Gagnon, C., Leblanc, M., & Larivée, S. (1991). Can disruptive boys be helped to become competent? *Psychiatry, 54,* 148–161.

Tremblay, R. E., Pihl, R. O., Vitaro, F., & Dobkin, P. L. (1994). Predicting early onset of male antisocial behavior from preschool behavior. *Archives of General Psychiatry, 51,* 732–738.

Tsuchida, I. (1993). *Teachers' motivational and instructional strategies: A study of fourth grade U.S. and Japanese classrooms.* Unpublished doctoral dissertation, University of California, Berkeley School of Education.

Tugwell, P. T., Bennett, K. J., & Sackett, D. L. (1985). The measurement iterative loop: A framework for the critical appraisal of need, benefits and costs of health interventions. *Journal of Chronic Disease, 38,* 339–351.

UNICEF. (1993). *Central and Eastern Europe in transition: Public policy and social conditions.* Florence, Italy: UNICEF International Child Development Centre.

UNICEF (1994). *Central and Eastern Europe in transition: Crisis in mortality, health and nutrition.* Florence, Italy: UNICEF International Child Development Centre.

Vagero, D., & Lundberg, O. (1989). Health inequalities in Britain and Sweden. *Lancet, ii,* 35–36.

Valkonen, T. (1989). Adult mortality and level of education: A comparison of six countries. In J. Fox (Ed.), *Health inequalities in European countries* (pp. 142–160). Aldershot, UK: Gower.

van Aalst, J. (1999). *The content of science and computer supported collaborative learning.* Unpublished doctoral dissertation, University of Toronto, Toronto, Ontario, Canada.

Ventura, S. J. (1995). *Births to unmarried mothers: United States, 1980–1992* (NCHS Series 21, No. 53, U.S. Department of Health and Human Services). Washington, DC: U.S. Government Printing Office.

Vitaro, F., & Tremblay, R. E. (1994). Impact of a prevention program on aggressive–disruptive children's friendships and social adjustment. *Journal of Abnormal Child Psychology, 22,* 457–475.

Vitaro, F., Tremblay, R. E., & Gagnon, C. (1992). Adversité familiale et troubles du comportement au début de la période de fréquentation scolaire. *Revue Canadienne de Santé Mentale, 11,* 45–62.

Vygotsky, L. (1978). *Mind in society: The development of higher psychological processes.* Cambridge, MA: Harvard University Press.

Vosniadou, S., & Brewer, W. F. (1987). Theories of knowledge restructuring in development. *Review of Educational Research, 57,* 51–67.

Waaler, H. T. H. (1984). Height, weight and mortality: The Norwegian experience. *Acta Medica Scandinavica, 1,* S679.

Wachs, T. D., & Gruen, G. E. (1982). *Early experiences and human development.* New York: Plenum.

Wald, N. J., & Hackshaw, A. K. (1996). Cigarette smoking: Epidemiological overview. *British Medical Bulletin, 52,* 3–11.

Wannamethee, G., Whincup, P., Shaper, G., & Walker, M. (1996). Influence of father's social class on cardiovascular disease in middle-aged men. *Lancet, 348,* 1259–1263.

Warriner, C. C., Lemmon, W. B., & Ray, T. S. (1963). Early experience as a variable in mate selection. *Animal Behavior, 11,* 221–224.

Wasik, B. H., Ramey, C. T., Bryant, D. M., & Sparling, J. J. (1990). A longitudinal study of two early intervention strategies: Project Care. *Child Development, 61,* 1682–1696.

Weber, L. (1971). *The English infant school and informal education.* Englewood Cliffs, NJ: Prentice-Hall.

Weinberg, M. K., Tronick, E. Z., Cohn, J. F., & Olson, K. L. (1999). Gender differences in emotional expressivity and self-regulation during early infancy. *Developmental Psychology, 35,* 175–188.

Weinberger, M. (1967). *Michelangelo, the sculptor.* New York: Cambridge University Press.

Weinman, D. K., & Rothman, A. H. (1967). Effects of stress upon acquired immunity to the dwarf tapeworm, *Hymenolepsis nana. Experimental Parasitology, 21,* 61–67.

Weisner, T. S. (1984). Ecocultural niches of middle childhood: A cross-cultural perspective. In W. A. Collins (Ed.), *Development during middle childhood: The years from six to twelve* (pp. 335–369). Washington, DC: National Academy of Sciences.

Weiss, J. M. (1984). Behavioral and psychological influences on gastrointestinal pathology. In W. D. Gentry (Ed.), *Handbook of behavioral medicine* (pp. 174–195). New York: Guilford Press.

Werner, E. E. (1989). Children of the garden island. *Scientific American, 260*(4), 106–111.

Wiekart, D. P., Kamii, C. K., & Radin, N. (1994). *Perry preschool progress report.* Ypsilanti, MI: Ypsilanti Public Schools.

Wilkinson, R. G. (1992a). Income distribution and life expectancy. *British Medical Journal, 304,* 165–168.

Wilkinson, R. G. (1992b). National mortality rates: The impact of inequality. *American Journal of Public Health, 82*(8), 1082–1084.

Williams, F. (1975). Family resemblance in abilities: The Wechsler Scales. *Behavior Genetics, 5,* 405–409.

Williams, J. R., Insel, T. R., Harbaugh, C. R., & Carter, C. S. (1994). Oxytocin administered centrally facilitates formation of a partner preference in female prairie voles (*Microtus ochragaster*). *Journal of Neuroendocrinology, 6,* 247–250.

Willms, J. D. (1985). The balance thesis: Contextual effects of ability on pupils' O-grade examination results. *Oxford Review of Education, 11*(1), 33–41.

Willms, J. D. (1986). Social class segregation and its relationship to pupils' examination results in Scotland. *American Sociological Review, 51,* 224–241.

Willms, J. D. (1992). *Monitoring school performance: A non-technical guide for educational administrators.* Lewes, UK: Falmer Press.

Willms, J. D. (1996). School choice and community segregation: Findings from Scotland. In A. C. Kerckhoff (Ed.), *Generating social stratification* (pp. 133–153). Boulder, CO: Westview Press.

Willms, J. D. (1997). *Literacy skills of Canadian youth* (Report prepared for Statistics Canada). University of New Brunswick, Fredericton, New Brunswick, Canada: Atlantic Centre for Policy Research in Education.

Willms, J. D. (1998). *District and provincial assessment: Can it be useful to principals and teachers?* (Policy Brief 1). University of New Brunswick, Fredericton, New Brunswick, Canada: Atlantic Centre for Policy Research in Education.

Willms, J. D., & Chen, M. (1989). The effects of ability grouping on the ethnic achievement gap in Israeli elementary schools. *American Journal of Education, 97*(3), 237–257.

Willms, J. D., & Echols, F. H. (1992). Alert and inert clients: The Scottish experience of parental choice. *Economics of Education Review, 11*(4), 339–350.

Willms, J. D., & Jacobsen, S. (1990). Growth in mathematics skills during the intermediate years: Sex differences and school effects. *International Journal of Educational Research, 14,* 157–174.

Willms, J. D., & Kerckhoff, A. C. (1995). The challenge of developing new social indicators. *Educational Evaluation and Policy Analysis, 17*(1), 113–131.

Willms, J. D., & Kerr, P. D. (1987). Changes in sex differences in Scottish examination results since 1976. *Journal of Early Adolescence, 7*(1), 85–105.

Willms, J. D., & Shields, M. (1996). *A measure of socioeconomic status for the National Longitudinal Study of Children* (Report No. 9607). Fredericton, New Brunswick: University of New Brunswick, Atlantic Center for Policy Research.

Willms, S., & Gilbert, L. (1990). *Healthy community indicators: Lessons from the social indicator movement.* Vancouver: University of British Columbia, Centre for Human Settlements.

Wilson, W. J. (1987). *The truly disadvantaged: The innercity, the innerclass, and public policy.* Chicago: University of Chicago Press.

Wilson, W. J. (1991). Studying inner-city social dislocations: The challenge of public agenda research. *American Sociological Review, 56*(1), 1–14.

Wilson, W. J. (1996). *When work disappears: The world of new urban poor.* New York: Knopf.

Winkleby, M. A. (1992). Socioeconomic status and health: How education, income, and occupation contribute to risk factors for cardiovascular disease. *American Journal of Public Health, 82,* 816–820.

Wolfson, M., Rowe, G., Gentleman, J., & Tomiak, M. (1991). *Career earnings and death: A longitudinal analysis of older Canadian men.* Canadian Institute for Advanced Research, Population Health Working Paper No. 12, Toronto.

Womack, P., Jones, D. T., & Roos, D. (Eds.). (1990). *The machine that changed the future.* New York: Macmillan.

Woodhead, M. (1996). *In search of the rainbow: Pathways to quality in large-scale programmes for young disadvantaged children.* The Hague: Bernard van Leer Foundation.

World Bank. (1993). *World Development Report 1993: Investing in health: World development indicators.* New York: Oxford University Press.

World Health Organization. (1986). *Charte d'Ottawa pour la promotion de la santé.* Ottawa: Association Canadienne de la Santé Publique.

Wynn, K. (1992). Addition and subtraction by human infants. *Nature, 358,* 709–750.

Yin, R. K. (1994). *Case study research: Design and methods.* Beverly Hills, CA: Sage.

Young, M. E. (1997). Policy issues and implications of early child development. In M. E. Young (Ed.), *Early child development: Investing in our children's future* (Proceedings of a World Bank conference on early child development: Investing in the future; pp. 323–330). Amsterdam: The Netherlands: Elsevier.

Youth Court Statistics. (1996). *Juristat, 16* (Table 3.7). Canadian Centre for Justice Statistics, Ottawa.

Zelazo, P. D., Carter, A., Reznick, J. S., & Frye, D. (1997). Early development of executive function: A problem-solving framework. *Review of General Psychology, 1,* 198–226.

Zigler, E., & Muenchow, S. (1992). *Head Start: The inside story of America's most successful educational experiment.* New York: Basic Books.

Zuboff, S. (1988). *In the age of the smart machine: The future of work and power.* New York: Basic Books.

Zuravin, S. J. (1989). The ecology of child abuse and neglect: Review of the literature and presentation of data. *Violence and Victims, 4,* 101–120.

Zuravin, S. J., & Taylor, R. (1987). The ecology of child maltreatment: Identifying and characterizing high-risk neighborhoods. *Child Welfare, 6,* 497–506.

Index